Home Health Care

ILLUSTRATED GUIDE TO

Home Health Care

Springhouse Corporation
Springhouse, Pennsylvania

Staff

Executive Director, Editorial
Stanley Loeb

Publisher
Barbara F. McVan, RN

Art Director
John Hubbard

Project Clinical Editor
Mary Ann Foley, RN, BSN

Clinical Editors
Patricia Graeff, RRT; Joan Mason, RN, MEd

Editor
Barbara Hodgson

Designers
Stephanie Peters (associate art director), Mary Ludwicki (book designer),
Elaine Ezrow, Janice Nawn, Amy Smith

Illustrators
Jackie Facciolo, John Gist, Bob Jackson, Bob Neumann, Judy Newhouse

Typography
Diane Paluba (manager), Valerie Rosenberger

Manufacturing
Deborah Meiris (director), T.A. Landis

Editorial Assistants
Maree DeRosa, Mary Madden, Dianne Tolbert

Production Coordinator
Margaret Rastiello

IGHH-020295
ISBN 0-87434-745-9

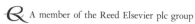 A member of the Reed Elsevier plc group

Library of Congress Cataloging-in-Publication Data
Illustrated guide to home health care
p. cm.
Includes index.
1. Home nursing. I. Springhouse
Corporation.
[DNLM: 1. Home Care Services. 2. Nursing
Care—methods.
WY I 295 1994]
RT61.I44 1994
362.1'4—dc20
DNLM/DLC   94-23124
ISBN 0-87434-745-9   CIP

Contents

Chapter 4: Hygiene

Chapter 5: Comfort Measures

Chapter 6: Hospital Beds

Chapter 7: Feeding the Sick

Chapter 8: Giving Medications

Chapter 9: I.V. Therapy

Chapter 10: Incontinence

Chapter 11: Pressure Ulcers

Chapter 12: Dressings and Bandages

Chapter 13: Crutches and Canes

Chapter 14: Exercises

Chapter 15: Walkers and Wheelchairs

Chapter 16: Oxygen Therapy

Chapter 17: Suctioning

Chapter 18: Tracheostomy Care

Chapter 19: Respiratory Therapy

Chapter 20: Feeding Tubes and Pumps

Chapter 21: Cast Care

Chapter 22: Urinary Catheters and Nephrostomy Tubes

Chapter 23: Dialysis Care

Chapter 24: Stoma Care

Chapter 25: Special Problems in Adults

Introduction

Each year, nurses, home health aides, physical therapists, occupational therapists, medical social workers, and other health care professionals make more than 2 million home health care visits. Increasingly, patients are elderly and homebound, and many have chronic illnesses, including circulatory system disorders, worsening arthritis, or cancer. Others are recovering from acute conditions, such as stroke, or from major surgery.

In the home setting, nurses and other professional caregivers typically have less time available than they would like for care and teaching. Spouses, adult children, and friends who care for others at home also have problems with time and usually have few or no resources for teaching. For all these caregivers—and for many patients too—*Illustrated Guide to Home Health Care* can help make care more thorough and teaching more manageable and understandable. Furthermore, this book can be an invaluable resource for motivating the patient to participate in personal care and strive for reasonable progress.

For these three groups of users of *Illustrated Guide to Home Health Care*, the same pages will function differently. Specifically:

If you're a nurse or other home health care professional, this book will help you:
• manage patient care and teaching tasks
• show and explain procedures that are new to the patient or family
• encourage patient compliance and record keeping.

If you're the primary caregiver for a spouse, parent, child, other relative, or friend, this book will teach you:
• what you need to know about caring for the patient at home
• how to perform care procedures with skill and confidence
• how to manage your time effectively and cope with your loved one's illness.

If you're the patient, this book will help you:
• understand why a procedure is important to you

- safely perform certain tasks yourself
- recognize danger signs so that you can get timely help.

The book's content is wide-ranging, as a glance at the table of contents shows. It begins with advice for the caregiver, providing self-awareness and encouraging an organized approach to care. Then it moves to care basics, danger signs, hygiene, and comfort measures—topics that apply to all patients. Next, it addresses such vital and practical topics as hospital beds, medications (including intravenous infusions), incontinence, pressure ulcers, dressings and bandages, crutches and canes, and walkers and wheelchairs. The book also covers such special procedures as oxygen therapy, suctioning, tracheostomy care, total parenteral nutrition, stoma care, and emergencies.

Throughout, the book presents its information step-by-step, enhanced by many illustrations. Technical language is used minimally. This presentation will save you time, build your confidence, and increase your understanding of what you're doing and why you're doing it. In turn, your patient will also understand more of the *how*'s and *why*'s of the care you're administering.

Illustrated Guide to Home Health Care meets a pressing need for a large and rapidly growing population of caregivers. It accommodates those with a wide range of skills, those who are unfamiliar with certain procedures, and those who are just beginning to give care to a relative or friend. For all these users, it will help by providing a systematic, clearly presented approach to care.

1   Help for the Caregiver

Learning about home care

The person you are caring for was in the hospital. You and he have decided—with your doctor's help—to continue care and treatment at home with you as the primary caregiver. The decision is the first step, but where do you go from here?

First, relax and identify your role and your sources of help. Recall your visits to the hospital. No one person took care of all your loved one's needs. You won't be alone either. You'll be part of a home care team sharing in the delivery of his care.

Home care team

Depending on your abilities and the needs of the person you're caring for, your home care team may include the following members:

• The *person you're caring for,* a central team member. He should do as much for himself as possible. He should work with you to create and keep a positive atmosphere.

• *Family members and friends.* Train and rely on them to help care for the person's many needs. They're the secret ingredient that makes home care so different from hospital care.

• The *doctor,* the medical leader of the home care team. Decide early on if the doctor supports your home care decision, keeps you informed about the person's condition, and answers all your questions. If your current doctor isn't willing to work with you, find another doctor who is.

• *Other health care professionals,* such as a nurse, nutritional consultant, speech or other therapist. They may join your home care team either as regulars or as occasional members, depending on the person's changing needs.

• *Community agencies.* Local offices of national groups offer counseling and support—for example, the American Cancer Society and Family Service America. Local groups provide specific services, like Meals On Wheels. Call on them—that's why they exist!

Preparing to go home

After the person you're caring for leaves the hospital, you may have to perform care measures that usually are handled by a health care professional. You can get ready for this responsibility by reading about the person's condition and its treatment and by talking with the doctor and the discharge planner. Be sure to write down any questions you have in advance, and take notes so you remember the answers. Ask for explanations when you don't understand an answer.

Find out about the person's condition

Before the person leaves the hospital, ask the doctor what to expect during recovery—both short term and long term. For instance, you might ask:

• Will the recovery be complete?
• How long will the recovery take?
• What impairment or limitations can be expected?
• About how long will they last?
• Will the condition worsen?
• What treatment does the care plan include?
• How often will follow-up checkups be needed?
• What medicines will be prescribed, and can the person use a generic (less expensive) form?

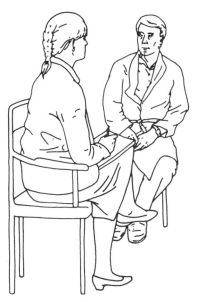

Getting answers to your questions

Discuss home health services

A home care program may emerge as a schedule of daily routines, procedures, medications, and visits with the doctor, nurse, aide, or therapist. The discharge planner will outline what needs to be done and help decide what you can and can't take on yourself. The discharge planner will also help coordinate the efforts of the home care team. Plan to talk with her about Medicaid, Medicare, or other insurance coverage. She can answer such questions as the following:

• How does the person apply for Medicare benefits?
• What services are available from non-

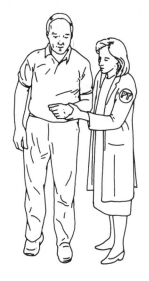

profit home care providers (such as the Visiting Nurse Association, whose rates are based on income)?
• What services are available from commercial home nursing services (whose rates are fixed)?
• Which organizations can I contact for help or information?
• Which therapists (such as physical, respiratory, or speech therapists) will come to the home?

Consider pharmacy services
The pharmacist can tell you about drug actions and effects and whether or not the person can safely take an over-the-counter drug. You might also ask:
• What kind of service can be expected?
• Does the pharmacy deliver?
• Is it close by?
• Is the staff cooperative?
• Does the pharmacist keep a file of the person's prescriptions?
• How will the pharmacy bill the person?

Obtain supplies and equipment
The discharge planner may be an excellent resource for learning about special supplies and equipment the person may need. She can probably help with such questions as:
• Should special equipment, such as a hospital bed or a wheelchair, be rented, borrowed, or purchased?
• How long will this equipment be needed?
• Over this period, what is the estimated cost of renting the equipment? Of buying it?
• Can the equipment be paid for in installments?
• Does Medicare, Medicaid, or other insurance cover the cost in full? In part? (For instance, the insurance may pay for 8 months of rental or 80% of a purchase.) Can the equipment be used for anything else?

Arrange hospital-to-home transportation
The doctor may recommend that the person go home in an ambulance or he may approve ordinary transportation. Depending on his response, you might need answers to the following questions:
• Can the local ambulance service be used? If so, how much

does it cost? If not, what private ambulance services are available, and at what cost? What services does the fee include?
• Can a friend or family member go with the person in the ambulance?
• For safe travel, what equipment is needed for the person to get in and out of a car or taxi?

Preparing the home

Most people don't realize how dangerous or inconvenient their homes can be, especially for someone recovering from an illness. Use the following list to pinpoint household areas that need to be adapted to the needs of the person in your care.

Bathroom
• Install grab bars in the shower and tub.
• Obtain a tub seat if the tub is hard to enter and exit.
• Buy a shower chair for sitting instead of standing to bathe.
• Install a raised toilet seat.
• Put nonskid strips or a tub mat in the bathtub.
• Attach a hand-held shower head for easy rinsing.
• Install easy-to-turn faucet handles.
• Hang mirrors, shelves, and racks at wheelchair level.
• Set water heater temperature no higher than 120° F (48.8° C).

Bedroom
• Keep a commode chair, urinal, or bedpan close to the bed.
• Secure a hospital-type bed (with side rails and attached trapeze).
• Install a bedside telephone.
• Provide a night-light or a bedside flashlight.
• Install a fire escape or portable ladder.

Kitchen
• Provide a working fire extinguisher.
• Lower kitchen counters, and reorganize storage areas.
• Install easy-to-reach stove controls.

Living room
• Add extra cushions to raise the seating level if the person has trouble rising from a low chair or sofa.

• Arrange furniture to permit free access.
• Remove electrical cords and wires from walkways.
• Provide a conveniently located telephone (either stationary or portable) with a long cord.

All areas
• Install smoke or heat detectors.
• Cover exposed heating pipes and radiators to prevent burns.
• Keep the indoor temperature no higher than 80° F (26.6° C) for maximum comfort.
• Provide good lighting.
• Install handrails along walls for support while walking.
• Provide low-pile carpeting for easy movement.
• Remove area and throw rugs, and keep floors free of clutter.
• Tape down loose carpet edges.
• Repair holes and rough floor areas.
• Install ramps over raised doorsills.
• Secure stair banisters and railings.
• Apply brightly colored tape on step edges.
• Widen door frames to at least 27 inches (69 cm) to accommodate a wheelchair.
• Provide a ramp leading into the house, and repair uneven spots on steps and sidewalk.

Addressing psychological and emotional changes

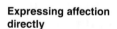

Expressing affection directly

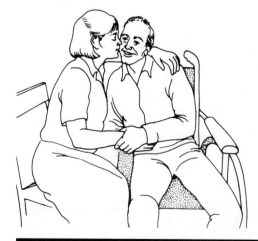

Taking care of a loved one who can't care for himself may be one of the most emotionally stressful challenges you'll encounter in your lifetime. Simply recognizing your emotions may offer relief when you're plunged into the situation.

Show your affection directly
Just as your home is still your home despite its adaptation to your family member's illness and treatment, your loved one is still your wife, husband, child, or parent, despite his or her condition. Affirm your loving relationship with the person directly; don't express your feelings only through the care you give.

Deal with your loved one's fear and guilt

Be as supportive and reassuring as you can, and contact groups that can provide information about his condition. He may also feel better talking to people with similar problems in a local support group.

Deal with your own fear and guilt

But what about your feelings—what kind of impact do they have? If the person's guidance and support people are frightened, his fear can spiral into anger and feelings of rejection. In addition, he'll lose confidence in the care you're delivering. This kind of chain reaction plays on your mental and physical health. Stress is exhausting. Beware! Fear and insecurity may wear you out before you've even begun your tasks. What can you do?

First, learn all you can about the person's condition, because changes that occur will then frighten you less.

Next, talk about your fears and moods with someone who can understand—not necessarily the person you're caring for. Talk to friends or other family members if you like. If not, find a community support group where you can share your feelings with other caregivers. Ask your local church or synagogue or the Visiting Nurse Association for support group contacts.

Don't deny your guilt feelings. Denial only makes them harder to deal with. When you start to think "I shouldn't feel this way" about your guilt feelings, fears, or moods, that's denial. To get rid of these feelings, recognize them right away and accept them. You may want to discuss them with someone you trust. Remain aware of and accept your other feelings as they arise. Take charge of your emotional life.

Expect role changes

Illness and care bring about role changes. Such changes are unsettling, and you'll need time to adjust to them.

Share these emotions with the person you're caring for when you can. Both of you are probably sensing the same changes from opposite sides of the picture. Expressing the feelings will make the role transitions seem less strange while relieving stress and reinforcing your emotional bond. Recognize that sadness and fear of loss spring from the same source as your love. Affirming your love for each other can energize your body and your spirit.

Trying to maintain normalcy

The concept of normalcy is central to home care. Normalcy is what you can offer your loved one at home that a hospital can't. Normalcy integrates home life and highly professional medical care. Equally important is the balance between caring for the person's needs and nurturing his independence.

Pay attention to family dynamics. The person you're caring for shouldn't become a dictator. Conversely, you and other family members shouldn't ignore his special needs for rest, peace and quiet, and timely attention to medical and personal needs.

Use normalcy and the knowledge that what affects him also affects you as two standards for decision making.

Choose a convenient location

When you decide where to place the person you're caring for in your home, figure out the effects of various options. Ask "How will this choice affect me? How will it affect him?" and "Will this choice help to create normalcy in our home?"

Integrating care and family dynamics

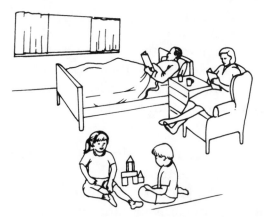

Each home is different. Don't assume anything. Keep an open mind. Discuss the choice of a location with the person you're taking care of and other family members. Try out various locations in your mind, including the family or living room. Ask:
• Is it close to a bathroom?
• Does it provide access to visitors?
• Is it convenient for you and comfortable for the person you're caring for?
• Can you control people traffic and noise when he needs rest?
• Can you create privacy with screens or by closing a door for rest, treatments, and procedures?

The best placement balances your loved one's needs with your own.

Try to maintain normal eating patterns

If possible, keep your normal mealtime schedule and include the person you're caring for when and where the family dines, even if he's on a different diet. This enriches his life and reduces the demands on your serving time.

Eating with a person who's in bed

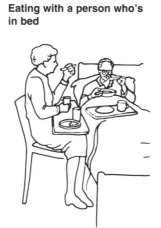

Eating with the family

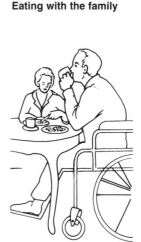

If the person can't join the whole family at the dinner table, various family members can eat their meals in his room. They can give you a break by serving and feeding him then, too.

Discuss sexual activity

Many couples hesitate to discuss their sex lives. Yet an adaptable and active sexual relationship may be a rejuvenating outlet for both, relieving the sense of isolation and offering comfort and contact.

If the doctor doesn't discuss sex in the meeting before your loved one leaves the hospital, don't hesitate to bring up the subject yourself. Ask the doctor to specify any limitations on sexual activity. Doubt due to unasked questions, such as "Is it OK to do this?" or "Will this be harmful to the person I'm caring for?" can inhibit healthy sexual interaction. Don't let limitations curtail your sexual activity. Explore alternative ways to express your sexual needs and feelings for each other.

Talking about sex is difficult for many people, even those who have shared a long-term sexual relationship. If you think that you and your loved one need help to open up the subject, seek the help of a counselor, especially one experienced with the problems of chronically or acutely ill people. Self-help groups can offer support and direction. Ask the doctor or the Visiting Nurse Association for sources.

Planning daily activities

Home care means a full schedule of daily activities, such as the following:
• Strictly adhering to the medication and treatment schedules the doctor's plan of care specifies
• Attending to your loved one's personal needs, including mouth care, daily baths, linen changes, and bathroom and urinal assistance or catheter maintenance
• Meeting nutritional needs by preparing and serving meals and snacks, adhering to a special diet, or administering a tube feeding and maintaining the feeding tube
• Keeping a record of the person's progress and measuring and recording vital signs
• Efficiently accomplishing supply shopping so you don't run out of the essentials.

And what about everyday chores, like dusting, vacuuming, and doing the laundry as well as taking a shower, shampooing your hair, and caring for your clothing?

Set reasonable goals and limits

How can you get it all done and still have the energy to be a sensitive and alert human being? The first means to that end is to set reasonable goals and limits for yourself each day. Easier said than done, perhaps, but you must learn to do it.

Schedule strenuous activities

Try to schedule activities that are strenuous for you and the person you're caring for so that they don't interfere with meals or rest. Physical exertion temporarily suppresses the appetite and stimulates the system, which could disrupt your schedule for nutrition and needed sleep.

Storing supplies conveniently

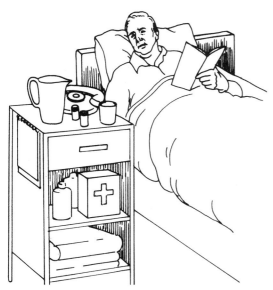

Plan ahead

In the end, you'll save time by taking the time to organize. Think geographically; map your excursions to minimize mileage. Do the same at home. Keep supplies conveniently located, and try to combine trips up and down stairs to reduce your steps.

Regular, ongoing lists help enormously. They're a wonderful tool—as long as you remember to look at them. Keep appropriate lists where you're sure to see them—on the refrigerator door, on the supply cabinet, and at the person's bedside.

Make sure you have the proper supplies for special treatments. If you need help locating an item, the discharge planner is a useful resource, as are the nursing staff, a physical therapist, and the equipment supplier.

Arrange for help

Don't try to do everything yourself; arrange to get help when you need it. You personally cannot and should not attempt to take on the whole load yourself.

Identify what kind of "people assistance" you need. A home health aide can help with the grocery shopping and tasks around the house as well as with care for your loved one. A nurse or an aide can relieve you of a task and monitor the person for signs you may not identify.

Sometimes, agencies and services can plug into your schedule. Meals On Wheels provides meals, even customized ones for special diets, such as diabetic or low-salt, for the homebound.

Local community groups, churches and synagogues, and the Visiting Nurse Association can refer you to homemaker support sources.

Respite hospital care is another possibility. Some hospitals open floors over weekends where they deliver maintenance care at reduced rates. Consult the doctor, and inquire at local hospitals.

Use a variety of helpers to get yourself out of the house. The alternatives—staying at home constantly or leaving the person unattended—are not acceptable. When do you leave the person, however, tell him when you'll return.

Avoiding burnout

Anyone who cares for a person who needs full-time supervision and care is a prime candidate for burnout. Seemingly endless responsibilities can leave you emotionally and physically drained with virtually no time for yourself. If you feel inadequate to handle an unexpected crisis, both you and the person you're caring for may suffer.

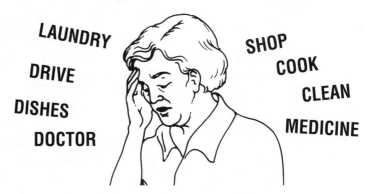

How can you cope? Start by learning the warning signs of burnout so you'll know if you're reaching your physical and emotional limits.

Ask yourself these questions:
• Do I have trouble getting organized?
• Do I cry for no reason?
• Am I short-tempered?
• Do I feel numb and emotionless?
• Are everyday tasks getting harder to accomplish?
• Do I constantly feel pressed for time?
• Do I feel that I just can't do anything right?
• Do I feel that I have no time for myself?

If you answered yes to these questions, you're probably suffering from burnout. If so, the tips that follow will help you meet your own needs so you can give better care.

Get enough rest

Exhaustion magnifies pressures and reduces your ability to cope. So the first step in combating burnout is to get a good night's sleep—every night, if possible. Here's how.

Decide how much sleep you usually need—say, 7 hours—and set aside this much time. Then, when you go to bed, try not to replay the day in your mind; this isn't the time to solve problems.

Rejuvenating rest

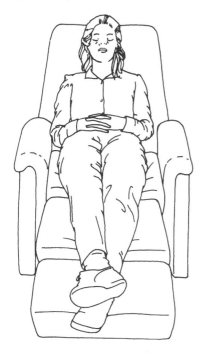

To help control disturbing thoughts, try relaxation techniques, such as deep breathing, reading, or listening to soft music. Or try dimming the bathroom lights and taking a warm bath or shower to relieve muscle tension and help you wind down.

Aerobic activity can encourage sleep by tiring you physically. It also increases your physical stamina, improves your self-image, brightens your outlook, and can get you out of the house.

If possible, hire a relief caretaker so you can attend aerobics classes, go for a brisk walk, or get some kind of exercise for at least 1 hour three times a week.

In addition, try to schedule three or four short breaks during the day.

Resting for 10 minutes with your feet up and your eyes closed can rejuvenate you and counteract the cycle of frantic activity that's probably keeping you up at night.

Finally, use sleeping pills and tranquilizers only as a last resort—and only temporarily. Both kinds of drugs have side effects that can cause more problems for you in the long run. Instead, to induce drowsiness, try drinking a glass of warm milk.

Eat well

Eating regular, well-balanced meals will help keep up your energy and increase your resistance to illness.

Skipping meals or eating on the run can cause vitamin and mineral deficiencies, such as anemia (a shortage of iron in the blood), that deplete your strength and make you feel exhausted.

Choose foods from the five food groups every day, avoid nonnutritious ("empty") calories, and unless you're overweight and the doctor advises it, don't diet—you need extra calories to fuel your increased activity.

Don't try to be superhuman

After you've been giving home care for several weeks, reappraise your earlier plans. How much can you really do? How much time do you need for yourself?

Delegate tasks. If possible, hire extra caretakers or someone to help with housework and shopping. Send out your laundry. Remember: You don't have to do it all yourself, or do it all today, or accomplish everything on your list. Do only what is necessary, and learn to set priorities.

Save some time for pleasurable activities. If you have 15 minutes' free time, listen to music or take a walk.

If you want to invite friends for dinner, go ahead. Just ask everyone to bring a course.

Confiding in a friend

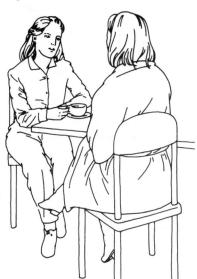

Confide in someone

A family member or close friend can help you resolve conflicts, be a sounding board for your anger and frustration, and offer emotional support. A support group can accomplish this too, as well as offer practical hints for home care.

Allow yourself some quality time alone

Free time won't happen automatically—you have to schedule it. In fact, the person you're caring for also needs time for himself. So allow yourself and him some personal space and private time. If you don't, you'll become too dependent on each other.

Try to keep your life as normal as possible. Continue to do things that you enjoy, either by yourself or with friends.

Remember: Meeting your own needs isn't selfish, even if the person you're caring for isn't homebound. If you continue to feel guilty about taking some time for yourself, seek counseling.

How much time alone is necessary? The answer depends

on you. At the least, you need to take the time to attend to your important personal needs.

At the other end of the spectrum, you might want or need to have a part-time or full-time job. If so, you'll need to arrange for a caretaker to fill in for you while you're working away from home.

Make sure this arrangement reflects your personality and your unique relationship with the person you're caring for.

What is your goal? To provide the best quality of life for the person without sacrificing your own. How you accomplish this goal is up to you. If you're happy with the arrangement and the person seems reasonably content, the arrangement is probably working.

Using good posture to protect your back

Good posture is a must whether you're standing, sitting, or lying down. It strengthens the abdominal and buttock muscles that support your hardworking back.

While practicing good posture, remember to maintain the natural curve of the spine by using muscle power, a pillow support, or a towel roll.

Correct posture   **Incorrect posture**

Standing and walking

When you're standing correctly, you should be able to draw an imaginary line from your ear through the tip of your shoulder, middle of your hip, back of your knee, and front of your ankle. You won't be able to do this if you stand with your lower back arched, your upper back stooped, or your abdomen sagging forward.

To correct your posture, stand 1 foot (30 cm) away from a wall. Then lean back against the wall with your knees slightly bent. Tighten your stomach and buttock muscles to tilt your pelvis back, and flatten your lower back.

Holding this position, inch up the wall until you're standing. Your lower back should still be pressed against the wall. This is the posture to assume when walking.

When walking, wear rubber-soled shoes with moderate heels, if possible. Avoid changing between low and high heels. When standing longer than a few minutes, put one foot on a stool or step, switching legs as necessary for comfort.

Sitting

If possible, sit on a hard, straight-backed chair. Place a towel roll or small pillow behind your lower back. Carry this back support with you when you travel.

To keep your back from tiring when you're sitting for a long time, raise one leg higher than the other by propping it on a footrest.

When you're seated reading or knitting, place a pillow on your lap to raise the work up to you. If you're working at a desk, slant a clipboard toward you, supporting it with books. Or sit at an artist's or a draftsman's table, if available.

When driving a car, support your neck with a towel roll or a neck rest. Build up the support if it feels too far back to support your neck comfortably. Position your seat low and close to the wheel, so your knees are level with your hips. You should be able to reach the pedals without fully extending your legs.

Lying down

Sleep on a firm mattress. If you must sleep on a soft mattress, support it with a bedboard or a piece of plywood placed underneath it.

The best position for sleeping is lying on your side with your knees bent and a pillow between them. This position prevents your spine from twisting when you drop your upper leg. Don't curl up excessively. This can put too much pressure on your back bones.

Sleeping on your back is OK if you keep a pillow under

Pillow placement when lying on your side

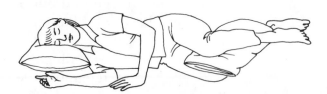

Pillow placement when lying on your back

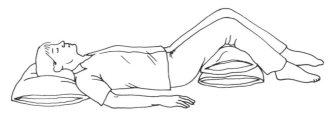

your knees or place a small pillow or rolled towel under the small of your back or both.

Avoid sleeping on your stomach or on high pillows. These positions can strain your back, neck, and shoulders. Also, avoid foam pillows because they don't allow complete resting support. If you read in bed, support your back and arms with pillows.

Picking up an object　　**Carrying an object**

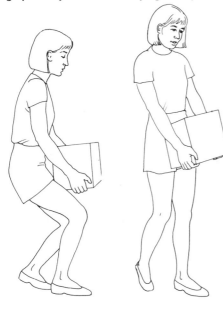

Lifting and carrying

Maintain the natural low back curve with your pelvis tucked in while lifting and carrying. Turn and face the object you want to lift. Keeping your feet flat and shoulder width apart, bend your knees, lower yourself to the object, and place your hands around it. Keeping your knees bent and your back straight, use your arm and leg muscles (instead of your back muscles) to lift the object. Avoid lifting heavy objects above your waist.

Carry the object by holding it close to your body. Avoid carrying unbalanced loads or anything heavier than you can easily manage. Get help to lift large or bulky items.

Pushing and pulling

Maintain the natural low back curve with your pelvis tucked in while pushing and pulling. When raking or vacuuming, bend your knees rather than bending or twisting your back. Avoid straining to open windows or doors, and don't attempt to move heavy furniture.

Preparing for an emergency

When an emergency occurs, quick thinking and action are necessary. It can be an extremely stressful situation at any time, especially if the emergency occurs with the person in your care. The guidelines and information that follow will help you ease the stress by being a prepared caregiver.

General emergency guidelines

• Keep a list of emergency numbers at each phone, including doctor, ambulance, fire, and police.
• Mark the national emergency number—911—on each phone in the home.
• Obtain special window stickers that indicate that a disabled person lives in the home.
• Notify local fire and rescue squads about the person's condition and the possibility that help may be needed in an emergency.
• Have a written description of the person's condition available to minimize confusion or miscommunication.

Medic Alert System

In an emergency, Medic Alert, a nonprofit medical identification service, informs caregivers of a subscriber's special medical needs. A Medic Alert necklace or bracelet identifies a special health condition—for example, allergies. Engraved on the necklace or bracelet is the person's identification number and Medic Alert's 24-hour hot line number.

Medic Alert identification bracelet

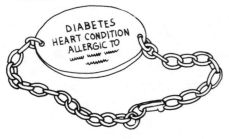
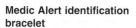

By calling the hot line and giving the person's identification number, the caregiver has access to important medical information. The service also records the names and telephone numbers of the doctor and people to contact in an emergency.

Who needs medical identification?

People with:
• allergies to drugs, venoms, or other substances
• conditions, such as diabetes, heart disease, or asthma
• medication regimens, such as insulin for diabetes
• devices, such as contact lenses or a pacemaker
• special instructions, such as organ donation.

How to obtain medical identification

You can obtain more information by writing or calling Medic Alert, Turlock, CA 95381-1009, (800) ID-ALERT.

Vial of Life

The Vial of Life program helps place a person's vital medical information—known medical conditions, medications, allergies, and blood type—at a rescue worker's fingertips. Here's how to set up this system.

Obtaining and using the kit

To participate in the Vial of Life program, all that's needed is a kit like the one shown below. The kit contains a plastic vial, a medical information form (designed to record information about two persons), a decal, and an instruction sheet.

A kit may be obtained through a pharmacist, a doctor, the Visiting Nurse Association, or a community services group. (If the Vial of Life program doesn't exist in your community, consider setting up such a program. Then advise emergency personnel of the program.) To obtain kits, contact Loral Packaging, Inc., 52 South Avenue, Garwood, NJ 07027.

Filling out the information form

Help the person fill out the medical information form, if necessary. The information should be as complete and detailed as possible. Write additional information on the back of the form.

Keeping the form secure

Now, roll up the form and place it inside the plastic vial. Firmly cap the vial.

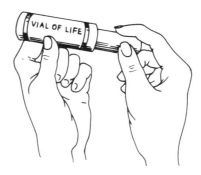

Attaching the vial to the refrigerator

Using a rubber band, attach the vial to the right side of the refrigerator's top shelf. Or hang it from the shelf's rung, as shown. To do this, place the slit in the ring on the cap's top against the rung, and press firmly until the ring snaps in place around the rung.

Why the refrigerator? Because nearly everybody has one, and most ambulance crews are trained to check it automatically for a Vial of Life.

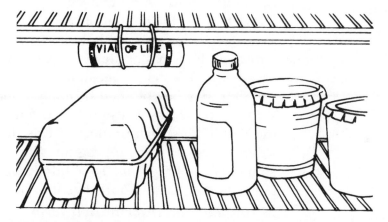

Attaching the decal

Firmly attach the decal to the outside of the refrigerator door. This tells the ambulance crew that a Vial of Life is inside. Take care not to cover the decal with a shopping list or note.

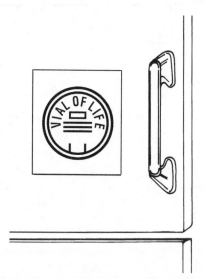

2 Care Basics

Providing safety and comfort

If you're caring for a relative or friend who is recovering from an illness, be sure to identify any household changes required for the person's safety and convenience. Give special attention to the rooms the person will be using the most often.

Adjust lighting, temperature, and humidity

• Install sufficient night-lights. Use light bulbs that are bright enough to compensate for impaired vision. Be sure stairways are well lighted.
• Keep room temperature at 68° to 72° F (20° to 22.2° C), or slightly warmer for elderly people and very young children. Set the hot water temperature at 115° to 120° F (46.1° to 48.8° C) to prevent accidental scalding.
• Maintain relative humidity at 30% to 60%.

Make it easier to use the phone

• Provide a phone with an enlarged dial (if the person has impaired vision) and an amplifier (if he has hearing loss). Locate phone cords away from household traffic.
• Post emergency numbers in large print by the phone.

Remove potential safety hazards

• Wipe up spills promptly. Keep floors free of clutter.
• Remove throw rugs or anchor them securely.
• Apply brightly colored tape to step edges.
• Provide sturdy chairs and stools with good support.
• Install handrails, if necessary.
• Make sure the heater is working and adequately vented.
• Keep electrical cords in good condition, and place them away from household traffic.
• Remove potential fire hazards; provide smoke detectors, and make sure they're in working condition.

Arrange the bedroom carefully

• If necessary, obtain an adjustable, hospital-type bed with side rails. Place the bed against a wall and lock its wheels. If the bed is not a hospital type, lock or remove its casters or wheels.
• Provide a bedside portable toilet, if necessary.
• Place a wastebasket lined with paper or plastic next to the

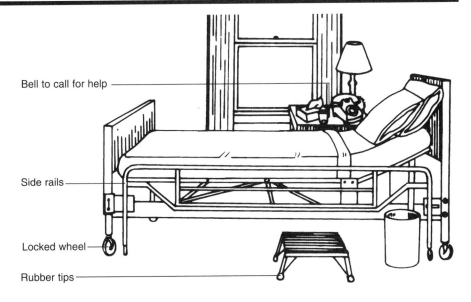

Bell to call for help

Side rails

Locked wheel

Rubber tips

bed for easy disposal of tissues and other waste items.
• Place personal items within easy reach, including a small
bell for summoning help.
• Adjust the ringer on a bedside phone to its lowest setting.
Keep in mind that the person may be unusually sensitive to
ordinary noises.
• If a footstool is being used, place rubber tips on the legs.

Take safety precautions in the bathroom
• Install grab bars in the tub and near the toilet. Also install
a raised toilet seat, if needed. Make sure the tub and shower
have nonslip bottoms and that bath mats are secure.
• Locate electrical outlets a safe distance from the tub.

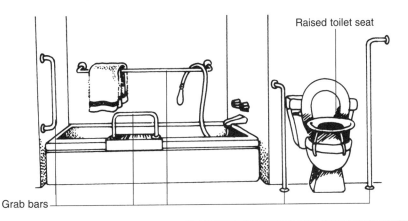

Raised toilet seat

Grab bars

Guard against falls in the kitchen
• Place often-used items within easy reach.
• Keep floors dry, nonslippery, and free of clutter.

Ease access to and from the outside
• Keep steps in good condition; mark the top and bottom steps with brightly colored paint or tape.
• Repair uneven areas on the sidewalk.
• Install a ramp leading into the house, if needed.

Preventing injury

Restraints can help prevent injury and provide protection. They can help keep a confused person from wandering, falling, or otherwise hurting himself.

Restraints serve many purposes. For instance, safety vests and safety belts prevent a person from falling out of bed or a chair. Limb holders prevent a person from removing dressings or catheters. Protective mitts prevent a person from injuring himself by scratching.

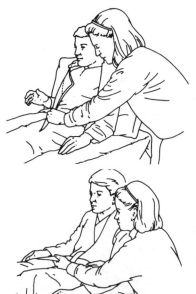

Putting on a safety vest

1 While holding the vest right side out, slip the person's arms through the armholes. Then pull the vest over his gown or pajamas. Crisscross the cloth flaps at the front, placing the V-shaped opening at the person's throat. (Never crisscross the flaps at the back because the vest may ride up and cause choking if the person becomes restless.)

2 Pass the tab on one flap through the slot on the opposite flap. Then adjust the vest for comfort. (You should be able to slip your hand between the vest and the person's stomach.) Wrapping the vest too tightly may restrict breathing. Tighten or loosen the straps so that the vest holds securely but doesn't restrict breathing. Loosen the vest often to let the person stretch, turn, and breathe deeply.

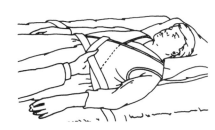

3 Now help the person lie down in bed. Tie the vest straps securely to the bed frame, out of his reach. Repeat on the other side of the bed. Leave 1 to 2 inches (2.5 to 5 cm) of slack in the straps to allow movement. (*Note:* If the bed frame is adjustable, be sure to tie the straps to the movable frame.) Use a knot or bow that can be released quickly in an emergency, like the ones shown here.

Applying a safety belt

1 Center the belt's flannel pad on the bed. Then wrap the belt's short strap around the movable part of the bed frame and fasten it under the bed.

2 Position the person on the pad, and then roll him slightly to one side while you guide the long strap around his waist and through the slot in the pad.

3 Wrap the long strap around the bed frame and fasten it under the bed. After applying the belt, slip your hand inside it to check that it's secure but comfortable.

Applying a limb holder

1 Pad the wrist or ankle with a washcloth before applying the limb holder. This prevents skin irritation.

2 Pass the strap on the narrow end of the limb holder through the slot in the broad end; or fasten the buckle or Velcro cuffs. Fasten the limb holder securely but not tight enough to restrict circulation. You should be able to slip one or two fingers inside it.

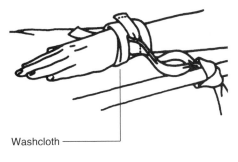

Washcloth

3 Tie the limb holder's long strap ends securely to the bed frame or to a chair beyond the person's reach. Bend his arm or leg slightly before securing the strap and leave 1 to 2 inches (2.5 to 5 cm) of slack. Always tie the straps with a knot that can be released quickly in an emergency. After applying the limb holder, make sure it doesn't obstruct circulation.

Putting on mitts

1 Wash and dry the person's hands. Then place a rolled washcloth or gauze pad in the person's palm and have him form a loose fist around it. Pull the mitt over it and secure the closure.

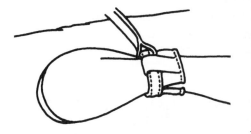

2 To restrict arm movement, tie the strap securely to the bed frame with a quick-release knot. When using mitts made of transparent mesh, check the person's skin frequently to make sure blood is circulating. At least once a day, remove the mitts to exercise the hands.

Performing proper handwashing

Everyday activities, such as petting your dog or sorting money, leave unwanted germs on your hands. These germs may enter your body and cause an infection. To prevent this, wash your hands several times daily—and always before meals. Here's how.

1 Wet your hands under running water. This carries away contaminants.

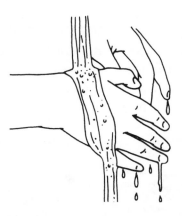

2 Lather your hands and wrists with soap. Although soap and water don't actually kill germs, they do loosen the

skin oils and deposits that harbor germs. While you're washing, give your fingernails a good scrub, too.

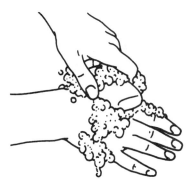

3 Now, thoroughly rinse your hands in running water. Make sure your fingers point downward. That way runoff water won't travel up your arms to bring new germs down to your hands.

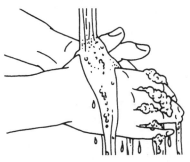

4 If you're at home, dry your hands with a clean cloth or paper towel. Don't dry off with a used towel, which may put germs right back on your hands. If you're in a public place, a hot-air hand dryer is best, but clean paper towels will do.

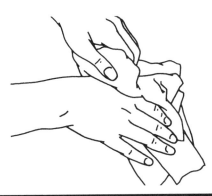

Help for dry hands

If your skin becomes dry or rough from frequent handwashing, apply hand lotion. And don't use strong soaps. They aren't needed for good hygiene, and they may cause drying or even allergic reactions.

Measuring vital signs

Vital signs include body temperature, pulse and respiratory rates, and blood pressure. They're measured to detect important changes in the body.

Temperature

Body temperature is the measure of heat within the body—the balance between heat produced and heat lost. Heat is produced by metabolism (the chemical processes that change food into energy and living tissue), exercise, and other factors. The body loses heat through the skin, lungs, and body wastes. When heat production balances heat loss, body temperature is normal. Oral temperature in adults normally ranges from 97° to 99.5° F (36.1° to 37.5° C).

Taking a temperature correctly

A fever usually means that your body is fighting an infection or some other illness. To find out if you or a family member

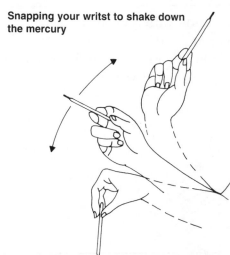

Snapping your writst to shake down the mercury

has a fever, you'll probably use a mercury or digital thermometer. You can take a temperature orally, rectally, or under the arm. A new device, a tympanic membrane thermometer, is now available that checks body temperature through the opening of the ear. Normal rectal temperature is about 1° higher and underarm temperature, 1° to 2° lower.

Using a mercury thermometer

Before using a mercury thermometer, wipe it with an alcohol-soaked gauze pad and rinse it off.

1 With your thumb and forefinger, grasp the thermometer at the end opposite the bulb.

Then quickly snap your wrist to shake down the mercury.

2 Next, hold the thermometer at eye level in good light and rotate it slowly until you see the mercury line clearly. Look for a reading of 95° F (35° C) or lower. Now you're ready to take a temperature.

3 To take an oral temperature, place the bulb of the thermometer under the tongue, as far back as possible. The person shouldn't bite on the thermometer or keep it in place with the teeth. This can affect an accurate reading. Leave the thermometer in place for 4 to 5 minutes—the time needed to register the correct temperature. Then remove the thermometer, and read it at eye level.

To make sure you get an accurate reading, never take an oral temperature right after smoking a cigarette or sipping a hot or cold beverage. Instead, wait for 20 to 30 minutes.

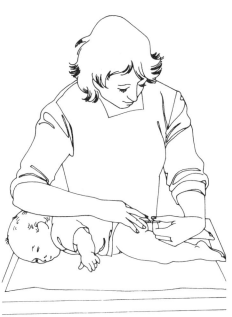

4 To take a rectal temperature, first dip the bulb end of the rectal thermometer in petroleum jelly. Then have the person lie on his side with the top leg bent. Gently insert the thermometer into the rectum about 1½ inches (3.8 cm) for an adult. If you are taking a infant's rectal temperature, position him on his stomach, as shown here, and insert the thermometer about ½ inch (1.3 cm). If the patient is a child, use the position used for adults and insert the thermometer about 1 inch. *Note:* To avoid accidents with a glass thermometer, consider using a tympanic membrane thermometer for infants and children.

Hold the thermometer in place for 3 minutes. Next, carefully remove it and wipe it with a tissue. Read the thermometer at eye level.

5 To take an underarm temperature, put the thermometer's bulb in one armpit and fold that arm across the chest. (This secures the thermometer.) Remove the thermometer after 10 minutes, and read it at eye level.

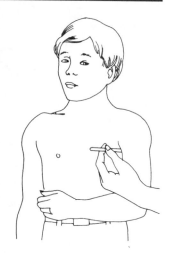

Using a digital thermometer

If you wish, you can use a digital thermometer instead of a mercury thermometer to take an oral temperature reading. Here's how.

1 Remove the thermometer from its protective case.

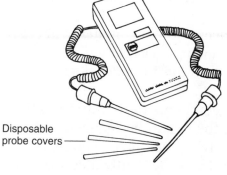

Disposable probe covers

2 Next, position the thermometer tip under the tongue, as far back as possible. Leave the thermometer in place for at least 45 seconds.

3 Remove the thermometer, and read the numbers displayed—this is the temperature. Clean the thermometer as the manufacturer instructs, and return it to its protective case.

Using a tympanic thermometer

If available, you can use a tympanic thermometer to take a temperature reading. Here's how.

Thermometer in unit base

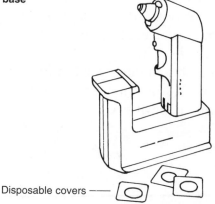

Disposable covers

1 Remove the device from the base unit.

2 Place a disposable cover snugly over the probe tip.

3 Insert the probe far enough into the opening of the ear canal to seal the opening.

4 Press and release the button to start the reading.

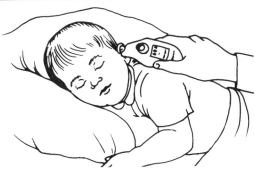

Inserting the probe into the ear canal

5 Remove the probe when you hear the beep. Read the numbers displayed—this is the temperature.

6 Press the release button to discard the probe cover. Return the device to the base unit.

Pulse

Every heartbeat produces a wave of blood that causes a pulsation through the arteries. The number of heartbeats per minute is called the pulse rate. The pulse rate is easy to find in the radial artery at the wrist, in the femoral artery in the

Pulse sites

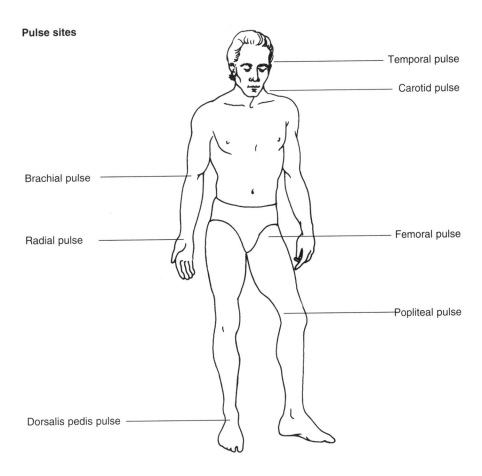

Temporal pulse

Carotid pulse

Brachial pulse

Radial pulse

Femoral pulse

Popliteal pulse

Dorsalis pedis pulse

groin, and in the dorsalis pedis artery in the foot. Other pulse sites are the temporal, carotid, brachial, and popliteal arteries.

The heart of an adult at rest normally beats 60 to 100 times per minute. The normal pulse rate varies with age, size, and weight. Men usually have a lower rate than women. Activity also affects the pulse rate. It's slower during sleep and faster after running, other vigorous exercise, or heavy physical work. Excitement, anger, fever, fear, and certain drugs (caffeine, for example) also increase the rate.

Taking a radial pulse

Before you begin, make sure you have a watch with a second hand.

Hand positions for taking a radial pulse

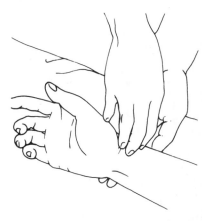

1 Have the person lie down or sit up with his arm placed comfortably at his side, palm facing upward. Then gently press your first, second, and third fingers on the radial artery inside the wrist. Don't use your thumb to take the pulse because it has a strong pulse of its own.

2 After you've located the pulse, count the beats for 30 seconds if the rhythm is regular. Then multiply by 2 to get the rate per minute. If the pulse is irregular, count for a full 60 seconds. If it's too fast (more than 100 beats per minute when the person is still) or too slow (less than 60 beats per minute when the person is still) for no known reason, call the doctor for advice.

Respirations

Respiration is the process of breathing—the exchange of oxygen and carbon dioxide between the atmosphere and the lungs. The respiratory rate is the number of breathing cycles (inhaling and exhaling) per minute.

A respiratory rate of 12 to 20 breaths per minute is considered normal. It may increase with excitement, exercise, pain, and fever. Rapid respirations indicate that the body is increasing its effort to maintain the right balance by taking deeper breaths. The respiratory rate decreases during sleep and relaxation. Although you can count your own respirations, you'll probably get a better reading if someone else counts them when you're not aware of it. Your respiratory rate may change if you're conscious of it.

Counting respirations

Count respirations right after checking the pulse. Here's how.

1 Observe the rise and fall of the chest during inhalation and exhalation. Count one rise and one fall as one respiration.

2 Count respirations for 30 seconds, and then multiply by 2 to get the rate per minute. If the rate seems abnormal, count for 60 seconds. Report an abnormal rate (below 12 or above 30) or an irregular rhythm to the doctor.

Taking blood pressure

A blood pressure reading indirectly measures the changing pressure that blood exerts on artery walls as the heart contracts and relaxes.

Blood pressure is highest with each heartbeat during contraction—the systolic, or maximum, pressure. The pressure diminishes as the heart relaxes. It's lowest when the heart is relaxed before it begins to contract again—the diastolic, or minimum, pressure. Normal blood pressure ranges from 100 over 60 to 140 over 90 in adults. (The first or top number—for example, 100—refers to the systolic pressure, and the second or bottom number—for example, 60—refers to the diastolic pressure.)

Blood pressure is measured with a blood pressure cuff and a stethoscope or with a digital blood pressure monitor.

Two rubber tubes extend from the cloth-covered blood pressure cuff. One tube is connected to a rubber bulb air pump. The other tube—the manometer—is connected to a glass tube that contains mercury or to a special gauge. If you're using this type of equipment to take a blood pressure reading, ask the doctor or nurse or your medical supplier for detailed directions.

Measuring your blood pressure

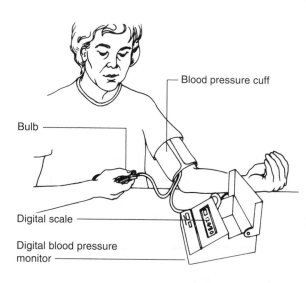

- Blood pressure cuff

Bulb

Digital scale

Digital blood pressure
monitor

Using a digital blood pressure monitor

Before you use a digital blood pressure monitor, thoroughly read the instruction book that comes with the unit. Operating steps vary with different units, so be sure to follow the directions carefully.

Taking your blood pressure

Take your blood pressure reading when you're relaxed and comfortable because physical exertion or emotional stress affects blood pressure.

1 Sit erect or lie down with your arm extended, well supported, and level with your heart. Apply the cuff over the brachial artery just above the elbow, as shown here. Wrap it firmly around the arm. Now, turn on the unit.

2 Inflate the cuff as the manufacturer directs until the digital scale registers about 160. Stop inflating the cuff. The numbers on the digital scale will start changing rapidly. When the numbers stop changing, your blood pressure reading will appear on the digital scale.

3 After you take the blood pressure reading and write it down, deflate the cuff, turn off the unit, and remove the cuff.

Taking another person's blood pressure

You can use a standard blood pressure cuff and stethoscope to take the blood pressure of the person in your care. If you're using an aneroid model, you may need to have it calibrated every 6 months. Just follow these steps.

1 Ask the person to sit comfortably and relax for about 2 minutes. Tell him to rest his arm on a table so that it's level with his heart. Use the same arm in the same position each time you take his blood pressure. While the person relaxes, hang the stethoscope around your neck.

2 Push up the person's sleeve, and wrap the cuff around his upper arm, just above the elbow, so you can slide only two fingers between the cuff and his arm.

3 Then, using your middle and index fingers, feel for a pulse in the wrist near the person's thumb.
When you find his pulse, turn the bulb's screw counterclockwise to close it; then squeeze the bulb rapidly to inflate the cuff. Note the reading on the gauge when you can no longer feel the pulse. (This reading, called the palpatory pressure, is your guideline for inflating the cuff.) Now, deflate the cuff by turning the screw clockwise.

Placing the stethoscope over the brachial pulse

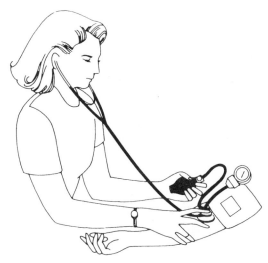

4 Place the stethoscope's earpieces in your ears. Then place the stethoscope's diaphragm (the disk portion) over the brachial pulse, in the crook of the person's arm.

5 Inflate the cuff 30 points higher than the palpatory pressure (the reading you obtained in step 3). Then loosen the bulb's screw to allow air to escape from the cuff. Listen for the first beating sound. When you hear it, note and record the number on the gauge: this is the systolic pressure (the top number of a blood pressure reading).
Continue to slowly deflate the cuff. When you hear the beating stop, note and record the number on the gauge: this is the diastolic pressure (the bottom number of a blood pressure reading).

6 Now, deflate the cuff completely and remove it. Record the blood pressure reading, date, and time.

Assisting elimination

The person who's confined to bed during an illness may need to use a bedpan and urinal. Follow these steps.

1 Warm the bedpan under running water and then dry it. If it's metal, check that it's not too hot because metal retains heat. Sprinkle talcum powder on the edge of the bedpan to reduce friction during placement and removal. Protect the bed from spills with linen-saver pads.

2 Raise the head of the bed slightly if the person has a hospital-type bed and the doctor allows it. Then rest the bedpan on the edge of the bed. Now, turn down the corner of the bedclothes, and ask the person to raise his buttocks by flexing his knees and pushing down on his heels. While supporting his lower back with one hand, center the curved, smooth edge of the bedpan beneath his buttocks. After placing the bedpan, raise the head of the bed further, if allowed, until the person is sitting erect. This position aids bowel movement and urination. Or tuck a small pillow or folded bath towel under the small of his back to support it. If the person can be left alone, provide toilet tissue and a bell so that he can signal when the bedpan can be removed. If the person is weak, stay with him.

3 Lower the head of the bed slightly if you have a hospital-type bed. Then ask the person to raise his buttocks off the bedpan. Support his lower back with one hand, and gen-

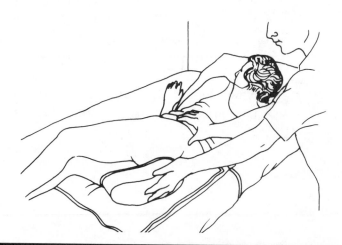

tly remove the bedpan. Cover the bedpan, and place it on a chair.

After a bowel movement, help clean the area, as necessary. Turn the person on his side, wipe carefully first with toilet tissue and then with a damp washcloth and soap, and dry well. If the person is female, clean from front to back.

Alternative method for placing the bedpan

If the person can't raise his buttocks from the bed, here's what to do: Roll him on his side, and position the bedpan against his buttocks. Then, holding the bedpan in place, roll the person on his back. After use, hold the bedpan securely to avoid spills, have the person roll to one side, and remove the pan. If necessary, ask someone to help you place and remove the bedpan.

Placing the urinal

If the person can't position the urinal himself, spread his legs slightly and hold the urinal in place while he urinates. Then carefully remove the urinal. The urinal shown on the left is for men; the one shown on the right is for women.

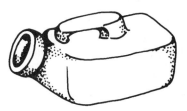 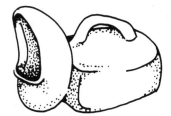

Cleaning up

End the procedure with these steps: Give the person a clean, damp washcloth for his hands and make him comfortable. Then take the bedpan or urinal to the bathroom. If the doctor has ordered it, measure the person's urine output. Then empty the bedpan, rinse it, and clean it thoroughly with a disinfectant, such as bleach diluted with water. Dry the bedpan and store it. If necessary, use an air freshener to eliminate odors.

Measuring fluid intake and output

The doctor may want you to keep a daily record of fluid intake and output. This record can help him judge the progress and response to treatment.

What are intake and output?

Intake includes everything you drink, such as water, fruit juice, and soda. It also includes foods that become liquid at room temperature, such as gelatin, custard, and ice cream. Intake even includes fluids, liquid medication, and solutions delivered through tubing into a vein (intravenously) or into the stomach.

Output includes everything that leaves the body as a fluid. It includes urine, drainage from a wound, diarrhea, and vomit.

Because intake should balance output, you need to keep accurate records. Whenever possible, measure fluids. Don't guess.

Measuring intake

Measure and record the amount of fluid you have with each meal, with your medication, and between meals. Pour any liquid first into a measuring cup or other graduated container and then into a glass or cup. Also, keep in mind that labels on cans and bottles indicate exact amounts.

Don't forget to subtract any amount you don't drink. The difference is the intake amount.

If you're receiving medication or nutrition intravenously or through a stomach tube, record the amount of fluid used.

Measuring output

1 Before discarding urine from a bedpan, urinal, or portable toilet, measure and record the amount. Keep a measuring container handy for this purpose.

2 If a drainage bag is in place, make sure to measure and record the amount of fluid in the bag before discarding it.

3 Measure and record vomitus or liquid bowel movements as output.

Common measures

Your doctor may want you to measure fluid intake and output metrically. To convert your household measure, use the information below.

To convert fluid ounces (oz) to the metric equivalent of milliliters (ml), multiply by 30. To convert milliliters to ounces, divide by 30.

APPROXIMATE EQUIVALENTS

Household	Metric
1 quart (32 oz)	1,000 ml
1 pint (16 oz)	500 ml
1 measuring cup (8 oz)	240 ml
2 tablespoons (1 oz)	30 ml
1 teaspoon	15 ml

3   Danger Signs

Learning about danger signs

Any marked change in a person's condition is a danger sign that could indicate a serious complication or deterioration in his health. Danger signs don't always signal a grave or an immediate threat, but they might. For example, a headache isn't a danger sign in a person who is known to suffer from migraine or tension headaches. And weakness usually isn't a danger sign in someone who's recuperating from major surgery, but sudden, profound weakness may well be a danger sign in such a person.

If you're caring for a person with a chronic illness, the doctor probably has already instructed you about the danger signs to watch for. He may also have told you what to do or what not to do when new signs occur.

But unless the doctor has clearly told you what to do, you should avoid treating the person in your care. For example, abdominal pain can have many causes. You could make a serious mistake if you give your favorite stomach remedy to a person with abdominal pain.

What should you do when a danger sign occurs and the doctor has not given you specific directions to follow? In that case, take these important steps.
• Make sure the person is comfortable and warm.
• Then call the doctor.
• In an emergency, take the person to the hospital. If you think that the danger sign requires quick action—for example, seizures, uncontrollable vomiting, pulse abnormalities, or crushing chest pain—and you can't immediately contact the doctor, call an ambulance and take the person to a hospital emergency department.

Establishing a baseline

You'll need to know what's normal and what isn't for the person you're caring for. (Remember, what's normal for one person may not be normal for someone else.) Certain indicators can help you establish the person's health baseline. Use the following guidelines.

Checking the skin

Have you noticed any change in the person's skin color and texture? Is he unusually pale or flushed? Does his face look puffy? How about skin texture? Look for any unusual red patches or swelling. Also note if the person's skin is rough or dry or shows poor elasticity.

To check elasticity, gently pinch a fold of the person's skin. Normally, the skin will resume its shape almost instantly. However, if it remains wrinkled for more than a few seconds, this shows poor elasticity.

Also, check the person's skin temperature by touch. In a cool environment, an elderly person may lose body temperature (hypothermia) without realizing it.

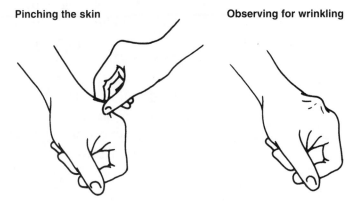

Pinching the skin   Observing for wrinkling

Testing strength

You can form a good idea of the person's baseline strength by knowing what tasks he can normally perform without difficulty; by watching his movements—for example, while eating or

Grasping the index and middle fingers

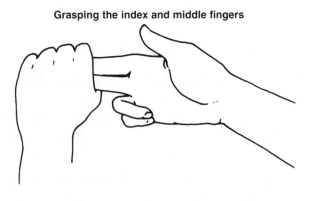

walking—and by testing his grip. To do so, ask the person to grasp your index and middle fingers firmly. Is his grasp the same in both hands?

Taking the temperature

Everyone's body temperature varies throughout the day and usually peaks between 5 p.m. and 10 p.m. Although 98.6° F (37° C) is considered normal, some people may have normal temperatures ranging from about 97.6° to 99.2° F (36.4° to 37.3° C).

Types of thermometers

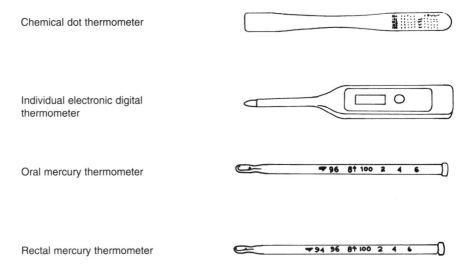

Chemical dot thermometer

Individual electronic digital thermometer

Oral mercury thermometer

Rectal mercury thermometer

The doctor will advise you about the best route for taking body temperature, depending on the person's age and condition. If the person is older than age 4, the temperature is usually taken orally (in the mouth) with a mercury thermometer. The temperature also may be taken in the armpit with a mercury thermometer if a person can't use the thermometer orally, but the reading is not as accurate. The thermometer must be left in place for 9 to 11 minutes. The temperature may be taken as well in the rectum with a rectal thermometer. Remember, never use oral and rectal thermometers interchangeably.

You'll need to establish the person's normal temperature by taking it regularly at the same time of day. For specific guidelines, see *Measuring vital signs*, page 28.

Checking the pulse

The pulse is a way of measuring heartbeats. A normal pulse rate may range from 60 to 100 beats per minute in an adult (at rest) and higher in a child or an infant. In some people, the pulse rate may be slower or faster at rest than the average, or it may be irregular. And many people have a natural pattern of heartbeats that's a little faster when inhaling and slower when exhaling. Ask the doctor what's normal for the person you're caring for. Then, to establish a baseline, take a resting pulse when the person has been at rest for 10 minutes or so.

Observing breathing

You can easily notice changes in the person's breathing. Watch for breathing that's rapid and shallow, for any sound of gasping or wheezing (whistling), or for other unusual sounds.

Check the person's breathing when he's at rest.

Noting the appetite

How much does the person in your care normally eat? Note the total amount eaten in an average day, including meals and snacks. Also, keep track of the person's normal fluid intake. A sharp increase or decrease may be important.

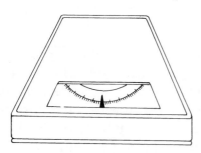

Checking weight

Always weigh the person at the same time of day. The best time is first thing in the morning, before breakfast but after he has urinated or had a bowel movement. Make sure he wears about the same amount of clothing each time, and always use the same scale.

Noting bladder and bowel habits

Any marked change in the person's bladder or bowel habits may be an important sign. Watch for changes in the number of times the person needs to urinate and the amount of urine he produces, and ask if urination is painful or difficult. Also, be alert for diarrhea and constipation. Note whether the urine or bowel movement has an unusual appearance.

Observing activity level and personality

What are the person's favorite activities? Reading? Watching television? Working at crafts or other projects? Keep in mind that a sharply reduced interest in his usual activities may indicate a worsening in his condition.

Also, be alert for mood changes and changes in his personality. For example, sudden irritability might be a danger sign if the person usually is good-humored but not if he's often out of sorts.

Finally, pay close attention to what the person in your care says about his condition. He'll usually be the first to notice such possible danger signs as a change in vision, difficulty swallowing, pain, numbness and tingling, and changes in bladder or bowel habits.

Identifying general signs

Don't let general signs, such as fever, headache, and loss of appetite, fool you. Although they commonly accompany minor illnesses, they can be danger signs in a person who's seriously ill.

Appetite loss

Loss of appetite can be a significant sign, particularly if it's new or a sign that doesn't improve. You may first notice the person's loss of appetite when he leaves food on the plate, asks for smaller portions, skips meals, or stops eating snacks. Tell the doctor about the person's loss of appetite. It may be a side effect of a new medication or an early sign of a serious disorder.

Seizures

Seizures—uncontrollable jerking motions of the legs, arms, head, or torso—are an emergency danger sign (unless you know the person is under care for a seizure disorder). Also sometimes called convulsions, seizures typically last from 2 to 5 minutes. If the person is having a seizure, you don't have to just stand by feeling helpless. Review the following guidelines for ways you can help.

• Remove any hard or sharp objects from the area.
• Place a pillow or rolled blankets around the person to prevent injury.

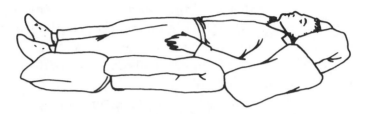

• Call the doctor or an ambulance.
• Never force anything into the person's mouth while he's having a seizure.
• Afterward, loosen any tight clothing and make sure he's breathing without difficulty.
• Also, write an accurate description of what you saw. This can help the doctor diagnose the type of seizure.

Dizziness

If the person you're caring for complains of dizziness, make sure he doesn't confuse dizziness with vertigo—two very different symptoms. Here's how to tell them apart.

Dizziness is a sensation of head spinning and unsteadiness. Vertigo is the feeling that the whole body is revolving in space or that objects are whirling around the body. A person with vertigo may even feel like he's being pulled sideways, as if by a magnet. Unlike dizziness, vertigo may be accompanied by nausea, vomiting, hearing loss, and noises in the ear. If dizziness seems to be a side effect of medication or if it doesn't stop, report it to the doctor. Dizziness usually lasts only a short time. And you may be able to correct it.

Positioning the head between the knees

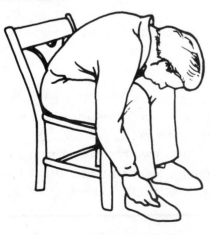

How to relieve dizziness

Follow the simple steps below.
• If the person feels faint, along with feeling dizzy, tell him to sit with his head between his knees until the feeling disappears.
• If the person you're caring for hasn't eaten

in a while, give him some orange juice or nondiet soda. Then offer him some high-protein food, such as cheese.

Fever

Fever usually is a sign that the body is fighting an infection. And during an illness or in an infection, a fever is normal and may help the body overcome the disorder. However, you should report to the doctor any fever that's:
• above 102° F (38.8° C).
• above 101° F (38.3° C) for 24 hours or more, especially if aspirin or acetaminophen has been used to control it.
• above 101° F (38.8° C) in a person age 65 or older.

Even fevers a degree or so above normal can be danger signs in people with chronic heart or lung disease—you'll want to recognize an infection as early as possible in such people.

Headache

Although a headache can be a danger sign of some disorder, in most cases, it results from muscle tension, allergies, minor illnesses, eye disorders, or migraine triggers. And most people with muscle tension or migraine headaches have had them before and know what they feel like. But regardless of previous headache experiences, you should call the doctor immediately and have the person you're caring for lie down if he suffers any of the following:
• a headache after a blow to the head
• a sudden headache that's not like any headaches he's had before
• a headache associated with a particular part of the head, such as an eye or an ear
• recurrent headaches in the same general area
• constant or persistent head pain or pressure that lasts for a day or more
• unusually severe head pain, possibly with a painful or stiff neck.

Lethargy and weakness

Does the person in your care seem lethargic—much less alert and active? Or does he describe feelings of weakness—losing strength, being fatigued, or having no energy? Both lethargy and weakness are changes in the person's usual energy level that may signal a health problem.

Lethargy refers to sluggishness that occurs when the person normally is wide awake. If the person in your care seems lethargic, first be sure to rule out normal causes. Did he sleep poorly the night before? Did he just wake up from a nap? If the person's normal activity level has decreased and lethargy has increased, notify the doctor.

Important: If you are unable to wake the person from sleep, call the doctor or an ambulance. Don't attempt to move a person who can't be awakened.

The person who experiences weakness may tremble or have a shaky voice or a weaker than normal grip. He may even drop things or have difficulty standing or sitting upright. Report any weakness to the doctor.

Light-headedness

Light-headedness is a feeling of wooziness and disorientation that's like dizziness but without the spinning sensation. It means that the brain isn't getting all the oxygen and blood it needs to work properly.

Moving legs to side of bed

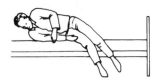

Never overlook light-headedness in the person you're caring for. It can also be a side effect of a medication or a sign of a heart disorder, an infection, or another serious problem. Tell the doctor if light-headedness follows the use of a prescribed medication, and have the person see the doctor right away if light-headedness occurs with signs of a heart disorder: chest discomfort, breathlessness, irregular heartbeat, and numbness or tingling in the arms or legs.

Dangling the legs

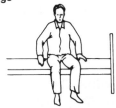

Light-headedness can also result from such simple things as abrupt changes in posture, diet, and temperature. If the doctor has ruled out a serious disorder, here are a few simple measures you can take when the person you're caring for feels light-headed.

Standing up slowly

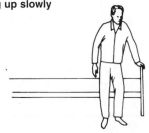

• If the person feels light-headed when he gets out of bed, tell him to move his legs over the side of the bed. Then help him sit up and let his feet rest on the floor or dangle. He should stay in this position for a few minutes. When he feels OK, he can stand up slowly.

• If the person who feels light-headed hasn't eaten in a while, give him some orange juice or nondiet soda. Follow this with cheese or another protein-rich food.

• Make sure he avoids extended time in the heat.

Numbness and tingling

A loss of feeling in any part of the body, tingling, or a "pins-and-needles" sensation—as if the part has fallen asleep—can be a danger sign unless it has an obvious cause, such as lying for too long on an arm or wearing tight shoes. Although some people with a chronic illness occasionally may experience numbness or tingling in their arms or legs, be sure to report it to the doctor if it's a new sign or if it's unusually severe or different in some way. Try to note:

• how the numbness progresses

• if the affected body parts change color

• what makes the numbness worse or better.

Pain

Pain is a common symptom that can arise from many causes. You'll usually have a good idea what caused a particular pain in the person you're caring for—for example, a recent injury or a known condition such as arthritis. But you should inform the doctor immediately of any lasting tenderness or unexplained, sudden, severe pain.

When the person you're caring for tells you that he's in pain, ask him to describe exactly how he feels, if possible.

Describing pain exactly

If the person finds it hard to describe his pain, learn more about it by asking him questions and writing down his answers. Use the questions on the next two pages to guide you. Remember that a detailed description of the person's pain can give the doctor clues about its cause and help him decide if it's a danger sign that requires prompt medical attention.

QUESTIONS	ANSWERS

Location

Where does it hurt? _____

Does the pain spread? If so, where does it hurt most
and where does it spread to? _____

What areas don't hurt? _____

Severity

How bad is the pain (mild, moderate, severe,
unbearable)? _____

How would you rate the pain on a scale of
1 (mild) to 10 (unbearable)? _____

Is it more severe than a toothache? _____

Is it more severe than stomach cramps? _____

Does the pain disrupt your usual activities? _____

Does it force you to lie down, sit down, or slow
down? _____

Does it seem to be getting better or worse, or
does it stay the same? _____

Quality

How does the pain feel? _____

Would you describe it as sharp, cramping, twisting,
squeezing, crushing, binding, stabbing, cutting,
burning, or dull; or as a soreness, numbness, or
pins-and-needles feeling? _____

Is the pain steady? _____

Has it changed? _____

| QUESTIONS | ANSWERS |

Timing
When did the pain start? _____

Did it begin suddenly or gradually? _____

How long does the pain last? _____

How often does it bother you? _____

What time of day does it
bother you most? _____

Does it wake you up when you're sleeping? _____

Does it ever occur before, during, or after meals? _____

Sources of relief and aggravation
What caused or happened just before the pain? _____

Does anything make it feel better, such as
changing diet, changing position, taking
medications, or resting? _____

Does distraction (for example, listening to
music) help relieve the pain? _____

Does anything make it feel worse, such as being
active, being in a certain position, coughing, or
touching the area? _____

Swelling

Tell the doctor about any new and unexplained swelling on the person's body. The person may complain of pressure, swelling, or bloating in her ankles, feet, stomach, or leg.

If the person you're caring for complains of fullness, aching, and tiredness in a leg—often with swelling and unusual warmth in part of the calf or thigh—take these steps:
• Tell her to lie down and raise the affected leg.
• Warn her not to walk around or rub the leg.
• Call the doctor.

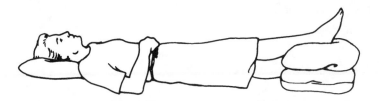

Identifying skin signs

Changes in the person's skin color and texture may be danger signs. Look for rashes, reddened or blotchy patches, loss of elasticity, recent swelling in the joints or elsewhere, new growths, and any change in a mole. Has the mole gotten bigger or changed color? Is it bleeding, ulcerated, or itching?

Also watch for the following skin signs.

Bluish or pale skin

Note bluish skin, usually seen in the fingernails and around the lips. If it's a new sign, it may indicate that the person's oxygen supply in his body cells and blood circulation are poor. Report bluish skin to the doctor.

Another sign of a circulatory problem, pale skin is an emergency sign if the skin feels cold, clammy, and accompanied by a fast, weak pulse and shallow breathing. Act immediately by:
• having the patient lie down with his feet slightly elevated and covering him with a blanket.
• calling an ambulance.

Pale skin that develops gradually—over a few days—isn't an emergency, but you should still bring it to the doctor's attention.

Reddened or darkened skin

Reddened or darkened skin over the body's bony areas may be the first sign of developing pressure ulcers—also called bedsores—in a person who's been bedridden for a long time. They're caused by continued pressure on certain skin areas, especially the body's bony parts.

For guidelines on preventing and caring for bedsores, see Chapter 11, Pressure Ulcers.

Recognizing mental status signs

Usually, you'll be the first to notice changes in the mental status of the person in your care.

Changes in personality

Is the person you're caring for less alert and no longer interested in his usual pastimes, such as reading, watching television, or some other hobbies? Is he neglecting personal hygiene? If so, bring these changes to the doctor's attention. Also report any personality or mood changes—sudden depression, irritability, even bizarre behavior. Sometimes, these changes result from medications or chronic diseases.

Confusion

A person who's confused may have trouble thinking and speaking. He may use the wrong words and have difficulty reading simple texts or performing easy mental tasks. Sometimes, confusion causes childish and unpredictable behavior. For example, the person may suddenly become listless or, in contrast, overactive. Report such episodes to the doctor or visiting nurse.

Memory loss

Memory loss, another danger sign, usually involves recent memory, especially of things that happen in the course of the day. The person may complain of difficulty concentrating on simple tasks, or he may repeatedly misplace books, clothing, or other articles. Tell the doctor about the person's memory loss.

Identifying eye signs

Vision changes aren't always obvious at first. Sometimes they develop over several months. But a sudden vision change, such as blurred vision, double vision, halos around lights, light flashes or sparks, or light sensitivity, is a danger sign. If the person in your care experiences a sudden vision change, don't try to move him, particularly if he also has a headache or a painful stiff neck. Have him lie down, make him comfortable, and call the doctor immediately.

Blurred vision

Blurred vision can arise from various conditions, some normal, some disease-related. If the person in your care has blurred vision with sudden, severe eye pain after an injury or with sudden vision loss, call the doctor right away.

Double vision

Double vision refers to seeing two images of the same object at the same time. This happens when the eye muscles fail to

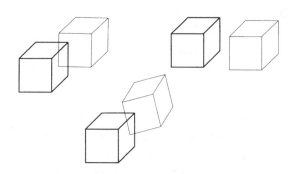

function equally. Depending on which eye muscles are affected, the two images seen by a person with double vision will appear in different locations. A few variations are shown here.

Double vision is a danger sign, especially if it's a new sign that's accompanied by severe headache or other signs.

Halos

Seeing halos refers to seeing rainbow-like rings around bright lights or bright objects. Sometimes a person may see halos if his eyes water excessively from wearing contact lenses too long, after an emotional upset, or if he's been exposed to intense light. But if the person suddenly sees halos, he should call the doctor right away if he's seeing them for the first time.

Light flashes or sparks

Light flashes or small, flashing sparks seen in front of the eyes ("seeing stars") may occur in people who suffer from migraine headaches. As with other visual signs, light flashes or sparks can be significant if they're a new sign. Is the person also experiencing eye pain or a headache? Contact the doctor at once.

Light sensitivity
A common sign, light sensitivity can range from mild to extreme intolerance of light. If pain and tearing accompany light sensitivity and last longer than a few hours, have the person see the doctor.

Dealing with heart and lung signs
Be alert for heart and lung signs, including breathing difficulty, changes in the pulse rate, chest pain, and coughing up sputum.

Breathing difficulty
Any breathing difficulty—shortness of breath, slow or fast breathing, and shallow breathing—usually is a danger sign. If the person you're caring for develops breathing difficulty, quickly take these steps:
• Call the doctor immediately.
• Have the person lie down, and make him comfortable—elevate his head and shoulders, loosen tight clothing, and keep him warm.

If the person develops rapid, shallow breathing along with a weak, racing pulse and cold, clammy skin, he may be in shock. Follow these steps:
• Have him lie down with his feet slightly elevated.
• Cover him with a blanket.
• Call an ambulance.

Wheezing, another type of breathing difficulty, may occur in people with chronic lung disease or asthma. But if wheezing is a new sign, contact the doctor.

Changes in the pulse
Call the doctor right away if the person you're caring for has any of the following pulse danger signs:
• A pulse rate below 60 beats per minute or above 100 when

Two pulse locations

Two pulse locations

Jugular pulse

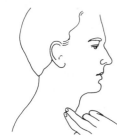

Radial pulse

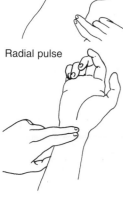

the person's at rest. A person with a pulse below 40 needs immediate medical attention.

• An unusually fast pulse rate, particularly one that doesn't slow down when the person is at rest.

• An irregular pulse—spotty, or speeding up and slowing down quickly. This danger sign may indicate an emergency. Take the patient to an emergency department or call an ambulance, whichever is faster.

Chest pain

Dull, continuous chest pain that's accompanied by a cough and sharp chest pain that increases while inhaling or coughing are both danger signs. Contact the doctor at once if the person you're caring for has either of these signs.

Squeezing or vise-like pain (or pressure) in the center of the chest, sometimes radiating to the neck, jaw, or shoulder or down the left arm, may occur in a heart attack. Although the pain of a heart attack can be similar to the pain of angina, anginal pain usually subsides quickly with rest; heart attack pain may continue for several hours. Take the person with these signs to an emergency department or call an ambulance.

Chest pain doesn't always mean a heart problem. A disorder that affects the lungs or ribs is also likely to cause chest pain.

Structures that can cause chest pain

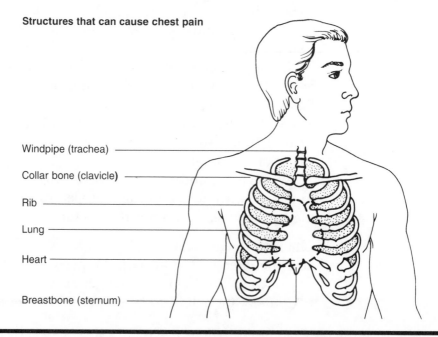

Windpipe (trachea)

Collar bone (clavicle)

Rib

Lung

Heart

Breastbone (sternum)

Coughing up sputum

A persistent, productive cough in someone who doesn't normally have a cough is a danger sign. Productive coughs bring mucus from the lungs to the mouth, creating sputum, a mixture of mucus and saliva. If a person with chronic lung disease coughs up sputum that is yellowish, greenish, or otherwise abnormal, you should consider it a danger sign. (A person with chronic lung disease usually produces clear to whitish sputum.) Sometimes a person with chronic bronchitis may cough up a little blood in the sputum, but you should still report it to the doctor. Also report any new cough that lasts longer than a week.

Pus-like sputum, sometimes yellowish, greenish, or rusty, may indicate an infection. A person with this danger sign should see a doctor quickly.

When the person you're caring for has a cough, coach him in deep-breathing and coughing exercises. (These exercises are explained in Chapter 19, Respiratory Therapy.) They can help expand and clear his lungs and prevent complications such as pneumonia.

Identifying and managing throat and digestive tract signs

Watch for throat and digestive tract signs. If they're new or persistent, they can signal a complication or a worsening of the person's condition.

Swallowing difficulty

Any difficulty swallowing—from the sensation of a lump in the throat, from pain, or from what seems to be muscle weakness—can be a danger sign. The person you're caring for may describe the difficulty as an inability to swallow or as a painful sensation that occurs when he does swallow. Or he may complain that food goes down his throat too slowly, particularly meat and bread. Does the person also have a fever or difficulty breathing? If so, call the doctor.

Vomiting

If the person begins to vomit, notify the doctor at once if:
• vomiting lasts longer than 24 hours.
• the person has recently had surgery.
• the vomit is dark, with a coffee-ground appearance.

Although you may not be able to make the person stop vomiting, you may be able to make him more comfortable. If the person asks for your help, support his forehead with your hand while he's vomiting. Afterward, give him water to rinse out his mouth and sponge off his face.

When vomiting has stopped, follow these guidelines to replace fluids and prevent further vomiting:
• Give a teaspoon of a clear liquid every 15 minutes until the person keeps it down. Liquids should be at room temperature and can include such things as tea, flat ginger ale, flat cola (unless he has diarrhea), and gelatin that's not jelled (any color except red, which can irritate the stomach). A child may suck on lollipops or ice pops.
• Progress to small sips of a clear liquid every 15 minutes.
• If the person doesn't vomit after 4 hours, give him larger sips of liquid and add dry toast or plain crackers.
• If these foods agree with his stomach, advance to a bland, light diet with such things as soft-boiled eggs, boiled chicken, and clear—not cream—soups.
• After 24 hours without vomiting, the person can begin to eat regular food as long as he avoids spices and overeating.

Abdominal pain

Pain in the area of the stomach or intestines is an especially common symptom. Occasional gas or indigestion isn't a danger sign. But if the person has abdominal pain that lasts 3 hours or more, contact the doctor immediately or take the person to an emergency department for an examination. You should also notify the doctor of abdominal pain that the person describes as abnormal or unusually sharp and intense. Then watch for changes in the pulse rate, breathing, and skin temperature.

Many people think that abdominal pain signals a stomach problem. But problems in other abdominal organs can also cause pain, such as gallbladder, kidney, or intestinal disease.

Blood in the stool

Notify the doctor if you find blood in the person's stool, which is always a danger sign whether or not the person has diarrhea. Blood causes dark, blackish stools, but may appear as clots or as bright red streaks.

Constipation

If the person you're caring for is constipated, he has a bowel movement infrequently and with difficulty. Constipation can be a normal or an abnormal condition. When constipation is a new sign, report it to the doctor.

People who have recently become bedridden often suffer from constipation. But unless the person experiences pain or extreme discomfort, this usually isn't a danger sign. Dietary changes, including more high-fiber foods and increased fluid intake, can relieve constipation. If the person can't eat high-fiber foods or increase fluids or the problem doesn't resolve itself, inform the doctor.

Diarrhea

Diarrhea is a condition of frequent loose or liquid bowel movements. You should quickly bring to the doctor's attention a violent attack of diarrhea, particularly when accompanied by pain, appetite loss, nausea, vomiting, or other unusual signs. Tell him what the person has eaten, and describe how long he's had diarrhea and how severe it is.

Identifying urinary signs

Urinary signs may indicate a disorder of the urinary tract, including all the organs involved in the production and elimination of urine from the body—the kidneys, ureters, bladder, and urethra.

Changes in bladder habits

People who have recently become bedridden commonly urinate more frequently than before. (Keep in mind that adults normally urinate four to six times daily.) But if the person suddenly needs to urinate every hour or half hour, this is abnormal. Unusually frequent urination can lead to too much fluid loss. The person may then feel weak and become dizzy when he stands up.

Urinating less frequently and in much smaller amounts than before is also abnormal. Note the amount of fluid the person drinks and the amount he urinates to decide if he's urinating more or less than usual.

Besides unusually frequent or infrequent urination, other changes in bladder habits include:
• waking at night to urinate (when it's a new sign)
• painful urination
• straining or difficulty urinating
• loss of bladder control (wetting).

Promptly report any change in bladder habits to the doctor. The more intense the symptoms, the sooner you should seek medical attention.

Changes in urine appearance and smell

Normally, urine varies in color from clear to deep yellow. But food colors and some medications can produce unusual colors. Red, rusty, or dark brown urine may mean that blood is present. So be sure to check with the doctor if the person's urine is an odd color.

Other abnormal signs include foul-smelling urine, milky urine, and urine that contains mucous threads or heavy reddish "dust" that settles quickly to the bottom of the toilet.

Keep in mind that normal color soon returns once the person stops taking medication or eating foods that change his urine color.

COLOR	DRUG OR FOOD
Brown	Macrodantin, used for kidney and bladder infections
Black	Iron pills, taken for anemia
Purple-red or red-pink	Phenolphthalein in Ex-Lax and Feen-A Mint, taken for constipation
Red	Beets or other red foods
Red-orange	Pyridium, used for urinary pain or irritation
Blue-green	Methylene blue, given for bladder and urethral infections

4 Hygiene

Importance of hygiene

Hygiene commonly refers to the everyday habits that keep the skin, hair, nails, and mouth clean. Most children learn personal hygiene habits from their parents, who teach them how and when to wash their hands, brush their teeth, and so on. In fact, the ability to care for one's own hygiene is considered an important step toward personal independence. This may be why many adults who are ill feel a loss of self-esteem when they must rely on someone else to attend to their personal hygiene.

So when you're caring for a person who's ill, encourage him to perform as much of his hygiene as possible. If he's too weak to do it himself, you'll need to handle it for him. Hygiene is too important to neglect because it does more than just keep a person clean.

It can:
• help keep the skin intact to fight infection and prevent injuries.
• help maintain a normal body temperature.
• remove from the skin substances in which bacteria will grow, reducing the risk of infection.
• keep the mouth and gums healthy, which makes eating easier and, therefore, promotes good nutrition.
• make the person more comfortable and relaxed.
• boost the person's morale. (When he looks his best, he may feel better both emotionally and physically.)

Giving a bed bath

When you're caring for someone who's confined to bed but fairly active, let her bathe herself as much as she can. This fosters independence and self-confidence. It's good exercise, too. She may just need you to gather the bath supplies and wash her back. If she's weak or not allowed to exert herself, you'll take charge of most or all of the bath.

1 Gather towels, a washcloth, a light cotton or flannel blanket, soap, lotion and other toiletries, and a basin. Fill the basin about two-thirds full with water at 120° F (48.8° C).

The water will cool to between 100° and 115° F (46.1° and 37.7° C) by the time it touches the body. If the water gets too cool or dirty during the bath, replace it.

To prevent drafts, close any doors and windows. (During the bath, avoid exposing the person to drafts by washing and then drying one area at a time.)

Next, wash your hands. You may want to replace the top bed sheet with a light flannel or cotton blanket. Help the person move near you, and help her remove her nightclothes. Cover her with a towel to provide privacy and warmth.

2 Wet the washcloth, but don't add soap. Wash one eyelid by wiping gently from the inner corner to the outer corner. Dry the eyelid. Then rinse the cloth and wipe and dry the other eyelid. Wash her face, neck, and ears with soap and water, unless soap irritates sensitive skin. Rinse well and pat dry.

Washing the arms

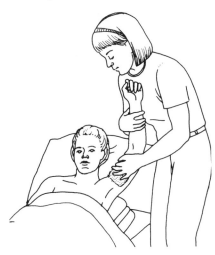

3 Place a towel under one of her arms. Using long, smooth strokes, wipe from her hand to her underarm. Wash, rinse, and dry thoroughly, giving special attention to the underarm area. Repeat these steps for her other arm. Then put the basin on a towel on the bed, and place the person's hands in the basin. Wash and dry one hand at a time.

4 Fold down the blanket or towel to expose the person's chest and stomach. Wash, rinse, and dry these areas. Be sure to dry creases and skin folds thoroughly. Then cover her chest and stomach with the blanket or towel.

5 Uncover one of her legs and put a towel under it. Using long, smooth strokes, wash, rinse, and dry each leg. Repeat these steps for the other leg. Then place the basin on a towel on the bed and soak and wash her feet.

Turning the person on one side

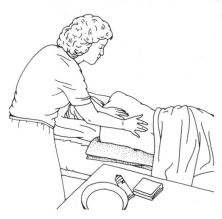

6 Get fresh, warm water. Then help the person turn onto her side, making sure she isn't too close to the bed's edge. Next, put a towel on the bed along her back. Wash, rinse, and dry her neck, shoulders, back, buttocks, and upper thighs. And rub her back with warm lotion.

7 The perineal, or pubic, area is the area between the thighs that includes the genitals. For more information, see *Giving perineal care to a woman*, or *Giving perineal care to a man*, which follow below.

Giving a partial bed bath

If a full bed bath each day makes the person's skin too dry, try giving a partial bed bath several days a week. Follow the steps for a complete bed bath, but wash only the person's face, hands, underarms, and perineal area.

Giving perineal care to a woman

Cleaning the perineum—the area between the thighs, including the genitals and anus—is a must with bathing and after episodes of bowel incontinence. Besides making the patient more comfortable, cleaning removes excretions that can cause irritation, skin breakdown, infection, and odor. Follow these steps.

1 Assemble the equipment: several washcloths, a clean basin, mild soap, a linen-saver pad, a bath towel, prescribed ointment or cream, toilet tissue or disposable wipes, and a trash bag.

2 Fill the basin two-thirds full with warm water. Then place it next to the patient's bed, along with the other items.

3 Wash your hands thoroughly. Then help the patient to lie on her back, and place a linen-saver pad under her buttocks.

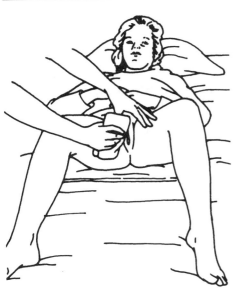

4 Ask the patient to bend her knees slightly and spread her legs. First, clean the vaginal area. After applying soap to the washcloth, separate her labia—the outer lips of the vagina—with one hand, and with the other hand, use gentle downward strokes to wash from front to back. Use a clean section of the washcloth for each stroke. Avoid touching the rectal area with the washcloth.

5 Rinse the vaginal area thoroughly with a clean washcloth to remove soap residue that can cause skin irritation. Pat the skin dry, paying special attention to skin folds. (Don't use powder—it may become caked.)

6 Now, clean the rectal area. Help the patient turn onto her left side with her right knee raised to expose the rectum. Remove excess feces with toilet tissue or disposable wipes. Then clean, rinse, and dry the area, wiping from front to back. Use a clean section of the washcloth for each stroke.

7 If the doctor orders it, apply ointment or cream to prevent skin breakdown or to heal irritation. Then tuck a pad between the buttocks to absorb oozing feces. Remove the linen-saver pad and then reposition the patient, straightening the bed linens to make her comfortable. Clean the basin for future use, and dispose of soiled articles.

Giving perineal care to a man

Cleaning the perineum—the area between the thighs, including the genitals and anus—is a must with bathing and after episodes of bowel incontinence. Besides making the patient more comfortable, cleaning removes excretions that can cause irritation, skin breakdown, infection, and odor. Follow these steps.

1 Assemble the equipment: several washcloths, a clean basin, mild soap, a linen-saver pad, a bath towel, prescribed ointment or cream, toilet tissue or disposable wipes, and a trash bag.

2 Fill the basin two-thirds full with warm water. Then place it next to the patient's bed, along with the other items.

3 Wash your hands thoroughly. Then help the patient to lie on his back, and place a linen-saver pad under his buttocks.

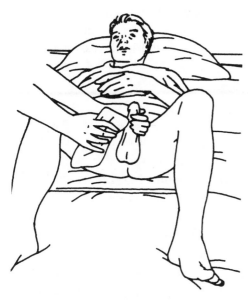

4 Have the patient spread his legs and slightly bend his knees. After applying soap to the washcloth, hold the shaft of his penis with one hand and clean with the other. Begin at the tip of the penis and work in a circular motion from the center outward. Use a clean section of washcloth for each stroke. Rinse thoroughly with a circular motion.

If the man is uncircumcised, gently retract the foreskin and wash underneath it. Rinse well, but don't dry because moisture prevents friction when replacing the foreskin.

5 Wash the rest of the penis, stroking downward toward the scrotum. Rinse well and pat dry. Then gently clean, rinse, and pat dry the scrotum.

6 Help the patient turn onto his left side with his right knee raised to expose the rectum. Remove excess feces with toilet tissue or a disposable wipe. Then clean, rinse, and pat dry the rectal area.

7 If the doctor orders it, apply ointment or cream to prevent skin breakdown or to heal irritation. Then tuck a pad between the buttocks to absorb oozing feces. Remove the linen-saver pad and then reposition the patient, straightening the bed linens to make him comfortable. Clean the basin for future use, and dispose of soiled articles.

Giving a tub bath or shower

When the doctor says the person you're caring for can take a tub bath, be sure sure to follow these safety tips:
• Consider installing sturdy grab bars on the tub or inside and outside the shower stall to help the person get in and out of the tub.
• Apply nonslip safety mats or treads to the bottom of the tub or shower to prevent falls.
• Place a nonskid bath mat—not a towel—on the floor in front of the tub or shower.
• Put a stool in the shower so the person can sit down while he showers.

Making a bathtub safe

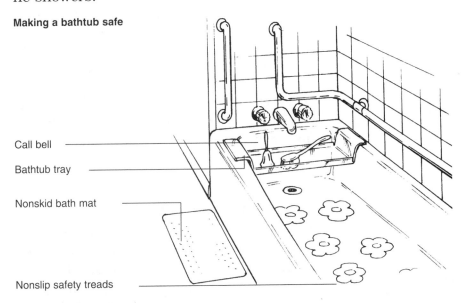

Call bell

Bathtub tray

Nonskid bath mat

Nonslip safety treads

• Check the water temperature.
• If you don't stay with the person during the bath, keep the bathroom door unlocked and stay close by in case of an emergency.
• Never turn on hot water when the person's in the tub.
• Place a bell or other signal device within his reach.
• Use devices that make bathing easier and safer, such as soap on a rope, a tub tray, and long-handled brushes; attach a hand-held shower hose to the shower head or faucet.

The person you're caring for may be able to take a tub bath by himself. But if he's weak, you can make bathing less strenuous by helping with these steps.

1 Make sure the bathroom is warm; close doors and windows to prevent drafts. Then fill the bathtub halfway with water that's about 105° F (40.5° C). Drape a light flannel or cotton blanket over the toilet or a nearby chair, so that the person can sit down and dry himself after the bath. Place the bath supplies within his reach.

2 Help the person remove his clothing, if necessary. As he enters the tub, support him by putting your hands under his armpits or on his waist. Or steady him as he sits on the edge of the tub, holds onto the grab bar, and eases himself into the water. If you have a mechanical lift, follow the manufacturer's instructions for helping someone into a tub. Once the person is in the tub, check on him every few minutes. If the doctor permits, he may soak for 10 to 15 minutes.

3 Let the water out of the bathtub, and then help the person out of the tub. Assist with drying, especially in hard-to-reach areas. (*Note:* He may feel weak and need extra help.)

Giving a sitz bath

Often used after rectal or perineal surgery, a sitz bath soaks just the perineal area and buttocks, relieving pain, promoting healing, preventing infection, and helping muscles relax in

Sitz bath setup

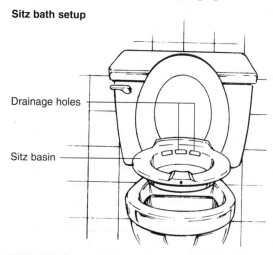

Drainage holes

Sitz basin

that area. Give a sitz bath as often as the doctor orders and add medications, as directed. The person you're caring for may be able to take a sitz bath by herself. But if she feels faint or weak, you'll need to help. Here's how.

1 Protect the person from drafts by closing any doors and windows. Raise the toilet seat and fit the sitz basin securely on the toilet bowl. Position the basin so that its drainage holes face the back of the bowl, as shown. When you've placed the basin correctly, you'll see a single slot in front. Fill

Soaking for 10 to 20 minutes

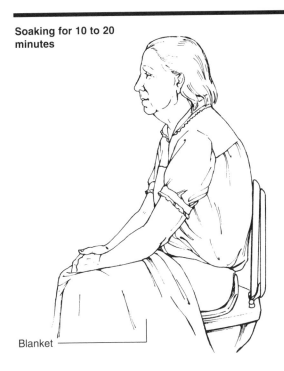

Blanket

the basin with warm water (100° to 115° F [37.7° to 46.1° C]), and add bath medication if the doctor prescribes it.

Note: If you don't have a portable sitz basin, fill the bathtub with 2 to 3 inches (5 to 7.6 cm) of water and the prescribed amount of medication. If the person has stitches or is in pain, have her sit on a rubber or plastic ring for comfort.

2 Help the person sit in the basin or tub. In the basin, the water should soak her perineal and rectal areas. In the tub, the water level should reach the top of her hips.

If the person feels chilly, wrap a light flannel or cotton blanket around her shoulders. Place a call bell within her reach.

Allow her to soak for 10 to 20 minutes, and add warm water, as needed, to keep the temperature constant. After the sitz bath, dry the person completely. If the doctor prescribes an ointment or a dressing, apply it after the person is thoroughly dried.

Providing hair care

Hair care can help a person look and feel much better, especially when she's ill. For quick and easy hair care, make sure the person you're caring for gets a good haircut in a simple style. Then follow these steps.

Brushing and combing

Daily brushing keeps hair in condition by stimulating blood circulation in the scalp and distributing oils evenly over the hair, which gives it a healthy shine. Daily combing also helps stimulate the circulation. When combing, work on one area at a time. To avoid pulling on the hair as you comb, hold the strands firmly, leaving some slack between the person's head and your hand.

Combing without pulling the hair

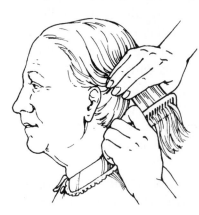

Coping with mats and tangles

As hair rubs against the mattress and pillow, mats and tangles can form. Regular brushing and combing is the best way to prevent them. Other good ways to control mats and tangles are:

• applying a cream rinse after shampooing
• loosely braiding long hair or tying it back
• using a wide-toothed comb to separate curly hair while it's wet.

To remove stubborn mats and tangles, apply alcohol to the person's hair with a gauze sponge. This should allow you to remove mats and tangles by combing the hair gently.

Shampooing the person's hair

A good shampoo cleans the hair and scalp and helps the person you're caring for look her best. If she can't move around well or the doctor says to avoid wet shampooing, try using a dry shampoo to remove dirt and excess oils. Most dry shampoo products are simple to use and easy to find in the drugstore. For best results, follow the directions on the container.

If the person you're caring for can move around well and the doctor permits shower or tub baths, you may help shampoo her hair during her bath. Otherwise, you can help her wash her hair at the bathroom sink.

Giving a shampoo in bed

Even the person who's confined to bed can enjoy a wet shampoo. Here's how.

1 After you gather the equipment, place absorbent towels and a waterproof sheet over the pillow. Put a shampoo basin or an inflatable sink on top of this. (These are available at some drugstores and medical equipment dealers.) If you don't have this equipment, roll a towel, bath blanket, or sheet into a log. Shape the log into a U and put it in a large plastic bag. Arrange the bag as shown to direct the flow of the water. Protect the floor with newspaper, and place a trash can or bucket on the floor to catch the rinse water.

Making a shampoo trough

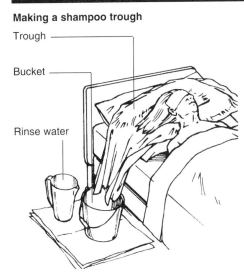

Trough

Bucket

Rinse water

2 Place a light flannel or cotton blanket over the person and help her move her head and shoulders to the edge of the bed. Pin a folded towel around her neck and put cotton in her ears. Make sure her head is turned away from the trough leading to the bucket. Before you begin to shampoo, place a folded towel over her eyes to protect them from the soapsuds.

3 Using a pitcher of warm water (105° to 110° F [40.5° to 43.3° C]), wet the hair well. Then apply shampoo and work it into a lather. Rinse thoroughly and repeat. Apply a cream rinse, if you like, to prevent tangles.

4 After the final rinse, remove the basin or trough and wrap a towel around the person's head. Then comb the hair, and towel or blow it dry.

Giving a shave

Many men like to shave every day. If the person you're caring for can shave himself, bring him the things he'll need, such as an electric razor or a safety razor, a bowl of water, shaving cream or soap, a towel, a mirror, and shaving lotion. If he can't shave himself, follow the manufacturer's instructions for an electric razor or follow these steps for a safety razor.

Holding the skin taut

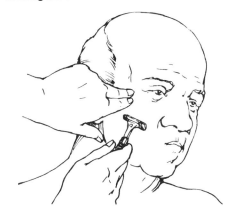

1 Tuck a towel under the person's chin, and wet his face by cradling it in a warm, moist washcloth. Apply shaving cream or shaving soap lather.

2 Hold the skin taut and, using short strokes, draw a sharp razor across the skin in the direction of the hair's growth. Ask the person to purse his lips or angle his chin, so that you can shave these areas safely.

3 After shaving, wash off any lather that's left on the face. Dry the skin gently. Apply shaving lotion, if desired.

Helping with mouth care

Mouth care, or oral hygiene, means keeping the whole mouth—the teeth or dentures, tongue, roof of mouth, and gums—clean and healthy. The keys to good oral hygiene are regular dental checkups, good nutrition, and frequent brushing and flossing. Mouth care is important because it:
• prevents tooth decay and bad breath.
• prevents mouth infections that can spread to other parts of the body.
• stimulates the gums to help prevent gum disease.
• keeps the mouth and lips moist.
• makes the mouth feel clean and fresh, which can boost the appetite and improve nutrition by making eating more enjoyable.

Follow these basics of good mouth care.

Tooth brushing

Some dentists recommend brushing after every meal. Others, even more often. But all agree that people should brush their teeth at least twice a day. Even a person who must stay in bed usually can do his own mouth care. Here's how you can help.
• Bring the person you're caring for a soft toothbrush, toothpaste or tooth powder (with fluoride unless your drinking water is fluoridated), a glass of cool water, a small basin, and a towel. *Note:* If the person's hands are weak or don't move easily, offer him an electric toothbrush. It's easier to grip and moves by itself.
• Help him sit up in bed, and tuck the towel under his chin. If he is unable, dip his toothbrush in the water and then apply toothpaste to it.
• Tell him to brush the surface of each tooth with 8 to 10 strokes, moving from the gums to the tooth crowns. He should also use short,

Brushing surfaces

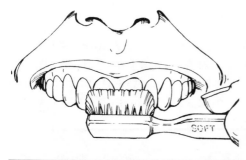

Vibrating at the gum line

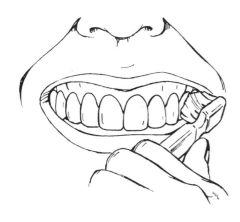

Sliding the floss between teeth

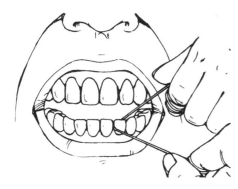

vibrating strokes where the gum meets the tooth.

• Remind him to brush his tongue and the roof of his mouth. This will help remove thickened saliva that can collect there.

• Remove the toothpaste foam and loosened food particles by giving the person some cool water so he can rinse his mouth. Then give him the basin to spit in. Wipe away any excess with the towel.

Flossing the teeth

To remove plaque and debris completely between the teeth, the person should floss his teeth after brushing. Here's how you can help him.

• Gather the equipment.

• Give him a 12- to 18-inch (30- to 46-cm) piece of dental floss and a floss holder, if he finds it helpful.

• Next, he should wrap the floss around his index fingers or load it into the floss holder.

• Then, he should slide the floss between two teeth, ease it back and forth between the gum and tooth, and repeat until he's flossed between each tooth.

Rinsing

After brushing and flossing, the person will need a final rinse with a commercial mouthwash or warm tap water. To prevent chapped lips, apply lanolin or a petrolatum ointment.

Caring for dentures

Caring for dentures is just as important as caring for natural teeth. In fact, for best results, dentures need brushing—or at least rinsing—after every meal and before bedtime. Most people prefer to remove, clean, and insert their own dentures, but you can do this, if necessary.

Loosening the upper plate

Grasp the inner and outer surfaces of the plate on both sides. Insert your forefingers over the upper edge of the plate, and press until the seal breaks between the denture and the gums.

Breaking the seal

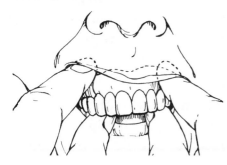

Removing the upper plate

If the plate isn't loosened fully, wiggle it slightly to break the seal that holds it to the roof of the mouth. Then pull the upper plate forward and out. Put it in a container until you can remove the lower plate.

Removing the lower plate

To remove a full lower plate, grasp its inner and outer surfaces with the thumb and forefinger. Then turn it slightly and pull it up and out. To remove a partial plate, apply equal pressure on each side close to the gum. *Note:* Don't pull on the clasps to remove a partial plate—you could bend or break them.

Cleaning dentures

Put a washcloth in the bottom of a basin that's half filled with water. (This cushions the dentures if they fall.) Then, using a stiff brush, scrub the dentures carefully with toothpaste and rinse them in cold water. Be sure to rinse the mouth while the dentures are out. If the person is going to sleep, soak his dentures overnight in a covered container filled with water and peppermint oil, lemon juice, or a denture cleanser. *Note:* Be sure to keep the dentures in a safe place.

Inserting dentures

Wet dentures form a stronger seal with the gums than do dry dentures, so rinse them in cool water before inserting them. Apply even, gentle pressure on both sides of the upper plate to work it into place in the person's mouth. Then insert the lower plate. Remember: Unless the doctor tells you to leave the dentures out, insert them every morning. This prevents gum swelling and changes that could make the dentures fit poorly.

Giving hand and nail care

Good nail care can prevent torn cuticles and dirty nails, which can easily lead to infection. And well-groomed nails look good. If the person you're caring for can't manage daily nail cleaning and weekly manicuring by herself, here's how you can give her good nail care.

Using an orangewood stick

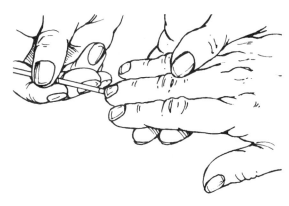

Caring for the cuticles

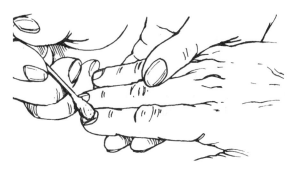

Cleaning under the nails

If you'll be doing a manicure, remove old nail polish. If the person's hands haven't been wet recently, place them in a basin and wash them with warm, soapy water to loosen dirt and soften the cuticle. Let them soak for 3 to 5 minutes, if you'll be doing a manicure. Then use the pointed end of an orangewood stick to clean under the nails. Pat the hands dry.

Softening the cuticles

Moisturize the nails and cuticles to keep them soft and to prevent cracking or tearing. To do this, rub the moisturizer into the sides of the nails. The massaging action stimulates blood flow, preventing calluses and keeping the cuticles healthy.

Pushing back the cuticles

Using a cotton-tipped applicator, such as a Q-tip or an orangewood stick wrapped in cotton, gently push back the cuticles as shown. *Caution:* Avoid chafing or poking the cuticles; this can cause hangnails and introduce infection.

Cutting the nails

To cut the nails, use sharp clippers or nail scissors, and follow the contour of each nail. If you see a torn cuticle, cut off the loose skin. Never cut off more skin or the cuticle could thicken and become infected.

Smoothing rough edges

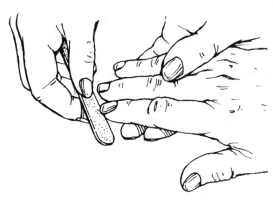

Filing the nails

Hold an emery board at a 45-degree angle to the nail and remove any rough edges. As you file, remember to stroke in one direction, rather than sawing back and forth.

Handling the final touches

Rinse and dry the fingers thoroughly. Finally, apply hand cream.

Giving foot care

Daily cleaning and regular trimming are important parts of foot care. They help prevent infection, control foot odor, and stimulate blood flow to the feet. They also keep the feet healthy and comfortable, preventing foot pain that can lead to fatigue, muscle aches, and limited movement.

If the doctor permits the person you're caring for to take tub baths, you can easily clean her feet by soaking and washing them during the bath. Afterward, you can apply lotion or powder to her skin. If she must stay in bed, follow these steps.

1 Fill a basin about halfway with soapy water that's between 88° and 95° F (31° and 35° C). Put a towel on the bed to keep the sheets dry. Then place the basin on it. Help the person flex one knee and put her foot in the basin. Put a pillow under her knee for support, and cushion the rim of the basin with a towel to prevent pressure. Wash the foot thoroughly, and let it soak for 10 to 15 minutes.

Note: If you don't plan to follow foot washing with a pedicure, you may wash both feet at the same time.

Soaking one foot

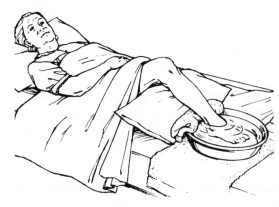

2 After soaking, rinse the foot, remove it from the basin, and place it on the towel. Gently blot the foot dry, and be sure

to dry thoroughly between the toes. As you dry, look for any abnormalities, such as redness, cracking, corns, calluses, and ingrown nails. Tell the doctor if you find any problems. Empty the basin, refill it with warm water, and wash and soak the second foot.

3 While the second foot is soaking, pedicure the first foot. Using a Q-tip or other cotton-tipped swab, carefully clean the toenails. Gently remove any dirt under the toenail with an orangewood stick. Rub a pumice stone on the heels, soles, and sides of the foot to remove dry, dead skin.

Properly trimmed toenails

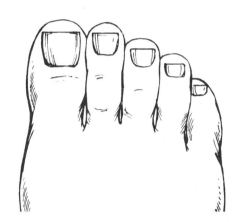

4 To prevent ingrown toenails, trim the nails by cutting straight across. Clip the nail, starting at one edge and working across. Then file trimmed toenails with an emery board to smooth rough edges.

Note: Don't try to cut the toenails if they are thick or tough or if the person has diabetes or a problem with his blood circulation. Instead, ask the doctor about calling in a foot specialist for help.

5 After you finish working on the feet, apply lotion to moisten dry skin or lightly dust powder between the toes to absorb moisture. Put on clean socks or stockings. *Note:* If the person has diabetes, put cotton or lamb's wool between the toes.

5 Comfort Measures

Importance of being comfortable

When you're comfortable, you'll usually feel at ease with yourself and your surroundings. When you're not comfortable—for example, when you're ill or in pain—you'll probably have trouble feeling good, mentally or physically. So when you're sick, or when the person you're caring for is sick, take whatever steps you can to increase comfort. During an illness, most people feel more comfortable if they get the right amount of these essential things:

• uninterrupted sleep
• rest and relaxation
• relief from pain
• appropriate amount of movement, exercise, and activity.

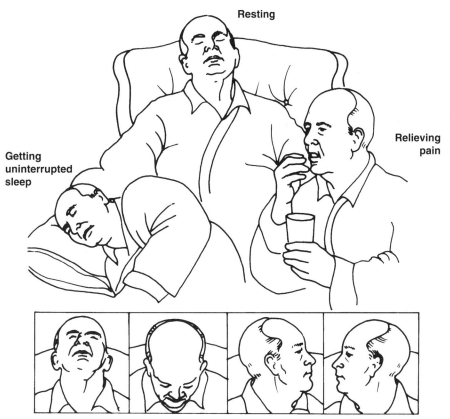

Resting

Relieving pain

Getting uninterrupted sleep

Performing relaxation exercises

Repositioning a person in bed

You'll use three positions when turning and repositioning a person in bed: back, side, and stomach. Follow these instructions.

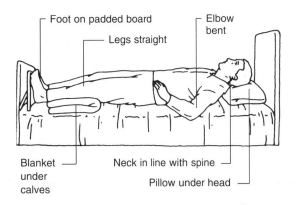

Foot on padded board — Elbow bent — Legs straight — Blanket under calves — Neck in line with spine — Pillow under head

Back position

Place a flat, firm pillow under the person's head so that his neck is straight and in line with his spine. Then lift his heels slightly by placing a thin blanket under his calves. Slightly bend his elbows, and rest his hands on his hips. Straighten his legs, and place his feet (toes pointing up) on a padded board resting against the foot of the bed at a 60-degree or 90-degree angle.

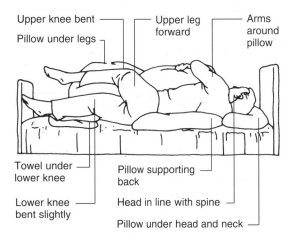

Upper knee bent — Pillow under legs — Upper leg forward — Arms around pillow — Towel under lower knee — Pillow supporting back — Lower knee bent slightly — Head in line with spine — Pillow under head and neck

Side position

After you've turned the person onto his side, place his head in line with his spine. Support his head and neck with a flat, firm pillow. Next, support his back with a pillow, and have him wrap his arms around another pillow. Then move his upper leg forward until his knee is bent, to raise it above his lower leg. Place a pillow under this leg to keep it at hip level. Slightly bend the lower knee, and place a folded towel (or blanket or piece of foam rubber) under it to keep his ankle off the bed.

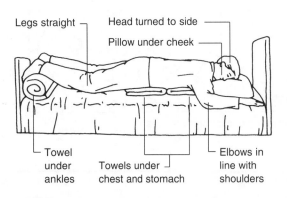

Legs straight — Head turned to side — Pillow under cheek — Towel under ankles — Towels under chest and stomach — Elbows in line with shoulders

Stomach position

After turning the person onto his stomach, turn his head to one side and place a pillow or folded towel under his cheek. Then move his arms up so that his bent elbows are in line with his shoulders. Next, place folded towels beneath his chest and stomach. Finally, straighten his legs. Support his ankles and raise his toes off the bed by using a rolled towel or small rolled blanket.

Helping a person get out of bed

If the person you're caring for has been resting in bed for several days or weeks, use caution the first few times she gets out of bed. You can help her get out of bed by following these steps.

Helping the person sit up

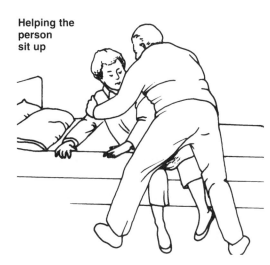

1 If you're using a hospital bed, lock the bed's wheels and lower the side rails. Now, move the person's legs over the side of the bed and grasp her shoulders, standing with a wide base of support. Ask her to push up from the bed with her arms. Shift your weight from the foot closest to her head to the other foot as you raise her to a sitting position.

2 While she gets used to sitting upright and dangling her legs, stand in front of her in case she falls. If you have an overbed table, place a pillow on top of it, and move it in front of her to help her support herself.

3 After she can sit up and dangle her legs without feeling dizzy or tired, put shoes with non-slip soles on her feet. If she's alert and fairly strong, put her feet flat on the floor and ask her to try to stand. Be ready to support her if she loses her balance.

Helping the person stand

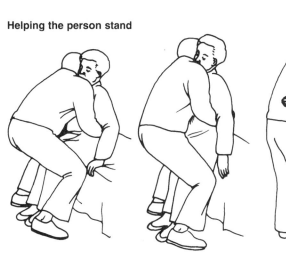

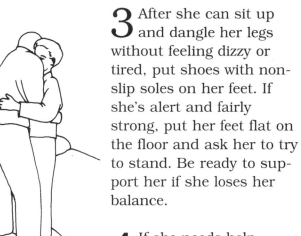

4 If she needs help standing up, position

your knees on either side of hers. Bend your knees, put your arms around her waist, and have her push up from the bed with her arms. Straighten your knees, and pull her with you while you stand.

5 Pivot and lower the person into a straight-backed chair with armrests or a wheelchair. Place her lower back against the chair's back, with feet on the floor, hips and knees at right angles, and upper body straight. Rest her forearms on the armrests.

Walking

If she can walk but needs support, stand behind her, placing one hand under her elbow and the other around her waist. Walk slowly and stop to rest as needed.

Reviewing massage techniques

An effective massage can make a person feel good all over. A back rub relaxes tense muscles in the neck, shoulders, and back, promoting rest. A foot massage helps to reduce swelling and increase flexibility in the feet, making standing and walking more comfortable. Both types of massage increase blood circulation to the skin.

Before actually performing massage, you'll need to understand massage techniques. Massage manipulates specific muscle groups to help relieve pain. The two basic techniques are effleurage and petrissage. Effleurage uses one or both thumbs or hands to make long, deep, or superficial strokes. In petrissage, the hands may be used to apply pressure to muscles.

Besides pressing, petrissage consists of kneading. This involves grasping a portion of one muscle group in

Stroking the back (effleurage)

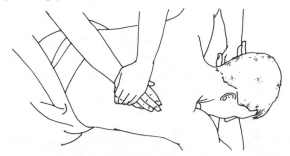

Using one hand over the other to press back muscles (petrissage)

Kneading the back (petrissage)

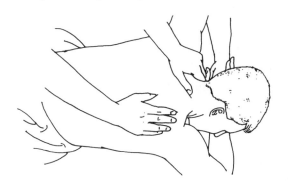

each hand and gliding one hand toward the other as you squeeze.

When giving any massage, keep these basic guidelines in mind.

• Make each hand movement slow and deliberate. Keep your strokes firm, smooth, and even; short, uneven strokes cause discomfort.

• Be thorough. Use overlapping strokes to cover the entire area, giving equal treatment to both sides of the body.

• Keep both hands on the person's body at all times, and make smooth transitions from one stroke to the next. Avoid removing your hands and reapplying them.

• When massaging arms and legs, always work toward the heart. Such movements help return blood from the arms and legs to the heart.

• To help the person relax and enjoy the massage, keep talking to a minimum. When you do speak, use a soothing voice.

Giving a back massage

Before giving a back massage, make sure your nails are trimmed and your hands are warm. Then follow these steps. (You can also use these techniques on other body areas.)

1 Position the person on his stomach or side with his back exposed. The room should be comfortably warm so that he doesn't become chilled.

2 Apply a nonoily lotion to the person's skin to reduce friction. Warm the lotion first by placing the bottle in a bowl of warm water.

Tell the person to imagine his muscle fibers stretching and relaxing as you massage.

3 Start with gentle strokes and gradually apply pressure, as tolerated. Using a circular thumb stroke, massage from the buttocks to the shoulders. Then, using a smooth stroke, return to the buttocks. Be sure to keep your hands in line

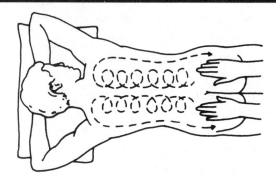

with the spine to avoid tickling the person.

4 Next, using your palms, stroke from the buttocks up to the shoulders, over the upper arms, and back to the buttocks. Use slightly less pressure on downward strokes.

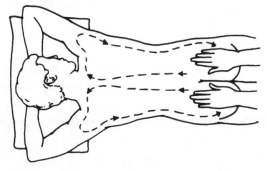

5 Using your thumb and forefinger, knead and stroke the left side of the back

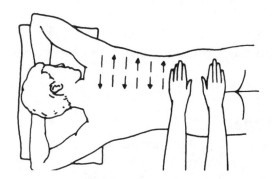

and the upper arm, starting at the buttocks and moving toward the shoulder. Then knead and stroke the right side of the back, rhythmically alternating your hands. Massage for 3 to 5 minutes or longer, as tolerated.

Giving a foot massage

Put a bottle of lotion in a basin of warm water to warm the lotion. Then position the person comfortably in bed or in a chair. Cover your lap with a towel, and support one of his feet between your knees or rest it on your lap. Apply lotion generously to the foot.

1 Steady the foot with one hand, and use the knuckles of your other hand to make small, firm circles over the entire sole, including the heel, as shown below. Massage firmly; too light a touch could tickle the person.

Now, support his foot with the fingers of both hands while you use your thumbs to make small circles over the sole.

Massaging the sole with your knuckles and thumbs

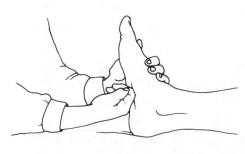

Massaging the foot's upper surface

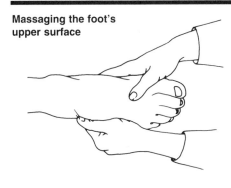

Squeezing the foot

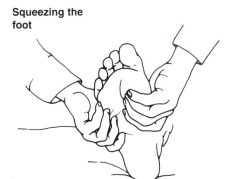

Stretching the toes

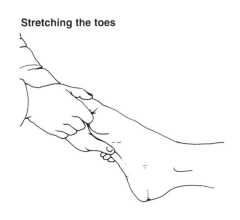

2 Next, place one hand under his ankle and gently lift his foot. With your other hand, move your fingertips and thumb in small, firm circles over his sole.

3 Locate the long tendons that run from the base of the ankle to each toe on the foot's upper surface. Now, as you support his heel with one hand, firmly but gently run the thumb of your free hand between each tendon groove and off his foot between his toes.

4 Grasp the person's foot with both hands, with your fingers under his sole and the heels of your hands on the top of his foot. Squeeze the foot firmly between your fingers and the heels of your hands, as shown here. Then slide your hands toward the foot's edges. Repeat this motion three times.

5 Use one hand to steady the person's foot. Grasp the base of his big toe with the thumb and forefinger of your other hand. Gently stretch and rotate the toe, using a corkscrew motion until your fingers slide off the tip of his toe. Repeat for each toe.

6 Complete the massage by cradling his foot between your hands for several seconds. Then gently place this foot next to his other foot. Repeat the massage on his other foot. (*Note:* Always wash your hands thoroughly after giving a massage.)

Learning to control pain

You can control pain with medication and with techniques such as distraction, relaxation, and guided imagery. If you're using pain medication, be sure to follow the doctor's orders. If you're trying distraction, relaxation, or guided imagery, practice the technique in between pain episodes so that you'll be prepared when pain occurs. Here's how each technique helps control pain.

Pain medication

The doctor may prescribe an analgesic drug or recommend a nonprescription analgesic (for example, aspirin). An analgesic affects the nervous system so that you feel less pain.

Distraction

With distraction, you learn to focus your attention on something other than pain—for example, listening to music. This activity becomes the center of your awareness.

Relaxation

With relaxation, you learn to change the way your body responds to the stress of being in pain. Normally, when a stressful condition like pain occurs, muscles tense, the heart beats faster, blood pressure rises, and breathing becomes faster and more shallow. These responses intensify pain. Relaxation can lessen pain by minimizing these responses and reducing anxiety.

Guided imagery

With guided imagery, you learn to create mental images that make pain less intense. Guided imagery affects how the body perceives and responds to pain. It helps control the message the mind sends to the body.

Using pain medication

If the doctor prescribes pain medication, be sure to follow his orders. These guidelines will help you get the most relief from pain medication.

• Take the medication regularly, as directed by the doctor. Don't wait until you're in a lot of pain or the medication may not effectively control the pain.

• If the pain seems particularly intense when you wake up in the morning, you may have had too little medication in your bloodstream to last through the night. To help, take the medication one or more times during the night, as needed, at the same dosage intervals as during the day. For example, if you take the medication every 4 hours and you go to bed at 10 p.m., set your alarm for 2 a.m. and take another dose. If necessary, reset your alarm for 6 a.m. and take another dose then.

• If you've been taking medication for 2 weeks or longer, don't suddenly stop taking it without the doctor's consent—even if you no longer have pain. The body may have become used to the medication. Stopping it suddenly may cause unpleasant or dangerous side effects.

• You may find that you can cope with pain better in a quiet, soothing environment. Try to avoid jarring or irritating surroundings—for example, bright lights or loud noise from a television or radio.

• To help prevent side effects, follow the doctor's advice about avoiding certain foods, alcohol, or other drugs while taking pain medication.

When to call the doctor

Eventually, you may notice that the pain medication no longer seems to work as well as it did before. If this happens, call the doctor so that he can find new ways to control the pain. Also call the doctor if:

• the medication makes you groggy or sleepier than usual.

• you develop a new pain or the pain seems different.

• you become constipated during treatment.

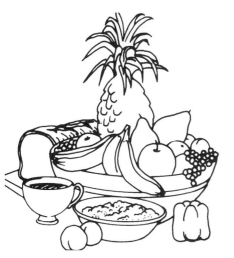

What to do about constipation

If you're taking a narcotic pain medication, you may become constipated. The following guidelines can help avoid this.

• Eat more high-fiber foods, including raw fruits and vegetables, whole-grain breads and cereals, dried fruits, and nuts. For snacks, choose high-fiber foods, such as date-nut bread, oatmeal cookies, and granola. Add 1 or 2 tablespoons of bran to cereal or eggs.

• Drink warm or hot beverages to stimulate bowel activity.

• Avoid hard cheeses and refined grain products, such as white rice and macaroni.
• Get more exercise, if possible.
• Follow the doctor's suggestions about modifying the diet, drinking extra fluids, and taking a mild laxative. Notify him if constipation persists.

Using distraction techniques

Use the following techniques to help distract you from your pain.

Listening to recordings

Consider getting a tape recorder with headphones and cassettes of your favorite music, comedy routines, or stories. Then sit or lie down in a comfortable position, with legs and arms uncrossed and relaxed, while you listen to the cassette through the headphones. Close your eyes and concentrate on the recording or stare at a nearby object. To make this tech-

Using recorded music as a distraction

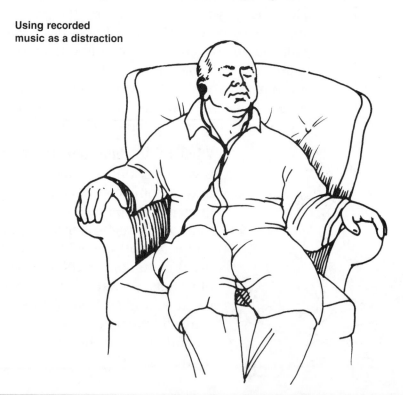

nique more effective, try any of these ideas:

• Combine music therapy with guided imagery by imagining yourself floating or drifting with the music. Or focus on a pleasant scene or on images suggested by the music. When listening to a story, try to imagine every detail the storyteller describes.

• Rhythmic movement can also serve as a distraction. Keep time with the music by slapping your thigh, tapping a finger or foot, or nodding your head.

• Keep your finger on the recorder's volume control dial. If the pain gets worse, turn up the volume. Then, when the pain subsides, turn the volume back down.

Singing

Select a song you like. Then mouth the words, exaggerating lip movements, while you sing it in your mind or aloud. Concentrate all your attention on the song's words and rhythm. (Closing your eyes may help.) Sing faster or louder when the pain gets worse; sing slower when the pain diminishes.

Rhythmic breathing

Stare at an object or a person while you inhale slowly and deeply. Then exhale slowly. Continue breathing slowly and comfortably (but not too deeply) while you count silently: "In, 2, 3, 4—out, 2, 3, 4."

While performing this exercise, concentrate on how the breathing feels. You may want to close your eyes and imagine the air moving slowly in and out of your lungs. Continue to count silently to keep breathing comfortable and rhythmic. If you begin to feel breathless, breathe slower or take a deep breath.

If rhythmic breathing alone doesn't distract you enough to relieve pain, add other elements. For example, try lightly massaging the painful area with a stroking or circular motion as you breathe. Or, if your condition permits, raise your arm as you inhale and lower it as you exhale. You might also try inhaling through your nose and exhaling through your mouth.

Using massage to relax muscles

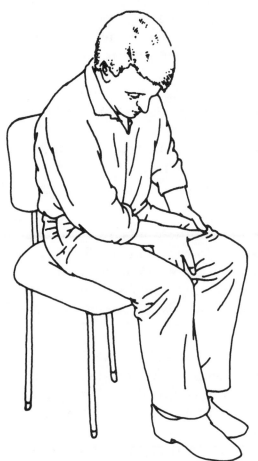

Using muscle relaxation

You can relax your muscles with a technique called progressive muscle relaxation. This technique helps to relieve the muscle tension that accompanies pain. By learning to tense and relax your muscles one by one, you'll find that you can relax your entire body. Follow these steps to relax your muscles.

1 Get comfortable and close your eyes. Now, starting at the top of your body, tense your forehead and face and hold this tension for 5 to 10 seconds.

2 Next, relax your forehead and face. Hold and enjoy this relaxation for 10 to 15 seconds.

3 Now, work toward your feet. First, tense and relax your jaw muscles. Proceed to the muscles in each shoulder, arm, and hand; then to your stomach and buttocks; and, finally, to each thigh, lower leg, ankle, and foot.

   If you have trouble relaxing some muscles or if the tension brings on pain, gently massage that body part until the muscles relax and feel comfortable.

4 To complete the exercise, open your eyes, stretch, and relax your entire body. Take a few deep breaths as if waking up from a deep sleep. Don't engage in any activity until you're alert.

Using breathing relaxation exercises

Special breathing techniques can help you cope with stress or pain. You can use it anywhere and at any time. You can also combine it with other techniques to help control pain. Try to

**Inhaling
slowly**

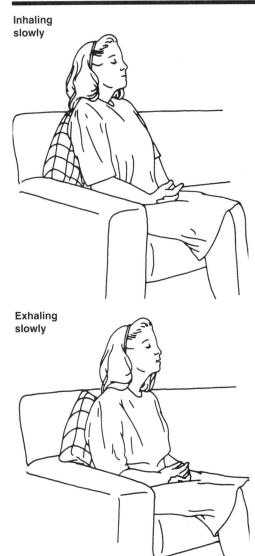

**Exhaling
slowly**

practice these simple breathing techniques daily. Follow these steps to perform relaxation breathing exercises.

1 Close your eyes. Inhale slowly and deeply through your nose as you count silently: "In, 2, 3, 4." Notice how the stomach expands first, then the rib cage, and, finally, the upper chest. Now, exhale slowly through your mouth as you count silently: "Out, 2, 3, 4, 5, 6." Pretend you're breathing out through a straw to lengthen exhalation. Let your shoulders drop slightly as your upper chest, rib cage, and stomach gently deflate. Repeat this exercise four or five times.

2 Inhale for 4 seconds and hold your breath for the count of 4, but don't strain. Then exhale through your mouth for 6 to 8 seconds. Practice this exercise four or five times.

A few tips

Perform these breathing exercises as long as needed during painful periods. You may vary the rhythm, but always exhale 2 to 4 seconds longer than you inhale.

If you feel light-headed or your fingers tingle, you may be breathing too deeply or too fast. Reduce the depth and speed of your breathing, or breathe into a paper bag until the feeling goes away.

Using imagination to control pain

Using imagination can help you cope with stress and pain. Following these steps will help you to use your imagination.

1 Begin by focusing on your breathing. Spend a few minutes breathing slowly and smoothly.

2 As you breathe, slowly count backward from 5, sinking deeper and deeper into a state of relaxation. Say to yourself, "I feel deeply relaxed."

3 Next, imagine a pleasant place that you can return to whenever you need relaxation or pain relief—for example, a warm, quiet beach or a tranquil, fragrant garden. Close your eyes to help you concentrate.

4 "Experience" the place with all your senses—sight, touch, smell, hearing, and taste. Remain there for about 5 minutes or longer, depending on the time needed for pain relief.

Let your imagination run free. Try to name the colors you see. Or trace the shapes of the flowers blooming in the garden. Breathe in the sweet fragrance of the blossoms, listen to the birds chirping, and feel the sun warm your skin. Now, sip a cool beverage before you step along the garden path and greet a friend.

5 Slowly let the image you've chosen fade from the center of your attention as you focus again on your breathing. Maintain a relaxed feeling. When you're ready, count slowly to 5 and open your eyes.

Using other ways to relieve pain

Four other techniques can help you deal with stress or pain.

Hypnosis

An altered state of consciousness, hypnosis requires focused concentration and minimal distraction. A hypnotized person becomes receptive to suggestions from a trained hypnotherapist. Hypnosis can help a person block his awareness of pain or interpret it in a positive way. Hypnosis can also be used to "move" the pain to a smaller or less significant body part (for instance, to transfer migraine headache pain to the little finger).

No one knows exactly how hypnosis relieves pain. But the method can provide long-lasting results without interfering with normal activities. Because hypnosis requires active participation, it usually changes a person's attitude toward pain and illness. By creating a feeling of control, hypnosis helps relieve the hopelessness and anxiety that can intensify pain.

Heat and cold therapy

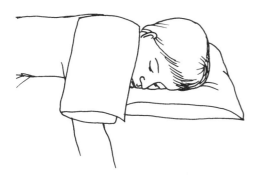
Applying dry heat directly to the skin

Different types of pain respond best to heat or cold therapy. The doctor will tell you whether to apply heat or cold or to alternate them.

Heat therapy. By using a covered electric heating pad or heat lamp, you can apply dry heat directly to the skin over painful areas. For moist heat treatment, use a hot pack, hot water bottle, or hot bath. Or use a heating pad to apply moist heat by laying a moist towel over the painful area, covering it with insulation (for example, plastic wrap), and placing the heating pad on top.

Cold therapy. Most cold therapy techniques require ice. Use an ice pack or wrap a large ice chunk in a washcloth and rub it over the painful area. To treat a large area, such as the lower back, soak a towel in ice water, wring out excess moisture, and apply it to the painful area.

If the injury's too sensitive to touch or if bandages prevent you from reaching the injured area, you can still use cold therapy by applying ice to the opposite side of the body. Called contralateral stimulation, this technique works because sensory input from both sides of the body influence nerve impulses that travel to the brain.

Biofeedback

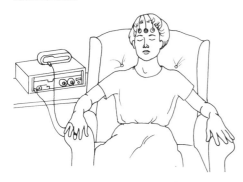
Relaxing while the biofeedback machine records data

This method can help control pain from muscle tension and stress. During a biofeedback session, the therapist connects the person to a machine that monitors body functions, such as body temperature, muscle tension, and heart rate. As the person tries to relax, the machine provides constant feedback in the form of noises, lights, or digital readings. This feedback tells the person immediately when she begins to relax. After learning through biofeedback which relaxation strategy works best for her, she can use this strategy the next time she feels tense.

Acupuncture meridians

Acupuncturists believe that life forces flow through meridians in the body. An acupuncturist inserts needles along these meridians—each associated with a major organ, body part, or energy pattern. Pain runs along the meridian path for a specific organ. For example, cardiac pain travels along the heart meridian, which runs down the inside of the arm.

Locations of several major meridians

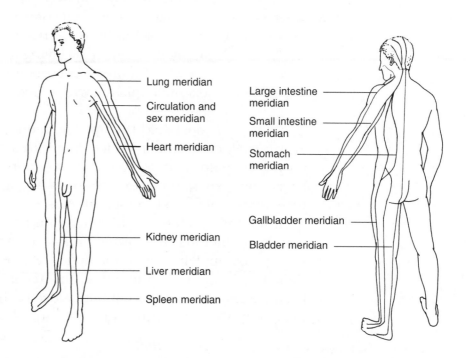

Lung meridian

Circulation and sex meridian

Heart meridian

Kidney meridian

Liver meridian

Spleen meridian

Large intestine meridian

Small intestine meridian

Stomach meridian

Gallbladder meridian

Bladder meridian

Learning about TENS

The doctor may order transcutaneous electrical nerve stimulation (also called TENS) for you to help relieve pain.

How TENS works

A small, battery-powered device sends safe electrical signals through wires and into the body by way of electrodes, which are attached to the skin.

Where to place the electrodes

A TENS therapist will show you where to attach the electrodes. Ask the therapist to label the sites with a marker. If necessary, use a mirror to help you see them.

If the electrodes require conductive jelly, spread it in a thin layer across each electrode before applying the electrode.

Placing electrodes on the wrong sites probably won't harm you, but avoid placing them on your belly if you're pregnant, on the sides of your neck, and on the voice box area.

Using TENS

The knobs on the unit are adjustable. The doctor will tell you what settings to use for the AMP/A, rate, and pulse width as well as how long and how often to use the unit.

You should feel a pleasant sensation while the machine is working. If you develop muscle spasms, contact the TENS therapist. The AMP may be set too high, or you may have placed the electrodes in the wrong places.

If your pain is increasing, follow the directions the TENS therapist gave you to change the settings on the TENS unit.

Safety tips

Follow the therapist's instructions carefully for the length of time you should leave the TENS unit on. Don't get into water with the unit on, and don't sleep with it on.

Skin care

Take good care of your skin. Prevent local skin irritation—redness and rash—by cleaning your skin before attaching the electrodes. Watch for signs of irritation.

If your skin does become irritated, don't place electrodes on those areas. Keep the skin clean and dry until it heals. If it's still irritated after a week, contact the doctor.

If you repeatedly develop local skin irritation from the electrodes, contact the TENS therapist to discuss an alternate wearing schedule or another type of electrode.

Caring for the TENS unit

Clean the TENS unit weekly by wiping it lightly with rubbing alcohol.

6 Hospital Beds

Learning about hospital beds

Hospital beds enhance home care. They ease the caregiver's tasks and add comfort for the person who is ill. Most people being cared for at home need some amount of bed rest. Bed rest helps injured tissues heal, helps relieve pain, and reduces stress on weakened body systems. A hospital bed lets a person who's weak or injured elevate the head or feet without physical effort or a caregiver's help, and this improves breathing and circulation. A hospital bed is higher than a regular bed, saving the caregiver's back and shoulders from strain. Also, it rolls easily on wheels.

Three types of hospital beds are available: manual, semi-electric, and fully electric. On each type, manual or electric controls adjust the bed frame height and position; the mattress moves with the bed frame. The bed moves from a low position (convenient for getting in and out of bed) to a waist-high position that eliminates stooping during bed making and while providing in-bed care. Different parts of the bed slant in various ways to suit the person's condition or to make him more comfortable.

Four different bed positions

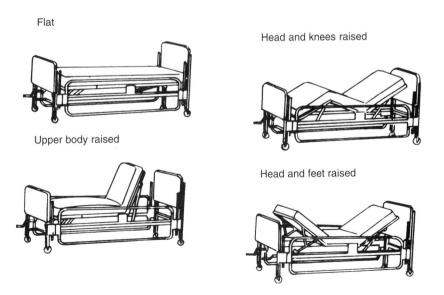

Flat

Head and knees raised

Upper body raised

Head and feet raised

Manual bed

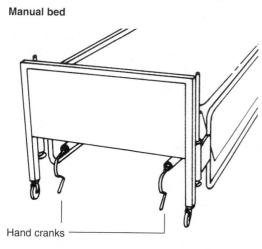

Hand cranks

Electric bed

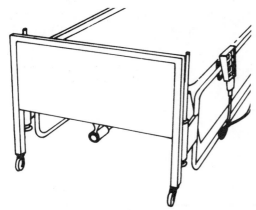

The head and knee sections of manual beds adjust by turning hand cranks at the foot or head of the bed. A manual bed may not adjust into as many positions as an electric bed. Bed height is fixed at waist level on some models; on others, bed height adjusts by turning a hand crank on the side of the bed.

Mattress positions on electric and semi-electric beds adjust electrically. Even a person who's unable to move can change the mattress's position by pushing buttons on a hand-held control. Bed height can be adjusted by a hand crank on semielectric beds and by control buttons on electric beds.

Choosing a hospital bed

Which type of hospital bed should you choose? Consider both the person's and the caregiver's needs. People who can't get out of bed or who are weak or injured need a semielectric or electric bed so that they can make adjustments themselves. Also, both the person who requires frequent repositioning and the caregiver will find a manual bed inconvenient. And a caregiver who is unable to use hand cranks—because of weakness, arthritis, or a sore back, for instance—will need fully automatic controls. The choice may be limited to what the person's insurance covers, as determined by his diagnosis; check with the insurance carrier.

Placing a hospital bed

Don't assume that the bed belongs in the bedroom. The person's regular room may be upstairs and removed from your home's activity center. If you place the bed there, everyone has to climb stairs, the person misses out on family interaction, and the caregiver spends too much time just getting to and from the person. Instead, consider a downstairs living room, family room, or den—somewhere centrally located that can still provide privacy and quiet when required. The main area of household activity may not be a good choice, however, for the person who requires a lot of rest.

Place the bed away from walls so that it's easy to reach on either side. Be sure the surroundings are clean, attractive, and interesting.

Learning about mattresses

A firm mattress is most comfortable. Firm, level support enhances blood circulation, maintains the best spine and body position to relieve backache and joint pain, and distributes body weight evenly.

A hospital bed purchased or leased from a medical supply company should include a waterproof mattress. If the mattress isn't waterproof, protect it with a waterproof mattress cover; a fitted one is easiest to keep in place, but a tucked-in plastic sheet will also do the job.

A regular (not water, air, or foam) mattress stays most comfortable and wears evenly if you remember to turn it once a week. One time, keep the mattress flat and turn it from end

Turning the mattress from end to end

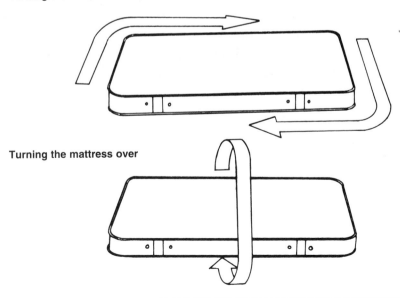

Turning the mattress over

to end; next time, lift the mattress and turn it over from side to side. Because this can only be done when the person is out of bed, mattress turning isn't an option for a bedridden person. When you turn a waterproof mattress, wipe it with a disinfecting solution of 1 part bleach to 10 parts water. (Once a month, wash the bed with this solution also.) Be sure to unplug an electric bed before cleaning the bed or the mattress.

Choosing a mattress pad

You'll need a standard mattress pad made of soft or quilted material to cover the mattress surface for the person's comfort and for mattress protection. Some mattress pads are fitted and tuck under; others have elastic loops that anchor the pad at the corners. The pad must fit snugly and without wrinkles. Be sure the pad is easy to wash and dry. The pad should be changed whenever it's wet or soiled or once a week if the person's almost always in bed; once a month is usually enough if the person occupies the bed less than half the day. If wetting is a problem, you can buy waterproof mattress pads that have plastic on their undersurface.

You may also need a special type of mattress pad—a pressure-relief pad—if the person spends a great deal of time in bed. Such a person can develop pressure ulcers (also called bedsores) from pressure on the skin, particularly on bony areas such as the heels, elbows, lower back, and shoulders. (People who are elderly, thin, weak, or obese or who have poor skin tone and circulation are at greatest risk to develop pressure ulcers.)

Learning about bed boards

If a mattress isn't firm enough, you can place a bed board between the bedsprings and the mattress. A bed board strengthens the bedsprings, firms up the mattress, and prevents it from sagging. But it won't make a bad mattress a good one.

You can purchase a bed board ready-made or make one

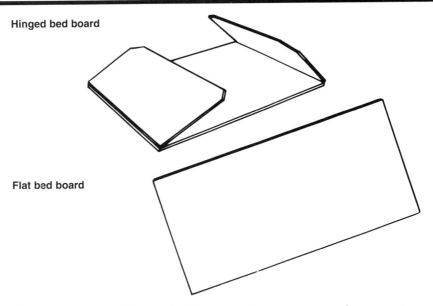

Hinged bed board

Flat bed board

from one-inch plywood. If you make your own, be sure to sand it smooth so that it doesn't snag the mattress. The board should run the length and width of the mattress. For a hospital bed, you'll need either a hinged bed board that conforms to the various bedspring positions or a board cut in three sections. Ask your medical equipment dealer if he can supply one. Remember to center the board over the bedsprings so that it doesn't jut out and cause accidental injury.

Pressure-relief devices

Special pads, mattresses, and beds can help relieve pressure on the skin for the patient who is confined to one position for long periods.

Gel flotation pads

These pads disperse pressure over a wide surface area.

Water mattress or pads

A wave effect continuously provides even distribution of body weight.

Alternating-pressure mattress

Alternating deflation and inflation of mattress tubes changes areas of pressure.

Convoluted foam mattress or pads

Elevated foam areas cushion skin, minimizing pressure. Depressed areas relieve pressure.

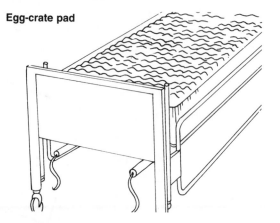

Egg-crate pad

Spanco mattress

This mattress, made of polyester fibers with silicon tubes, decreases pressure without restricting position.

Sheepskin pad

This type of pad prevents pressure and absorbs moisture. It must be in direct contact with the skin.

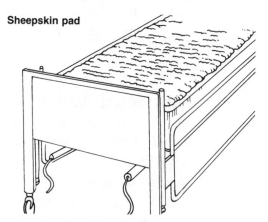

Sheepskin pad

Foam rubber

Cut to just the right size and shape, foam rubber cushions individual areas.

Clinitron bed

This bed contains beads that move under an airflow to support the patient, thus eliminating shearing force and friction.

Stryker or Foster frame and CircOlectric bed
These devices relieve pressure by turning the patient.

Lift sheet and mechanical lifting device
A lift sheet and other devices prevent shearing by lifting the patient rather than dragging him across the bed.

Mechanical lifting device

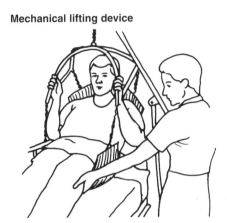

Padding
Pillows, towels, and soft blankets can reduce pressure in body hollows.

Foot cradle
This device lifts the bed linens to relieve pressure over the feet.

Using bed attachments
You can buy or make various devices to keep the bed linens from touching the person, to prevent footdrop, and to support the person's back when he's sitting up.

Bed cradle
A bed cradle is a frame that keeps the bed linens off the person. Bed cradles can be used for people with burns, open wounds, infections, wet casts, circulation problems, or extreme sensitivity to touch. Not only do cradles relieve the bedding's weight or even touch, which can lead to skin irritation and breakdown, but they also promote air circulation

and dry, perspiration-free skin.

Bed cradles come in different sizes. A foot cradle lifts bedding off a person's lower legs and feet. Several of these smaller frames used together can keep bed linens off larger body areas. Commercial foot cradles slip under the mattress.

An overbed cradle, a cagelike frame on top of the mattress, keeps bed linens off the person's whole body. Commercial overbed cradles slip under the mattress and are held by the mattress or attach to the bedsprings.

Foot cradle

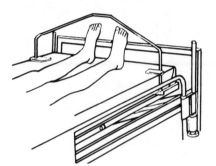

Overbed cradle

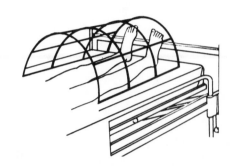

You can buy a bed cradle or make one in the size you want. A strong cardboard box with two sides cut out makes a fine cradle. You can use several together if you need a whole-body cradle. If the "box cradle" has rough edges, cover them

Making a bed cradle

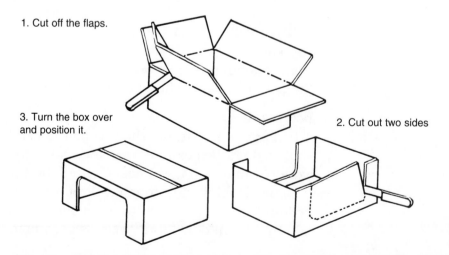

1. Cut off the flaps.

3. Turn the box over and position it.

2. Cut out two sides

with soft material such as old sheeting or moleskin. Punch some holes in the box to improve air circulation.

You may want to tape such a homemade frame to the bottom sheet to keep it in place. Then place the top sheet over the frame and tuck it in at the foot of the bed. Position and secure cradles with the person in bed, and remove cradles before he gets out of bed.

Footboard

A person who's confined to bed for a long time can develop a condition called footdrop, in which the foot points from the ankle instead of remaining flexed. A footboard is a removable

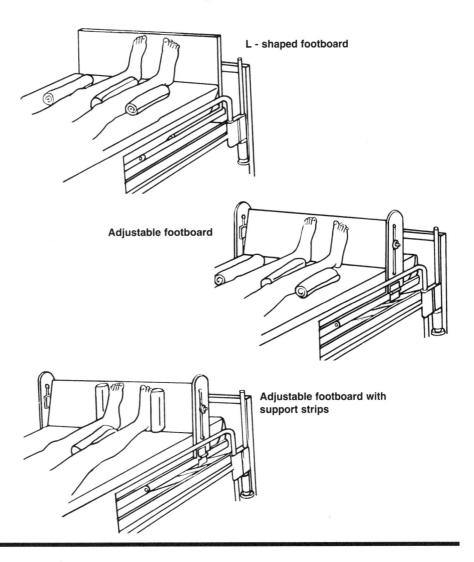

L - shaped footboard

Adjustable footboard

Adjustable footboard with support strips

device, usually a board, that prevents footdrop by keeping the feet upright. It also serves as a cradle by keeping bed linens from pressing on the feet and lower legs.

Whatever type you choose, position the person comfortably and then adjust the footboard so that the person's feet rest firmly and comfortably against it. If the footboard isn't padded, pad it with a towel or bath blanket. If you can't adjust the board, tuck a folded bath blanket between it and the person's feet. Place a pillow, rolled towel, or sandbag beside each foot so that the feet don't turn outward. Also make sure the person's heels are padded or protected. If the person's legs are long enough, position the heels over the mattress edge. Finally, fold the top sheet over the footboard and tuck it under the mattress. Even with a footboard, you'll still need to exercise the person's feet and legs.

Backrest

Firm support makes sitting up in bed much more comfortable. A hospital bed provides this support when the head of the bed is elevated. You can also buy an adjustable backrest or mattress raiser from a medical supply company or many department stores. Or you may make one yourself.

Here's one homemade backrest you can use in a bed that has a headboard or that's up against a wall. Arrange two firm pillows in a V shape so that they cross at the top, with the bottom edges touching; lay a third pillow crosswise over them under the person's head and shoulders.

Or turn a straight-backed kitchen chair upside down with the top resting on the mattress and the legs in the air. Cover the chair with pillows. The chair's back supports the person's back. A folded-up card table makes a good prop, too, if you tie it to the head of the bed.

Pillow backrest

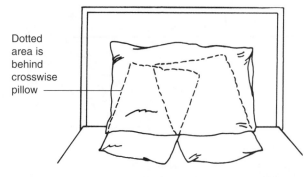

Dotted area is behind crosswise pillow

Chair backrest **Card table backrest**

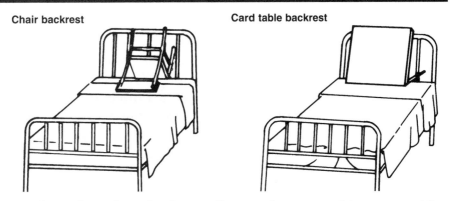

If you have beach chairs, flat-on-the-ground types provide a ready-made adjustable backrest.

In addition to backrests, a small pillow or pad tucked under the small of the back can relieve lower back strain for the person who's sitting up in bed.

Overbed table

The standard hospital-type overbed table rolls easily and is hard to tip over. The height adjusts easily. Some models feature tilting trays, and some include undertray storage for small items such as pencils, tissues, eyeglasses, and writing tablets.

Hospital-type overbed table **Homemade overbed table**

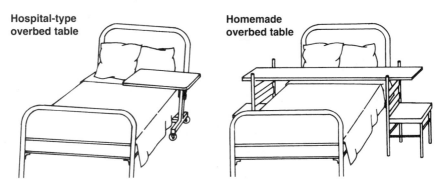

Insurance may not pay for an overbed table—it's considered a convenience, not a medical necessity. So you may want to make your own overbed table. To do this, place two straight-backed wooden chairs on either side of the bed and lay a sturdy plank, closed ironing board, or dining room table leaf across the chair backs. If you use a plank, sand it smooth or cover it with plastic or washable shelf paper so you can clean it easily.

Bed tray

An over-the-lap bed tray or table may be used instead of the overbed table. It's a handy way to serve meals. You can buy one with folding legs. You can also make one by sawing off the legs of an old card table to the right height. Or recycle a sturdy cardboard box, one with a strong, unopened bottom. Here's how: Remove the top flaps, cut out most of the two long sides, and reinforce the bottom, if necessary. Make sure it has no rough edges, and cover the box with plastic so that it's easy to clean.

Homemade bed tray   **Commercial bed tray**

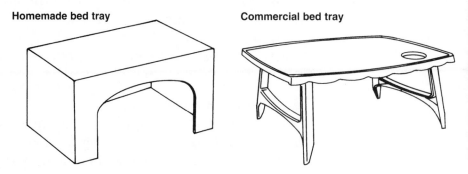

Bedside table

Besides an overbed table, you'll need a standard bedside table to hold such items as a lamp, water pitcher and glass, tissue box, clock, and books. Most important, the table should hold a telephone and a call bell. A bedridden person must have a means of communication. A bell reduces the person's sense of isolation and increases his sense of security. A bedside telephone keeps the person in contact with friends and the outside world. A call bell and a bedside telephone are also important safety features.

Rubber-tipped footstool

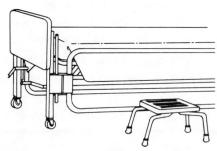

Footstool

Even with a hospital bed as low to the floor as possible, a person may need a footstool to get in and out of bed. Be sure it's sturdy; the legs should be widely spaced, with rubber tips, so that the stool doesn't tip or slide. The stool's surface must be nonskid, too: commercial bedside stools have grooved rubber tips for maximum traction.

Making a bed

Bed making involves more than linen changes. You'll need to know how to choose appropriate bedding and how to use bed-making techniques that keep the person comfortable and prevent skin breakdown.

Bed height

Be sure to take advantage of the hospital bed's adjustable feature: raise the bed to about waist level so that you have a comfortable working height and avoid back strain from working in a bent-over position.

Drawsheets and turning sheets

Always make the bed with a drawsheet—an extra sheet folded lengthwise that lies across the bed, directly under the person. You can change a soiled drawsheet more easily than the whole bed. If the drawsheet's plastic, cover it with a second drawsheet.

A drawsheet can also serve as a turning sheet for a person who can't help move or turn himself. Here's how. With the drawsheet under the person from shoulders to knees, grasp the sides to form handles. With someone standing on the opposite side of the bed, you can use the sheet to make a

Using a drawsheet for turning

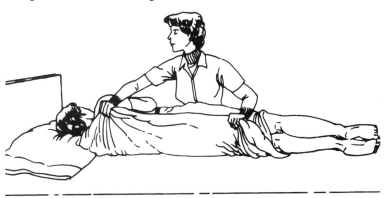

sling; you can move the person without straining him or you or wrinkling the bottom linens. A drawsheet may help prevent the person from sliding up and down in bed.

A drawsheet helps you turn a person yourself. To use it, stand at the side of the bed. Reach over the person and firmly grasp the sheet's opposite rolled edge. Then pull the rolled edge carefully toward you, turning the person. *Caution:* Keep the side rails up while turning the person. After turning, reposition the person comfortably; then tuck the drawsheet back in.

Hem positions

Always keep the rough side of the sheet's hem away from the person. Face the bottom sheet's rough side down, toward the mattress. Face the top sheet's rough side up and then turn the top sheet down over the blanket and bedspread at the head while tucking it under at the foot. Keeping the hem's rough side away from the person ensures that it doesn't rub against the person's heels or arms, thus eliminating a possible source of skin irritation.

Bedmaking technique

1 Push the mattress to the head of the bed before making the bed. Adjusting it later loosens the bed linens.

2 Use a fitted bottom sheet if possible. Don't use a regular twin fitted sheet; it's too small for a hospital bed mattress. Buy a fitted sheet that's made for hospital bed use.

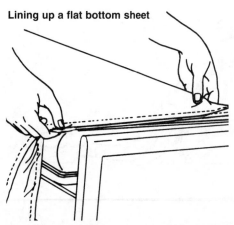

Lining up a flat bottom sheet

3 Flat sheets pull out easily from under the mattress, especially at the foot of the bed. So line up a flat bottom sheet with the end of the mattress rather than tucking it under. And be sure the sheet is wide enough to tuck well under along the sides.

4 Miter the corners to keep them firmly tucked under the mattress. To miter the top edge of a bottom sheet, tuck the end evenly under the mattress at the bed's head. Then lift the side of the sheet edge about 12 inches from the mattress corner and hold it at a right angle to the mattress. Next, tuck in the sheet's bottom edge hanging below the mattress. Finally, drop the top edge and tuck it under the mattress.

Making a mitered corner

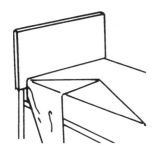

1. Lift the side of the sheet and hold it at a right angle to the mattress.

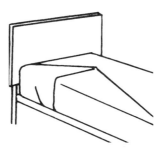

2. Next, tuck in the sheet's bottom edge.

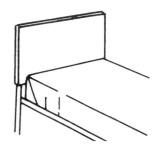

3. Finally, drop the top edge and tuck it under the mattress.

5 After fitting all corners of the bottom sheet or tucking them securely, pull the sheet at an angle from the head toward the foot of the bed. This tightens the linens, making the bottom sheet smooth.

• Because a drawsheet is smaller and has longer ends, it tucks in securely, usually stays smoother, and straightens out more easily than the bottom sheet.

Bedding

Give special attention to the type of bedding the person requires.

• Use bedding that's soft and easy to wash. Synthetic fabrics may feel too warm, may not absorb sweat, and may stain. Blankets and bedspreads should be warm but lightweight and, again, washable; thermal blankets are a good choice. Old sheets are softer than new ones. Don't use strong detergents or bleach when washing; they can irritate the skin. Fabric softener helps keep bedding soft but may cause allergic skin reactions.

• Make sure all bedding is long and wide enough to tuck well under while easily covering the person completely.

• Make sure to have extra sets of sheets and pillowcases so that spares are on hand during laundering and emergencies. You'll also need several extra sheets to fold in half lengthwise as drawsheets.

Extra pillows

Provide extra pillows. They have many uses. Three pillows make a good backrest, as explained earlier in this chapter. Several pillows together can prop up a heavy cast. Rolled-up pillows under body areas such as the knees and back promote comfort, help circulation, and relieve pressure. Pillows tucked around arms, legs, and sides help maintain body support; they're particularly effective for a person in a side-lying position.

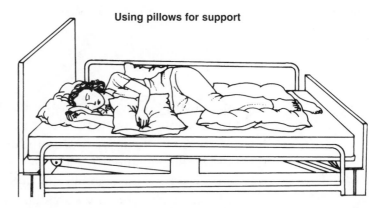

Using pillows for support

Making an occupied bed

Don't worry if the person you're caring for can't leave the bed; making a bed with someone in it isn't difficult. The basic idea is to strip and remake half the bed at a time. To become an expert occupied-bed maker in no time, follow these steps.

1 Remove bedside accessories (such as tables and trays). Wash your hands and then assemble clean linen:

• two sheets
• two drawsheets
• pillow case
• blanket
• linen-saver pad (optional).

2 Explain to the person what you're going to do, and suggest ways in which he can help. Be sure the side rail on the side opposite you is raised so he won't fall out of bed. Lower the head of the bed, if the person's condition permits, to ensure tight-fitting, wrinkle-free sheets. Raise the bed's height to your waist level so you won't strain your back.

Remove extra pillows. Then remove blankets or spreads and loosen the top sheet. For warmth and privacy, drape the top sheet over the person. While you're stripping the bed, watch for items the person may have dropped in the bedding.

Rolling up the bottom sheet

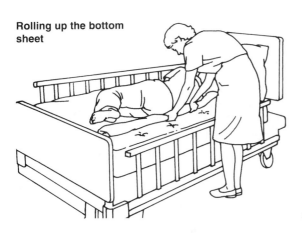

Applying the clean sheet

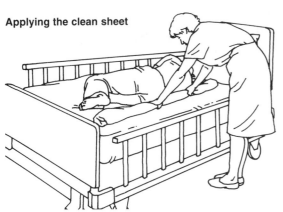

3 Roll the person to the side opposite where you're standing. Loosen the bottom sheet on your side. Roll it up tightly toward the center of the bed, tucking it under the person's back.

4 Place a clean bottom sheet, folded lengthwise, on the bed with the fold along the person's back in the center of the mattress. Line up the end of the sheet with the mattress foot, hem down. Now, roll or fold the top half of the clean bottom sheet tightly against the person's back. Tuck in the other half at the head and side, smoothing out any wrinkles.

5 Place a linen-saver pad, if needed, in the center of the bed, tucked under the person. Then cover the pad with a folded drawsheet. Roll or fold each sheet's top half and tuck it under the person. Tuck each sheet under the mattress on the side nearest you.

6 Raise the side rail on your side. Roll the person over the used and fresh linen to the bed's clean side. Then move to the other side and lower that side rail.

Moving the bedridden person

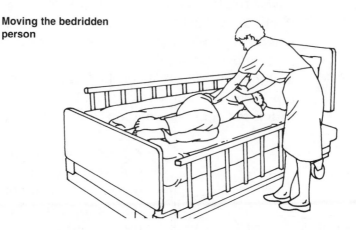

7 Remove the used bottom sheets. Unroll the clean bottom sheet, pad, and drawsheet. Pull the linens tightly to eliminate wrinkles, and tuck the fresh linen under the mattress.

8 Help the bedridden person into a comfortable position. Then remove the pillows, take off the used pillowcases, and slip on fresh ones. Replace the pillows.

Now, center a clean top sheet over the soiled top linens, unfolding to each side. Pull the used top linens out from under the clean sheet at the person's feet. If he is able, the

Changing the top sheet

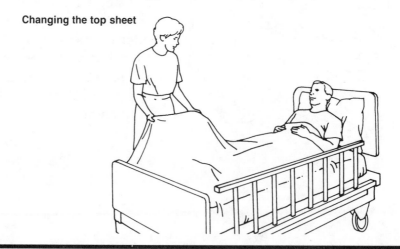

person can hold the clean top edge to help.

Place the blanket over the clean top sheet. Turn the top of the sheet over the blanket and miter the corners.

9 Raise the head of the bed to a comfortable position for the person. Remember to return the bed to the low position and to move the overbed and bedside tables back within easy reach for the person.

Making an unoccupied bed

Because you may be changing linens often, learn to do it efficiently: one side at a time.

1 Begin by removing all used linen and then assembling and folding clean linen lengthwise.

2 Center the bottom sheet's lengthwise fold on the mattress; then secure a fitted sheet at top and bottom or miter a flat sheet's top corner after lining up its end with the mattress foot. Next, center and tuck in a linen-saver pad (optional), then a drawsheet, then the top sheet with its wide hem even with the head of the bed, and, finally, the blanket and/or bedspread.

3 Switch to the bed's other side and repeat the steps.

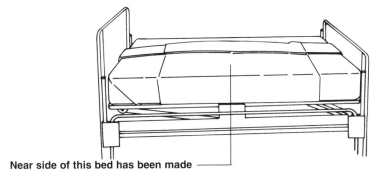

Near side of this bed has been made

7   Feeding the Sick

Learning about nutrition during illness

Everyone needs to eat a variety of foods each day for optimum health. But when a person's ill, fighting illness, or recovering from an injury or surgery, his need for a well-balanced diet increases dramatically. So does his need for certain nutrients, such as vitamin C, which the body uses more of during times of emotional and physical stress. What's more, certain drugs interfere with the body's production of necessary vitamins. For example, prolonged use of antibiotics suppresses the body's ability to produce vitamin K and some B vitamins. Several oral diabetes medications interfere with the absorption of vitamin B_{12}. And laxatives, diuretics, some anti-inflammatory drugs, and certain cancer drugs and treatments can upset the body's balance of vitamins and minerals.

Just when a person needs it most, a well-balanced diet can be hard to get if his condition makes eating difficult, painful, or unappealing. In addition to planning, preparing, and serving nutritious meals, you may need to help the person in your care eat—either by feeding him, providing him with special utensils so he can feed himself, or taking steps to improve his appetite and make mealtime more enjoyable.

Planning nutritious meals

When helping the person you're caring for plan nutritious and realistic well-balanced meals and snacks, think of adaptations he can make to accommodate possible problems, including dental problems, sensory problems, reduced energy, slowed GI function, and, if applicable, a limited food budget. Begin by stressing, however, that he can make his diet work effectively for him.

Emphasize the importance of eating the recommended number of servings each day from the six food groups shown on the Food Guide Pyramid on the next page. This is the best way to help the person in your care meet his dietary needs. If the patient eats a large dinner, suggest making lunch the most substantial meal because it provides energy for a more physically active time of day. Explain how he can fit nutritious snacks, such as raisins, fresh fruit, cottage cheese, celery, and cheese and crackers, into his meal planning.

Show the person how to keep a daily food diary by recording what he eats, when he eats, and how he feels during and

Food guide pyramid

Use the pyramid below to help you eat better. Remember to check food labels on prepared foods because fats, oils, and sweets can be added to many foods in the five major groups.

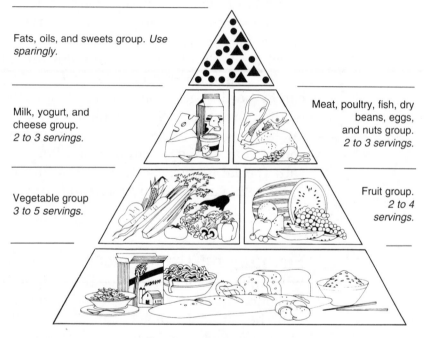

Fats, oils, and sweets group. *Use sparingly.*

Milk, yogurt, and cheese group. *2 to 3 servings.*

Meat, poultry, fish, dry beans, eggs, and nuts group. *2 to 3 servings.*

Vegetable group *3 to 5 servings.*

Fruit group. *2 to 4 servings.*

Bread, cereal, rice, and pasta group. *6 to 11 servings.*

Adapted from U.S. Department of Agriculture, U.S. Department of Health and Human Services.

shortly after eating. That way he'll know how various foods affect him physically and emotionally. Now, review the following general dietary goals with him.

Reducing fat intake

Advise the person to trim visible fat from meat and drain fat from food during cooking. Also remind him to avoid animal fat, such as lard and salt pork, for cooking. Tell him to cut back on fried foods and to substitute 1% fat or skim milk for whole milk.

Cutting down on cholesterol

Tell the person you're caring for to cut down on eggs, organ meats, and shellfish, such as shrimp, lobster, and crab. He should also consume less beef, dark-meat fish (such as mackerel and sardines), and nondairy cream substitutes.

Encouraging fruit intake

Urge him to eat fresh bananas, oranges, apples, grapes, peaches, pears, strawberries, and plums. Explain to him that these fruits supply vitamins A, C, and E as well as potassium and fiber. Also explain that fresh fruits help satisfy a craving for sweets. Suggest seasonal fruits; they're usually ripe and less expensive.

Tell him to refrain from eating fruits packed in heavy syrup. These contain excess sugar and calories.

Increasing vegetable intake

Point out that vegetables contain fiber, which prevents constipation and lowers serum cholesterol levels. To obtain maximum nutrients from vegetables, suggest that he eat them raw or steam them. Then he can drink the broth (which contains vitamins and minerals) or he can save it for use in soups and sauces, if he prefers.

Promoting intake of whole grains

Tell him that whole-grain cereals and breads contain fiber. Like vegetables, these foods help prevent constipation.

Eliminating refined sugar

Recommend that he substitute fresh fruits, nuts, seeds, and raisins for refined sugar. Inform him that sugar can cause headaches and anxiety. Explain that he'll get enough natural sugars from fresh fruits.

Reducing salt intake

Inform the person you're caring for that processed food contains large quantities of salt, which can cause water retention and irritability. Recommend that he read the labels on the products he uses. Suggest that he sprinkle herbs or lemon juice on vegetables and meat for added flavor or ask the doctor if he can use a salt substitute.

Increasing mineral intake

Encourage him to eat more low-fat dairy products, whole grains, nuts, and dark, leafy vegetables. Also tell him to drink fluoridated water, if possible. Explain that minerals, such as calcium, are vital to healthy bones and gums and help maintain mental equilibrium.

Ensuring adequate fluids

Tell him to drink plenty of fluids—at least 6 to 8 glasses or 48 to 64 ounces (1,440 to 1,920 ml), daily—unless contraindicated.

Stopping smoking

Inform him that smoking—whether a cigarette, cigar, or pipe—interferes with nutrient absorption.

Limiting alcohol

Emphasize that more than five drinks weekly will prevent proper vitamin and mineral absorption. If your patient's used to having a glass of wine with his meals, however, or the doctor's prescribes wine to stimulate his appetite, he should continue this pattern.

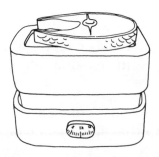

Measuring a serving

Most people estimate the size of a serving. But if you're caring for someone who must eat a special diet, the doctor may want you to measure serving sizes. If so, follow these tips.

Weighing portions

Invest in a small scale to weigh portions. For example, if the person's diet calls for a 4-ounce (113-gram) cooked hamburger, weigh the meat before and after you cook it: you'll see that it shrinks in size and weight after cooking. You can also use your scale to weigh out the correct serving of cereals, grains, and other foods.

Comparing sizes

Look at the size of produce carefully when you shop, and try to get an idea of medium or average sizes. For instance, an apple can be extra large—the kind you'd see in a "bon voyage" fruit basket—or it can be small—almost the size of a plum.

Measuring foods

Measure foods with a measuring cup and measuring spoons. For accuracy, don't use a heaping teaspoon or cup. Instead, level it off. If you're using a see-through measuring cup, hold it at eye level to measure precisely.

Preserving nutrients when you cook

Some preparation methods can strip foods of their nutrients. But you can preserve most of the vitamins and minerals if you follow these guidelines.

Preparing fruits and vegetables

Serve raw fruits and vegetables if the person can eat them. Cut or trim the food as little as possible and just before cooking or serving.

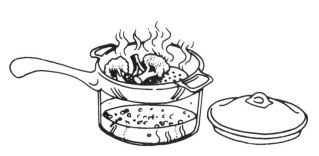

Rinsing and soaking foods properly

Rinse fresh produce just enough to remove dirt, and soak dried beans and peas only until they're slightly softened. That way, you won't rinse or soak away the vitamins and minerals these foods contain.

Steaming and stir-frying foods

Avoid boiling vegetables for a long time in lots of water, and make sure the water is boiling rapidly before adding them. Boiling, simmering, and pressure cooking can destroy vitamin C and other nutrients. Instead, try steaming vegetables, using a steamer like the one shown here. This process can double the amount of nutrients that remain in vegetables. Or stir-fry vegetables or meat—another nutrient-saving method. Remember to cook vegetables until they're tender in small amounts of liquid to prevent scorching.

Adding protein and calories to the diet

When a person's diet doesn't provide enough calories, his body draws on its stores of fat for fuel. Then it begins to break down protein, leading to tissue loss. This leaves the person very weak, prevents worn-out tissue from healing and rebuilding, and keeps the body from producing substances that help fight infection. As a result, the person will have a harder time getting well.

You can make up for changes in the sick person's normal eating patterns by adding protein and calories to each meal, if the doctor approves. People with certain illnesses—those that affect the kidneys, for example—may require a low-protein diet, so be sure to check with the doctor before changing the diet.

Adding protein

Here are some ways to add protein to the diet:
• Add diced or ground meat to vegetable dishes, sauces, casseroles, and soups.
• Add skim milk powder to hot and cold cereals, scrambled eggs, meat loaf, and baked desserts.
• Mix canned tuna or salmon and chopped hard-boiled eggs into sauces served with pasta, rice, and casseroles.
• Serve a high-protein dietary supplement, as described in the supplement chart that follows.
• Offer high-protein snacks, such as nuts, cheese, and peanut butter, if the person can eat these foods.

Adding calories

Here are some ways to add calories to the diet:

Encourage high-calorie snacks

Good choices include dried fruits, such as raisins and apricots; peanut butter or cheese spread on crackers, bread, fresh fruit, or raw vegetables; milk shakes made with ice cream, cream, powdered milk, or instant breakfast powders; and breakfast bars.

Add extra fats and sugar to food

Fats are a great source of calories, if the doctor permits them. But fat is difficult for people with cystic fibrosis to digest, so watch for signs of malabsorption to see if more enzymes are needed. Try the following suggestions:

• Put margarine or butter on bread, rice, noodles, potatoes, and vegetables. Use mayonnaise or margarine on sandwiches.
• Add sour cream to casseroles, or serve it with potatoes, vegetables, meat, and fruit.
• Serve meat, vegetables, and casseroles with cream sauces or gravy.
• Mix extra amounts of salad dressing in salads.
• Add whipped cream to hot chocolate, fruit, and desserts.
• Top ice cream with syrup or preserves.
• Spread bread, muffins, biscuits, or crackers with jam, jelly, or honey.
• Substitute half-and-half or cream for milk.
• Add cheese to scrambled eggs, sauces, vegetables, casseroles, and salads.
• Use extra eggs in sauces, casseroles, sandwich spreads, and salads. Add powdered eggs to milk shakes. (Don't use raw eggs—they can cause food poisoning.)
• Sprinkle chopped or ground nuts on ice cream, yogurt, frozen yogurt, pudding, breads, and desserts. (Children under age 4 shouldn't eat whole nuts because they might choke.)

Serve high-calorie supplements

If the person you're caring for has lung damage, repeated infections, or weight loss, try adding commercial, high-protein calorie supplements to his daily diet. Or use instant breakfast powders mixed with whole milk for about the same number of calories and nutritional value.

SUPPLEMENT & FORM	WHO CAN USE IT
Ensure Ready-to-use liquid or powder (mix with water)	People who need supplemental nutrition, especially if they're on a low residue diet
Ensure Plus Ready-to-use liquid	People who need supplemental nutrition, especially those who need increased calories but can't tolerate increased fluids
Isocal Ready-to-use liquid	People who need supplemental nutrition
Meritene Ready-to-use liquid or powder	People who need supplemental nutrition
Pulmocare Ready-to-use liquid	People with respiratory disorders, such as emphysema, who need supplemental nutrition; reduces production of carbon dioxide
Sustacal Ready-to-use liquid, powder (mix with milk), and ready-to-eat pudding	People who need supplemental nutrition

CHARACTERISTICS	SPECIAL CONSIDERATIONS
• Flavors: Vanilla, chocolate, and strawberry. Or mix vanilla with Vari-Flavors Flavor Pacs. • Nutrients: Nutritionally complete; high in protein; low in sodium and cholesterol; lactose-free	• Calorie content may be too low for some people. • Don't give to a person who requires a low-protein diet. • Possible side effects include vomiting, diarrhea, and cramps.
• Flavors: Vanilla, chocolate, coffee, and strawberry. Or mix vanilla with Vari-Flavors Flavor Pacs. • Nutrients: Nutritionally complete; high in calories and protein; lactose-free	• Don't give to a person on a low-protein diet. • Possible side effects include vomiting, diarrhea, and cramps.
• Flavor: Bland, unsweetened • Nutrients: Nutritionally complete; lactose-free	• Easy to digest
• Flavors: Vanilla and chocolate • Nutrients: Nutritionally complete; high in calories and protein; low in sodium; gluten-free; lactose-free if given as a liquid	• If given as a liquid, it's easy to digest. If given as a powder prepared with milk, it may cause diarrhea, vomiting, cramps, and abdominal distention.
• Flavors: Vanilla and chocolate • Nutrients: Nutritionally complete; high in calories and fat; low in carbohydrates and protein; lactose-free and gluten-free	• Easy to digest • Extra vitamins and minerals are necessary.
• Flavors: Vanilla, chocolate, eggnog, and butterscotch • Nutrients: High in calories and protein; lactose-free (liquid only)	• Don't give to a person who requires a low-protein diet. • Possible side effects include diarrhea, vomiting, and cramps. • Tell the person to sip it slowly through a straw. Don't use powder if the person is lactose-intolerant.

Planning a calcium-rich diet

The body needs calcium for strong bones and teeth. Eating calcium-rich foods is one way to make sure the body gets enough of this vital mineral.

What's enough?

How much calcium you need changes throughout your lifetime. For example, teenagers need extra calcium for their rapidly growing bones. Women need more calcium after menopause as well as during pregnancy and while breastfeeding.

Ask your nurse or doctor to help you determine exactly how much calcium you or the person you're caring for needs each day.

Where to get calcium

Dairy products (milk, cheese, yogurt, and ice cream) are potent calcium sources. If you're avoiding cholesterol or watching your weight, you can still have skimmed or powdered milk and fat-free yogurt.

If you have trouble digesting milk, you may still be able to eat yogurt, hard cheeses, acidophilus milk, or lactose-reduced milk. (Ask your grocery store manager to stock lactose-reduced milk if your store doesn't carry it.) Or ask the pharmacist about adding lactobacillus acidophilus to regular milk. Also called by such trade names as Bacid and Lactinex, this substance makes milk easier to digest.

Certain vegetables, such as collards, turnip greens, and broccoli, contain lots of calcium. Oysters, salmon, sardines, and tofu are other foods with a high calcium content.

Other tips

Some foods, especially very fibrous foods, can interfere with your body's uptake of calcium. So, to get the most calcium from the foods you eat, avoid eating calcium- and fiber-rich foods at the same meal.

Also, eat less red meat, chocolate, peanut butter, rhubarb, sweet potatoes, and fatty foods. And cut down on caffeine-containing drinks, such as coffee, tea, and colas.

Calcium's most effective when your body has enough vitamin D. Spending just 15 minutes in sunshine every day will fill your daily requirement. Besides, most manufacturers add vitamin D to milk and cereals. And egg yolks, saltwater fish, and liver also have this vitamin.

Avoid taking a vitamin D supplement, though, unless your doctor specifically tells you to do so. Too much vitamin D may do more harm than good.

Cutting down on salt

If your body is retaining water, you may need to cut down on salt. Reducing your salt intake isn't hard to do. The following information and suggestions will help you get started.

Facts about salt

- Table salt is about 40% sodium.
- Americans consume about 20 times more salt than their bodies need.
- About three-fourths of the salt you consume is already in the foods you eat and drink.
- One teaspoon of salt contains 2 grams (2,000 milligrams) of sodium—the recommended daily amount for people with high blood pressure.
- You can reduce your intake to this level simply by not salting your food during cooking or before eating.
- Some people are so sensitive to salt that even a moderate amount causes their blood pressure to rise.

Tips for reducing salt intake

Reducing your salt intake to 1 teaspoon or less a day is easy if you:
- read labels on medicines and foods.
- put away your salt shaker, or if you must use salt, use "light salt" that contains half the sodium of ordinary table salt.
- buy fresh meats, fruits, and vegetables instead of canned, processed, and convenience foods.
- substitute spices and lemon juice for salt.
- watch out for hidden sources of sodium—for example, carbonated beverages, nondairy creamers, cookies, and cakes.
- avoid salty foods, such as bacon, sausage, pretzels, potato

chips, mustard, pickles, and some cheeses.

Know your sodium sources

Canned, prepared, and fast foods are loaded with sodium; so are condiments, such as ketchup. Some foods that don't taste salty contain high amounts of sodium. Consider the values below:

Food	Milligrams of sodium
1 can tomato soup	872
1 hot dog	639
1 cheeseburger	709
1 tablespoon ketchup	156
1 dill pickle	928
1 cup corn flakes	256

Other high-sodium sources include baking powder, baking soda, barbecue sauce, bouillon cubes, celery salt, chili sauce, cooking wine, garlic salt, onion salt, softened water, and soy sauce.

Surprisingly, many medicines and other nonfood items contain sodium, such as alkalizers for indigestion, laxatives, aspirin, cough medicine, mouthwash, and toothpaste.

Eating potassium-rich foods

If your doctor has prescribed a diuretic (water-reducing pill), you may need to add potassium to your diet.

How much potassium do you need?

Doctors recommend 300 to 400 milligrams of potassium daily. Not enough potassium can cause leg cramps, weakness, paralysis, and spasms. Too much can cause heart problems and fatigue.

The chart that follows lists potassium-rich foods along with their potassium content (the number of milligrams in a 3½-oz [85-gram] serving). Because some of these foods are also high in calories, check with your doctor or dietitian if you're on a weight-reduction diet.

Meats	Milligrams of potassium
Beef	370
Chicken	411
Lamb	290
Liver	380
Pork	326
Turkey	411
Veal	500
Fish	
Bass	256
Flounder	342
Haddock	348
Halibut	525
Oysters	203
Perch	284
Salmon	421
Sardines, canned	590
Scallops	476
Tuna	301
Fruits	
Apricots	281
Bananas	370
Dates	648
Figs	152
Nectarines	294
Oranges	200
Peaches	202
Plums	299
Prunes	262
Raisins	355
Vegetables	
Asparagus	238
Brussels sprouts	295
Cabbage	233
Carrots	341
Endive	294
Lima beans	394
Peppers	213
Potatoes	407
Radishes	322

Vegetables *(continued)*	Milligrams of potassium
Spinach	324
Sweet potatoes	300
Juices	
Oranges, fresh	200
reconstituted	186
Tomato	227
Other foods	
Gingersnap cookies	462
Graham crackers	384
Oatmeal cookies	
with raisins	370
Ice milk	195
Milk, dry	
(nonfat solids)	1,745
Molasses (light)	917
Peanuts	674
Peanut butter	670

Preventing unnecessary weight gain

When a person's sick, reduced activity and overeating due to boredom can cause unnecessary weight gain. Although ideal weight standards vary, carrying extra pounds puts stress on the body and can lead to serious health problems. If the person in your care is gaining too much weight, check with the doctor. He'll tell you how to decrease fats and carbohydrates from the person's diet while keeping a proper nutrient balance for essential protein, vitamins, and minerals.

Preventing boredom

If the person is overeating out of boredom, try to find ways to keep him stimulated. Provide a supply of books, magazines, or crossword puzzles, along with paper and a pen or pencil. If possible, make sure he has access to a television, radio, or cassette player and tapes. Most important, spend time with the person, and encourage friends and other family members to visit him, if his condition permits.

Cutting calories

To prevent unnecessary weight gain, follow these tips:
• Serve chicken or fish instead of beef, and low-fat dairy products instead of whole milk products.
• Provide low-calorie snacks and desserts, such as sugar-free gelatin, fresh fruit, and ice milk, if the person can eat these foods.
• Offer low-calorie beverages, such as water, club soda or seltzer, 1% or skim milk, and vegetable juice cocktail, instead of high-calorie drinks or snacks.

Giving liquid supplements

If the person you're caring for has trouble chewing or the amount of food he eats can't meet his increased nutritional needs, the doctor may recommend a liquid nutritional supplement.

Regardless of the supplement you choose, keep these tips in mind. Chilling the supplement may make it tastier. Also, you should store any opened cans of supplement in the refrigerator. If they're not used within 48 hours, discard them.

Stimulating the appetite

Loss of appetite is common during illness. Try the following tips to stimulate a desire for food.

Make mealtime more enjoyable

• Create a pleasant dining atmosphere. Accompany meals with music, soft lights, a brightly colored table setting, or any

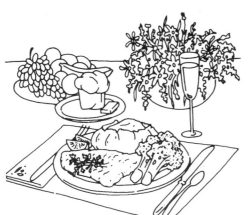

other atmospheric detail the person requests while eating. If permitted, include a glass of wine or beer with the meal.
• Arrange food attractively on the plate. Add a garnish, such as parsley or a slice of lemon, to make the food appealing.
• Ask family or friends to share meals with the person. Or try using television as company. Or read to the person during meals.

• Serve frequent, small meals instead of three large meals.
• Keep nutritious snacks on hand—nuts, fruit, and cheese, for example—for the person to eat whenever he feels hungry.

Be creative with your cooking
• Vary the diet and try new recipes. Experiment with spices and seasonings to make food more flavorful.
• If the person can tolerate dairy products, add margarine or butter to foods to improve flavor. Also try mixing canned cream soups with milk rather than water and adding cream sauce or melted cheese to vegetables.
• Serve milk shakes, eggnog, or prepared liquid food supplements between meals. You may want to enrich some beverages with eggs, honey, or powdered milk.

Overcome obstacles to eating
• If possible, the person should take a walk or exercise moderately before meals to help build appetite.
• If nausea discourages the person from eating, try to curb it by eating low-fat meals. Avoid overly sweet or spicy foods. Serve dry foods, such as toast or crackers, when the person gets up in the morning.
• Minimize mouth soreness or dryness by avoiding foods that are very salty, spicy, or hot. Instead, eat cold foods, such as ice cream, frozen yogurt, milk shakes, and cold soups. Ice chips, flavored ice pops, hard candies, lemon slices, and dill pickles help keep the mouth moist.
• If you or the person you're caring for lives alone, consider contacting Meals On Wheels or a similar community program when you don't feel like cooking.

Feeding a bedridden person
Mealtime may be the high point of a bedridden person's day. So before serving a meal, take a few minutes to ensure success.

Serve meals at peak appetite times. Typically, the person is hungrier in the morning because the body needs food for the day. In the evening, his appetite may wane as his needs decrease. Too much food can cause heartburn and disrupt sleep.

Avoid serving food when pain, medication, fatigue, or therapy diminishes appetite. And try to coordinate meals and treatment. For instance, certain medications must be taken with food; others require an empty stomach.

Serve small, balanced meals. Three to six meals throughout the day promote optimal digestion and calorie use.

Getting ready

Help the person use the bathroom, bedpan, or urinal, and wash his hands. (Always wash your own hands before caring for the person or handling the food you're serving him.)

Then tidy and air the room to remove clutter and odors. Help the person sit comfortably by raising the bed (if it's a hospital bed) or by supporting him with pillows.

Using special equipment

Ensure a level, steady eating surface by using a tray with raised sides (to confine utensils and contain spills) and support legs that fit over the lap.

Consider using plates that have compartments (to separate foods and flavors) and covered cups and straws for dripless drinking. Use a spoon rather than a fork to provide more control and lessen the potential for injuring the mouth.

Serving the meal

Stimulate the person's appetite by serving small portions. Prevent choking by serving bite-sized, tender foods, such as pureed fruit, chopped or grated vegetables, and thinly sliced or ground meats.

Promote easy swallowing by offering foods with the same texture served at room temperature. Pureed vegetable soup is easier to swallow than thin broth with vegetable chunks. Tepid foods are safer to swallow than those served steaming.

Arrange food so that the person can see it. Or tell him its location as it corresponds to the hours on a clock; for example, fish at 12 o'clock, broccoli at 6.

Encourage self-feeding so that the person feels more independent and less helpless. If the person tires easily, help him conserve his strength by assisting with feeding. Put food in

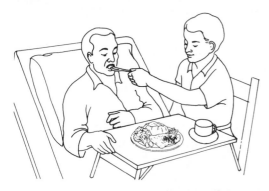

alternate sides of the person's mouth (unless one side is paralyzed). If the person drools, provide smaller spoonfuls. Blot his mouth as needed.

Don't rush. Rushing can spoil the person's appetite and interrupt digestion.

Using special feeding devices

Special glasses, cups, plates, and utensils can make eating easier and more enjoyable. Here are some tips on ways to use these devices.

Glasses and cups

If you or the person you're caring for has trouble holding a glass, use an unbreakable plastic tumbler instead. Plastic is lighter and less slippery than glass. Or use terry cloth sleeves over glasses to make them easier to grasp.

You can also choose from many specially designed cups. For instance, you can use a cup with two handles, which is easier to keep steady than a cup with one handle. You can try a pedestal cup or a T-handle cup, which is easy to grasp. You can also try a cup with a weighted base, which helps prevent spills.

T-handled cup with weighted base

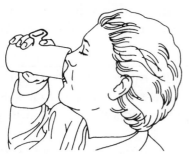

Cup with V-opening

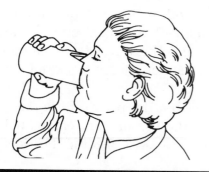

If you have a stiff neck, use a cup with a V-shaped opening on its rim. You can easily tip this cup to empty it without bending your neck backward.

If your hands are unsteady, you may find it easier to hold a cup with a large handle. Or drink from a lidded cup with a lip to help decrease spills. If you have decreased sensation or feeling in your hands, use an insulated cup or mug to avoid burning yourself.

Drinking straws

Flexible or rigid straws, either disposable or reusable, come in several sizes. Some straws are wide enough for you to drink soups and thick liquids through them. To hold the straw in place, use a snap-on plastic lid with a slot for the straw.

Dishes

If possible, try to use only unbreakable dishes. To keep a plate from sliding, place a damp sponge, washcloth, paper towel, or rubber disk under it. Consider using a plate with a nonskid base or place mats made of dimpled rubber or foam. Suction cups attached to the bottom of a plate or bowl also help prevent slipping.

You can consider using a plate guard. This helpful device blocks food from falling off the plate, so that it can be picked up easily with a fork or spoon. Attach the guard to the side of the plate opposite the hand you use to feed yourself.

A scooper plate has high sides that provide a built-in surface for pushing food onto the utensil. Eating from a sectioned plate or tray may also be convenient.

Dish with sides and suction cups

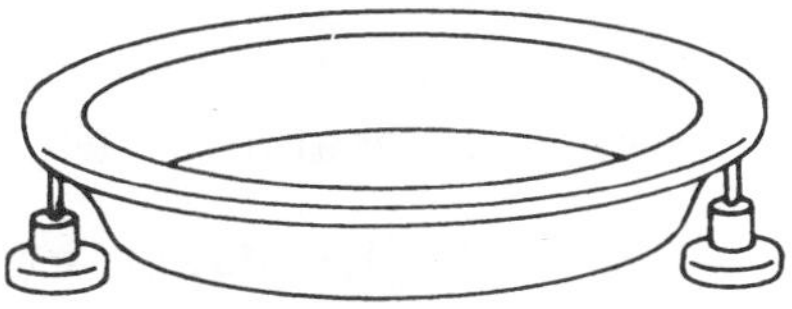

Plate guard

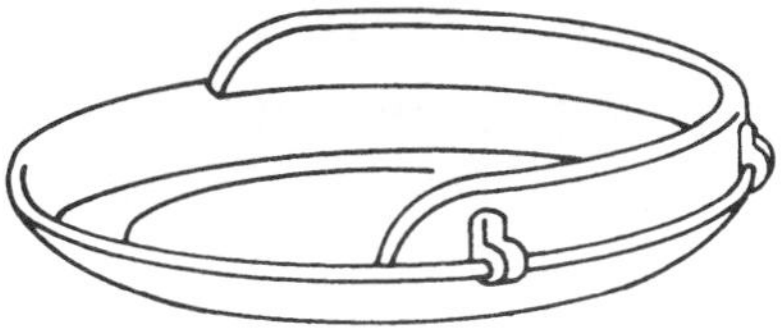

Scooper plate

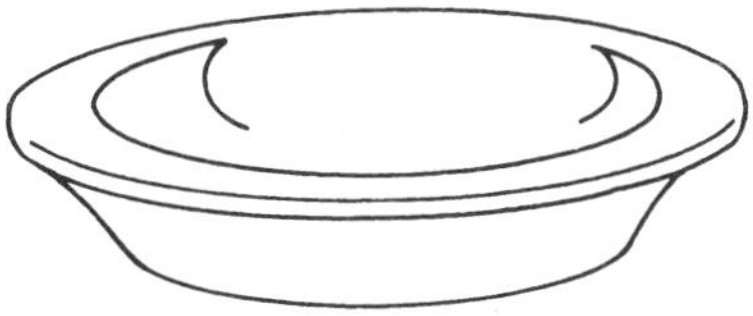

Flatware

If your hand is weak or your grip is shaky, you may want to try ordinary flatware with ridged wood, plastic, or cork handles—all easier to grasp than smooth metal handles. Or try building up the handles with a bicycle handlebar covering, a foam curler pad, or tape (this also works for holding pens and pencils, toothbrushes, and razors). You can also try strapping the utensil to your hand.

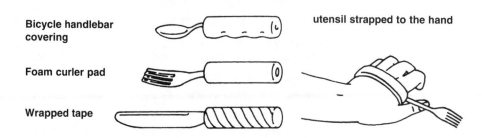

Bicycle handlebar covering

Foam curler pad

Wrapped tape

utensil strapped to the hand

Easing chewing and swallowing problems

If the person you're caring for has trouble chewing and swallowing food, you can still feed him a balanced diet. To ease these problems, follow these tips when you prepare the person for a meal and serve him his food.

Preparing the person for a meal

• Encourage the person to take his time when he eats and not to feel self-conscious about eating slowly. Tell him to concentrate on the process and to avoid talking.
• If possible, help the person sit in an upright position.
• Tell the person not to turn his head to the right or left while eating.

Serving food

• Put small amounts of food on the fork or spoon to prevent gagging.
• Avoid serving sticky foods, such as peanut butter.
• Serve liquids separately from solid foods because liquids are usually harder to swallow.
• Prepare foods so that they're easy to chew. For example, add meat tenderizer when you prepare meats, if the doctor

allows it. Puree cooked vegetables or fruits in a blender or food processor. Or grate raw vegetables or slice raw fruits into small, easy-to-chew pieces.

• Serve protein-rich foods that are easy to chew, such as eggs, beans, boneless fish, and milk products.

• Foods served at room temperature are easier to swallow than very hot or very cold foods. And foods with the same texture are also easier to swallow. For example, a vegetable puree soup is more comfortable to eat than vegetable soup with cubes of vegetables and meat.

• Thick liquids go down more easily than thin liquids. Milk shakes, partially frozen fruit juices, and thick soups, for example, are easier to drink than tea, regular fruit juices, and broths.

8   Giving Medications

Giving medications correctly

The doctor has prescribed medication to help treat the condition of the person you're caring for. This medication will help only if you give it correctly. Here's how.

Filling the prescription

• Have the prescription filled at the pharmacy the person ordinarily uses. That way, the pharmacist can keep a complete record of the person's medications. Tell him if the person is allergic to any drugs.

• If you need to refill a prescription, don't wait until the last minute. Refill it before you run out of medication.

Giving the medication

• Give the medication in a well-lighted room. Double-check the label to make sure you're giving the right medication. If you don't understand the directions, call the pharmacist or doctor.

• If you forget to give a dose or several doses, don't give two or more doses together. Instead, ask the doctor or pharmacist for directions.

• Don't stop giving the medication unless the doctor tells you to. And don't save it for some other time.

Storing the medication

• Keep the medication in its original container or in a properly labeled prescription bottle. If the person is taking more than one medication, don't store them together in a pillbox.

• Store the medication in a cool, dry place or as directed by the pharmacist. Don't keep it in the bathroom medicine cabinet, where heat and humidity may cause it to lose its effectiveness.

• If children are in the household, make sure the medication containers have child-proof caps. Always keep the containers beyond the reach of children.

Avoiding problems

• Keep the following information about each medication on index cards or a chart: the drug's name, its purpose, its appearance, how to take it, when to take it, how much to take, and special precautions or side effects. Remember most medications cause side effects.

• If you have questions about symptoms that seem to be related to the medication, call the doctor right away.

• If the person is pregnant or breast-feeding, talk to the doctor before giving any medication or home remedy. Some medications may be harmful to the baby.

• Never give medication that doesn't look right or after the expiration date printed on the label. The medication may not work. Even worse, it may harm the person.

• Don't give any nonprescription medications without first checking with the pharmacist. Sometimes, another medication can change the way a prescribed medication works.

• Alcohol and some foods also can change the way some medications work. Read the medication label. It may tell you what to avoid.

• Don't share your medication with family members or friends. They could be hurt by it.

Giving or taking oral medications

Most medicines are prescribed for the oral route—through the mouth. Oral medicines come in a wide variety of tablets, capsules, and liquids. In addition to the medicine itself, some tablets and capsules may include other ingredients, such as an enteric coating, which keeps the tablet or capsule intact until it reaches the small intestine, or a sustained-release coating, which allows small amounts of medicine to be released in the bloodstream over a longer time. Some uncoated tablets are scored so that you can break them easily if the dosage calls for one-half a tablet.

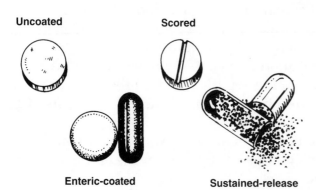

Uncoated

Scored

Enteric-coated

Sustained-release

Knowing the facts about medicines

Be sure to give any medicine exactly as prescribed. Know the name of the medicine and what it's for. Be sure you know what side effects normal dosage may cause, and tell the doctor if they occur. Also report all the drugs the person's taking, including nonprescription drugs. He can tell you if the person can continue to take them safely and if taking them will cancel or change the treatment effect of either medication. Give the drug at the right time. Ask if it should be taken with meals or between meals. If it can be taken with meals, know which foods the person should avoid or include. Warn him not to take the drug with alcohol or other drugs. Ask the doctor what to do about any missed dose.

Making tablets and capsules easier to swallow

When giving tablets or capsules, ask the person to drink some water or juice first. Then he should place the tablet or capsule well back on the tongue and swallow a full mouthful of water or juice. Usually, you may crush uncoated tablets and open soft, uncoated capsules. Then you can mix the drug in a beverage or a small amount of soft food, like applesauce or mashed potatoes. *Important:* Before mixing any drugs with food or a beverage, check with the doctor or pharmacist.

When giving tablets and capsules, take these precautions. Never crush or open coated tablets or hard or coated capsules or let the person chew coated capsules. The coating, or hard gelatin shell, makes swallowing easier and may disguise an unpleasant taste. If you destroy an enteric coating, the drug won't be absorbed properly.

If the doctor prescribes enteric-coated tablets or capsules, give them with plenty of water between meals so that they'll pass quickly into the small intestine. Don't give enteric-coated tablets with milk or antacids because these liquids will cause the tablets to disintegrate too soon. Don't crush or open prolonged-action, repeat-action, or sustained-release capsules. Opening these capsules may change the dose and increase the risk of overdose.

Storing tablets and capsules correctly

To avoid giving medicine that has deteriorated, follow these guidelines.
• Protect tablets and capsules from humidity, light, and air.
• Return to the pharmacy any medicine that looks discolored or smells strange. This indicates deterioration.

• Check the expiration date, and discard any outdated drug.

Measuring liquid medicine exactly

If you're using a disposable medicine cup, rinse the cup in water to prevent medicine from sticking to its sides. As you pour the medicine, keep the label pointed up so that spilled liquid won't hide it. Recheck the dose by setting the cup on a level surface at eye level. If you've poured too much, discard the excess.

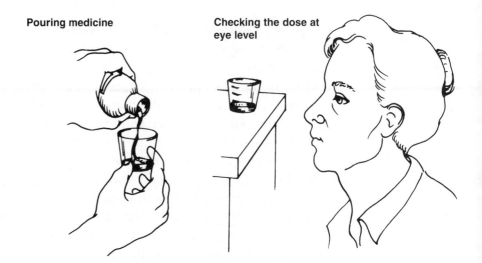

Pouring medicine

Checking the dose at eye level

Making liquid medicine more palatable

If the medicine has an unpleasant taste, try one or more of these tips.

• Dilute liquid medicine with water or juice, but be sure to ask the doctor or pharmacist if the medicine is compatible with other liquids.

• You can give ice chips to numb the taste buds before the person takes a medicine, or pour the medicine over ice and have the person drink it through a straw. (Avoid this method for small doses because it may affect dosage accuracy.)

• If the medicine is oily, chill it first. The person can hold his nose as he swallows.

• Relieve a bitter aftertaste by sugarless hard candy or chewing gum after taking the medicine. Or provide a gargle of water or mouthwash.

Making a medication clock

To help you remember to give medication at the right times, you can make a simple device called a medication clock. Using or copying the sample clocks shown below, write A.M. in the center of one clock and P.M. in the center of the other clock. Use a different color to label each clock so that you can easily tell them apart.

The rest is simple: just write the names of the medications you're supposed to give in the spaces for the hours when you're supposed to give them. Then be sure to check the clock often during the day, so you don't miss giving any medication.

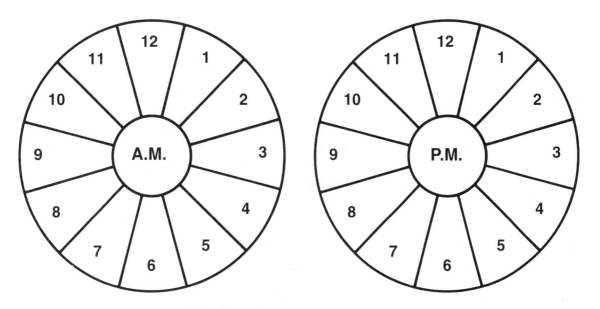

Giving sublingual and buccal medications

Some oral medications are made not to be swallowed but to be absorbed through the tissues of the mouth. Sublingual medications are absorbed through the membranes under the tongue; buccal medications are absorbed through the membranes in the cheek.

Note: Caution the person not to swallow either type of medication. This will reduce its effectiveness.

Positioning medications correctly

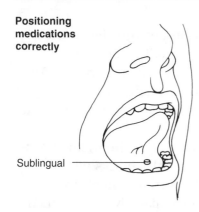

Sublingual

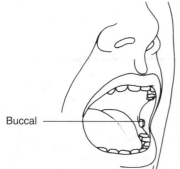

Buccal

Sublingual medication

Before you give a sublingual medication, read the instructions on the container's label. Then take out tablet, and place it under the person's tongue. He should hold it with his tongue until it's absorbed. Store the closed medication container safely.

Buccal medication

To give a buccal medication, first read the label instructions. Then take out a tablet, and place it between the person's cheek and teeth. He should close his mouth to hold the medication in place until it's absorbed. Store the medication container safely.

Applying topical medications

Topical medications are medications that you apply to the skin: powder, lotion, cream, paste, or ointment. With the exception of transdermal skin patches and nitroglycerin ointment, a topically applied medication is used for its local effect—the effect it has at the site where it's applied. In contrast, a medicine injected through the skin or administered through a body opening (such as the mouth or rectum) is intended to medicate the entire body.

Preparing the skin area

Before you apply any topical medication, make sure the skin area is clean and dry. If the doctor has instructed you to remove the residue of previous applications before applying fresh medication, do so.

Applying powder

Powder helps skin stay dry. It helps prevent skin irritation, too, by reducing surface friction from clothes or bed sheets. Apply powder to clean, dry skin. You can keep from inhaling powder particles by turning your head away from where you're applying the powder. Cover your mouth with a cloth if you're applying powder near to your face or neck, and exhale as you apply it.

Applying lotion

Lotion soothes, cools, and protects the skin. Be sure to shake the lotion container well. Warm the lotion so that the person won't be startled or become chilled. Be sure to check the skin for signs of irritation (redness, soreness, or itching) between lotion applications. If any occur, call the doctor for instructions.

Applying cream

Cream lubricates dry skin and reduces the amount of skin moisture that's lost. After applying a cream, check for signs of irritation: redness, soreness, or itching. If you see any occur, call the doctor for instructions.

Applying paste

The thick consistency of paste provides a uniform coating that remains on the skin, allowing longer medication contact. After applying a paste, cover it with a gauze pad to increase medication absorption and protect clothing or bed sheets.

Applying ointment

Ointment also provides longer medication contact. Apply a thin layer of ointment, and rub it in well.

Applying nitroglycerin ointment

1 Measure the prescribed amount of nitroglycerin ointment onto the special paper.

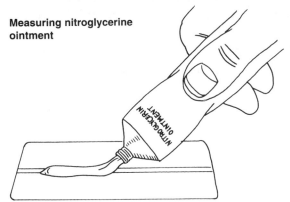

Measuring nitroglycerine ointment

2 Spread it lightly over the area specified by the doctor—usually the upper arm or chest. Don't rub it into the skin. For best results, spread the ointment to cover an area about the size of the application paper (roughly $3\frac{1}{2}$ by $2\frac{1}{4}$ inches [9 by 6 centimeters]).

3 Cover the ointment with paper and tape the paper in place. You may want to cover the paper (including the side edges) with plastic wrap to protect clothes from stains. If the person devel-

ops a persistent headache or feels dizzy while using the ointment, call the doctor.

Applying a transdermal patch to the upper arm

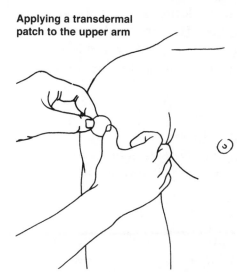

Applying transdermal patches

Transdermal patches, applied to the skin, contain medication that's absorbed into the body. How often you change a patch depends on the medicine that's in it. A patch should always be applied to a hairless area of the body—for example, behind the ear.

To apply the patch, open the packet, pull the strip off the back, and place the patch where the doctor has told you to.

The adhesive backing on the patch is strong, so the person can take a shower and continue other activities without concern.

Instilling eye drops

Here's how to instill drops in your eye:

Warming the medication

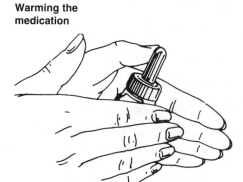

1 Begin by washing your hands thoroughly.

2 Hold the medication bottle up to the light and examine it. If the medication is discolored or contains sediment, don't use it. Instead, take it back to the pharmacy and have it examined.

If the medication looks OK, warm it to room temperature by holding the bottle between your hands, for 2 minutes.

3 Moisten a rayon cosmetic puff or a tissue with water, and clean any secretions from around your eyes. Use a fresh rayon puff or tissue for each eye.

Removing secretions

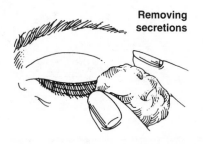

4 Now, stand or sit before a mirror or lie on your back, whichever is most comfortable for you. Squeeze the bulb of the eyedropper and slowly release it to fill the dropper with medication.

5 Tilt your head slightly back and toward the eye you're treating. Pull down your lower eyelid.

6 Position the dropper over the conjunctival sac you've exposed between your lower lid and the white of your eye. Steady your hand by resting two fingers against your cheek or nose.

7 Look up at the ceiling. Then squeeze the prescribed number of drops into the sac. Take care not to touch the dropper to your eye, eyelashes, or finger. Wipe away excess medication with a clean tissue.

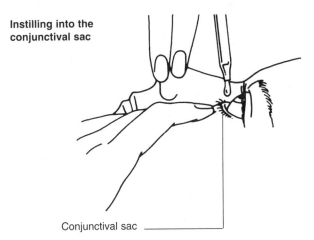

Instilling into the conjunctival sac

Conjunctival sac

Applying pressure

8 Release the lower lid. Try to keep your eye open, and don't blink for at least 30 seconds. Apply gentle pressure to the corner of your eye at the bridge of your nose for 1 minute. This will prevent the medication from being absorbed through your tear duct.

9 Recap the bottle, and store it away from light and heat. If you're using more than one kind of drop, wait 5 minutes before you use the next one. And remember, never put medication in your eyes unless the label reads "For Ophthalmic Use" or "For Use in Eyes."

Using eye ointment

1 Wash your hands thoroughly. Then hold the ointment in your hand for several minutes to warm it.

Wiping away secretions

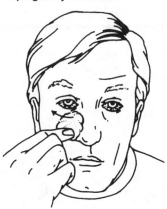

2 Moisten a rayon or cosmetic puff tissue with water, and clean any secretions from around your eye. Wipe outward in one motion, starting at the side near the nose. Remember to avoid touching the uninfected eye.

3 Now, stand or sit before a mirror or lie on your back, whichever is most comfortable.

4 Gently pull down your lower eyelid. Tilt your head back slightly and look at the ceiling.

5 Squeeze a small amount of ointment (about ¼ inch to ½ inch [0.6 to 1.3 centimeters]) inside the conjunctival sac between your lower eyelid and the white of your eye. Steady your hand by resting two fingers against your cheek or nose. Hold the tube close to its tip so that you don't accidentally poke your eye with the applicator tip.

Instilling the ointment

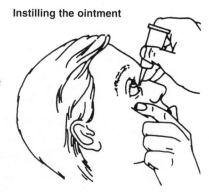

6 Without touching the tube's tip with your eyelashes, close your eye to pinch off the ointment. Roll your eyeball in all directions with your eyes closed.

7 Recap the medication. If you're using more than one ointment, wait about 10 minutes before you use the next one. Don't worry if your vision is blurred after you use the ointment; the blurring is temporary and is normal.

Instilling eardrops

To instill eardrops in another person, you'll need the medication in a bottle with a dropper tip or a separate dropper as well as some moist cotton balls.

Getting ready

1 Wash your hands thoroughly. Then examine the medicine. If it looks discolored or contains sediment, notify the doctor and have the prescription refilled. If it looks normal, you can proceed.

2 Warm the medicine by holding the bottle in your hands for about 2 minutes.

3 Then shake the bottle (if directed), open it, and fill the dropper by squeezing the bulb. Place the open bottle and the dropper within easy reach.

Giving eardrops

1 Have the person lie on his side to expose the ear you're treating. Now, gently pull the top of his ear up and back (down and back for a child). This will straighten the ear canal.

2 Position the filled dropper above—but not touching—the opening of the ear canal. Gently squeeze the dropper's bulb once to release 1 drop. Watch the drop slide into the ear canal. Or have the person tell you when he feels the drop enter his ear.

Instilling drops while holding the ear

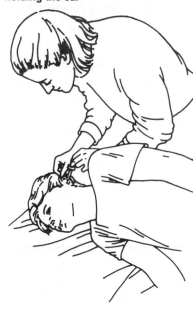

Then, gently squeeze the dropper's bulb to release the number of drops prescribed.

3 Continue holding the ear as the eardrops disappear down the ear canal. Now, massage the area in front of the ear. Ask the person to tell you when he no longer feels the drops moving in his ear. Then release the ear.

4 Tell the person to remain on his side and to avoid touching his ear for about 10 minutes. If the person is active, place an eardrop-moistened cotton plug in his ear to help keep the medicine in his ear canal. Don't use dry cotton because it may absorb the medicine.

If both ears require medicine, repeat the procedure in the person's other ear. Finally, return the dropper to the medicine bottle (or recap the dropper bottle).

Store the bottle away from light and extreme heat.

Instilling nose drops

To instill drops in your nose, you need only the medication in a bottle with a dropper tip or a separate dropper.

Precaution: Hold the medication bottle up to the light and examine the medication. If it's unusually cloudy or contains flecks, return the medication to the pharmacy.

1 If the medication looks OK, hold the bottle between your hands for 2 minutes to warm the medication. Open the bottle, and then squeeze the dropper to fill it with medication.

Tilt your head back, and gently push up the tip of your nose to completely open the nostrils.

2 Place the dropper about $\frac{1}{2}$ inch (1.3 centimeters) into your nostril and hold it level. Now, squeeze the dropper repeatedly until you've instilled the prescribed number of drops.

Keep your head tilted back for about 5 minutes. If any

medication runs into your throat, spit it out and tilt your head back again. If the doctor has instructed you to repeat this procedure in the other nostril, do so. Then recap the medication bottle, and store it safely.

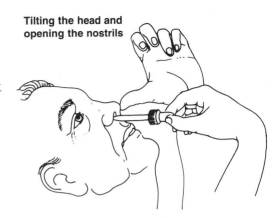
Tilting the head and opening the nostrils

Using an oral inhaler

Inhaling your medication through a metered-dose nebulizer will help you breathe more easily. Use it exactly as the doctor has directed. Here's how.

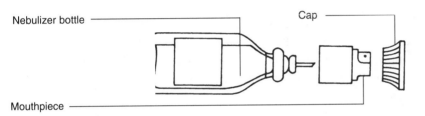

Nebulizer bottle —————

Cap ———

Mouthpiece —————

1 Remove the mouthpiece and cap from the bottle. Then remove the cap from the mouthpiece.

2 Turn the mouthpiece sideways. On one side of the flattened tip, you'll see a small hole. Fit the metal stem on the bottle into the hole to assemble the nebulizer.

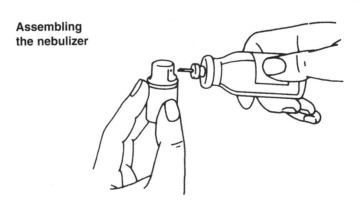
Assembling the nebulizer

3 Exhale fully through pursed lips. Hold the nebulizer upside down, as you see here. Close your lips and teeth loosely around the mouthpiece.

Positioning the mouthpiece before inhaling

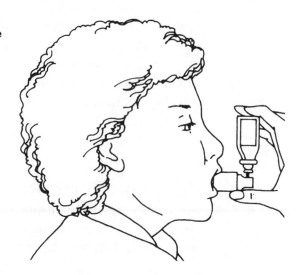

4 Tilt your head back slightly. Take a slow, deep breath. As you do, firmly push the bottle against the mouthpiece—one time only—to release one dose of medication. Continue inhaling until your lungs feel full.

Inhaling as you release a dose of medication

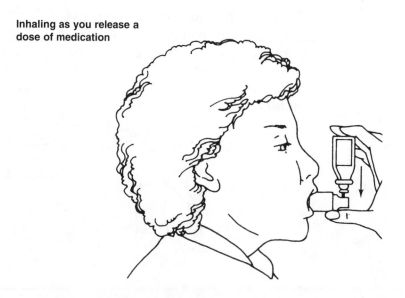

5 Take the mouthpiece away from your mouth, and hold your breath for several seconds.

Holding your breath

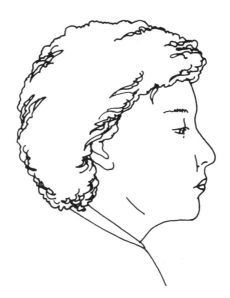

6 Purse your lips and exhale slowly. If your doctor wants you to take more than one dose, wait a few minutes and then repeat steps 3 through 6. Now, rinse your mouth, gargle, and drink a few sips of fluid.

Exhaling through pursed lips

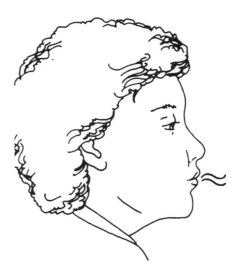

7 Remember to clean the inhaler once a day by taking it apart and rinsing the mouthpiece and cap under warm running water for 1 minute (or immerse them in alcohol). Shake off the excess liquid, allow the parts to dry, and then reassemble them. This prevents clogging and sanitizes the mouthpiece.

Precautions

Remember to discard the inhalation solution if it turns brown or contains solid particles. Store the medicine in its original container, and put it in the refrigerator, if the label directs. *Important:* Never overuse the oral inhaler. Follow the doctor's instructions exactly.

Inserting a rectal suppository

A rectal suppository can help stimulate regular bowel movements at the desired time.

Caution: Unless the doctor orders otherwise, don't use rectal suppositories or other laxatives routinely because you can become dependent on them.

You can learn to insert a rectal suppository quickly and easily by following these steps.

1 Wash your hands. Then gather the items you'll need: the suppository, a disposable glove, and a tube of water-soluble lubricating gel.

2 Put the glove on your right hand (or on your left hand if you're left-handed). Now, remove the foil wrapper on the suppository.

If you have trouble doing this, the suppository may be too soft to insert. Hold it under cold running water until it becomes firm, or put it in the freezer for 1 or 2 minutes before inserting it—just don't let it get too cold and hard. Better yet, store the suppositories in the refrigerator.

Lubricating the suppository

3 Once you've removed the foil wrapper, put a generous dab of lubricating gel on the

rounded end of the suppository. Hold the lubricated suppository in your gloved hand.

4 Now, lie on your side with your knees raised toward your
chest. Take a deep breath as you gently insert the suppository—rounded end first—into your rectum with your
gloved hand. Push the suppository in as far as your finger will
go to keep the suppository from coming back out.

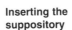

Inserting the
suppository

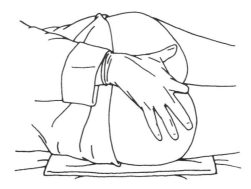

5 Once the suppository's in place, you'll feel an immediate
urge to have a bowel movement. Resist the urge by lying
still and breathing deeply a few times.

Try to retain the suppository for at least 20 minutes, so
that your body has time to absorb it and get the maximum
effect from the medication. After you have a bowel movement,
discard the glove and wash your hands.

Giving an enema

After washing your hands, assemble the equipment: about 8
ounces (.25 liter) of warm enema solution, an enema bag with
attached tube and clamp, a bedpan with a cover (optional), a
tube of water-soluble lubricating gel, a waterproof pad, a
glove, and some toilet tissue. *Note:* You can also buy prepared
disposable enema kits in adult and child sizes. If the doctor
tells you to use one of these, follow the instructions on the
package.

1 Clamp the tubing on the enema bag, and then pour the solution into the bag. To test the flow, unclamp the tubing and allow a small amount of solution to run through and out the end. If it runs through smoothly, reclamp the tubing, and resume the procedure. If it doesn't, check the tubing for kinks or a clog.

Have the person lie on his left side with his knees bent: this position will help the enema solution flow into his colon.

Position for having an enema

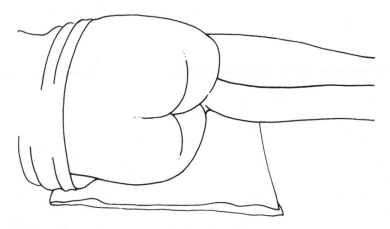

Tuck the waterproof pad under him to keep the bed sheet dry. Then expose his buttocks.

Now, squeeze some lubricating gel onto some toilet tissue, and roll the end of the tubing in it.

2 With your ungloved hand, separate the person's buttocks so that you can see his anus. Then ask him to take a deep breath. As he does so, gently insert the tubing about 4 inches (10 centimeters) into the rectum.

If you feel resistance, allow a little solution to flow in to relax the rectal muscles. If you still can't advance the tubing, remove it and call the doctor for instructions.

Inserting the tube

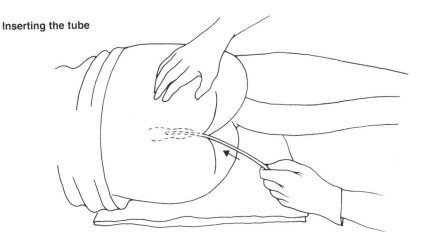

3 With the tube in place, hold the enema bag about 5 inches (12.7 centimeters) above the person's anus and release the tubing clamp. Let the solution flow into his colon by gravity: don't try to hurry it.

If the person gets stomach cramps or feels a need to have a bowel movement while the solution is in his colon, lower the bag or clamp the tubing closed to stop the flow, and tell him to breathe deeply. Rub his stomach gently to help him relax.

4 After most of the solution has flowed into the person's colon, clamp the tubing closed and remove it as the person takes a deep breath. (Don't let all the solution flow in; this could introduce air into the colon.)

Because the person's colon is full, he'll feel an urge to evacuate it—a defecation reflex. To help him retain the enema solution, hold his buttocks together until this urge passes.

Encourage him to retain the solution for about 30 minutes for an enema that needs to be retained and about 15 minutes for a cleansing enema. (The doctor will tell you which type to give.)

5 After the person has released the solution from his colon into the toilet or bedpan, wash and dry his buttocks, and remove the waterproof pad from the bed. Discard the pad along with the toilet tissue.

Rinse and dry the tubing, enema bag, and solution container.

Giving yourself an enema

If the doctor orders an enema for you, he'll tell you what brand of commercial enema to buy. Giving yourself an enema is a bit awkward, but it really isn't difficult.

Just be sure you're close to a toilet, and if possible, have the enema in the morning so that you won't need to use the bathroom during the night. Here's what to do.

1 Wash your hands. Then open the disposable enema package and read the instructions carefully.

2 Hold the enema bottle upright, grasping the grooved bottle cap with your fingers. Gently remove the protective shield with your other hand.

Right-knee-bent position

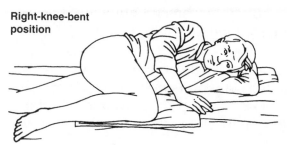

3 Now, lie on your left side with your right knee bent. This position helps the enema solution flow into your colon. Be sure to place a linen-saver pad under your buttocks to keep the bed dry.

Or you can lie in the knee-chest position.

Knee-chest position

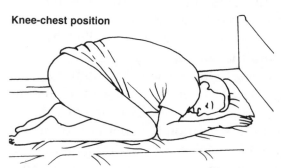

4 Gently insert the tip of the enema bottle about 4 inches (10 centimeters) into your rectum.

Take slow, deep breaths as you slowly squeeze the bottle to deposit the solution in your rectum. When the bottle is empty, remove the tip from your rectum.

5 Because your colon is full, you'll feel an immediate urge to have a bowel movement. Try to resist the urge, holding the solution in for 2 to 5 minutes for a cleansing enema and for as long as you can tolerate for an oil retention enema. Then expel the solution into the toilet.

6 After moving your bowels, clean the perineum carefully. Then put the used enema bottle in its original box.

Discard the box, the linen-saver pad, and other disposable articles.

Administering vaginal medication

If the doctor has prescribed a vaginal medication for you, follow these instructions to insert it.

1 Plan to insert the vaginal medication after bathing and just before bedtime to ensure that it will stay in the vagina for an appropriate amount of time.

Collect the equipment you'll need: the prescribed medication (suppository, cream, ointment, tablet, or jelly), an applicator, water-soluble lubricating jelly (such as K-Y Jelly), a towel, a hand mirror, paper towels, and a sanitary pad.

2 Next, empty your bladder, wash your hands, and place the towel on the bed. Sit on the towel, and open the medication wrapper or container.

3 Using the hand mirror, carefully inspect your perineum, which is the area between your anus and your genitals. If you see signs of increased irritation, don't insert the medication. Notify the doctor. He may change your medication.

Suppository

4 Place a vaginal suppository or tablet in the applicator, or fill the applicator with cream, ointment, or jelly.

5 To make insertion easier, lubricate the suppository or applicator tip with water or water-soluble lubricating jelly.

Now, lie down on the bed with your knees flexed and legs spread apart.

Spread apart your labia with one hand, and insert the applicator tip into the vagina with the other hand. Advance the applicator about 2 inches (5 centimeters), angling it slightly toward your tailbone.

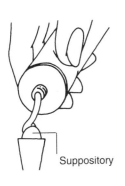

Suppository

Inserting the applicator

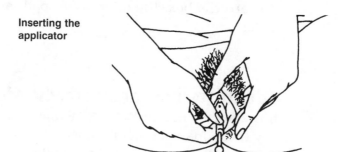

6 Push the plunger to insert the medication. Be aware that the medication may feel cold.

Inserting the medication

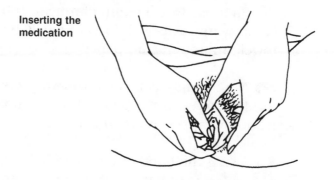

7 Remove the applicator and discard it if it's disposable. If it's reusable, thoroughly wash it with soap and water, dry it with a paper towel, and return it to its container.

Applying a sanitary pad

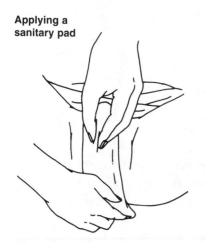

8 If the doctor prescribes it, apply a thin layer of cream, ointment, or jelly to the vulva (the area including the vagina, labia majora, and labia minora).

9 Remain lying down for about 30 minutes so that the medicine won't run out of your vagina. Apply the sanitary pad to avoid staining your clothes or bed linens.

Then check your vagina for signs of an allergic reaction. If the area seems unusually red or swollen, contact the doctor.

Learning about injections

Medication usually is ordered to be taken orally—by mouth. Sometimes, however, the doctor orders medication to be taken a different way, such as by injection. An injection, or shot, may be given for any of several reasons, such as the following:

• Taken orally, the medication would be irritating to the throat or stomach or would be destroyed by stomach acids before it could take effect.

• The medication isn't available as a pill, tablet, or drinkable liquid.

• The person receiving the medication can't or won't swallow it.

• The medication works better or faster when it's absorbed into the body through direct injection into skin or muscle.

Injection routes

As the doctor directs, you may be injecting medication into the subcutaneous skin layer or deeper, into muscle.

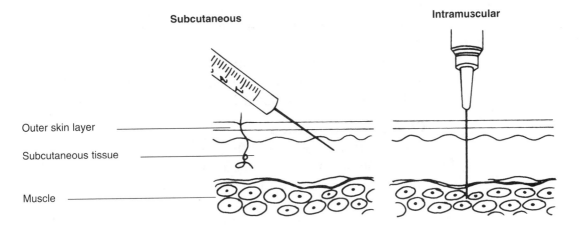

Subcutaneous

Intramuscular

Outer skin layer

Subcutaneous tissue

Muscle

How does the doctor decide which injection route to use for a particular person? Each route has certain advantages and disadvantages, but perhaps the most important difference between them is this: medication given intramuscularly takes effect quickly—usually within 10 to 30 minutes—whereas medication given subcutaneously takes effect more slowly (usually after 30 minutes). Basing his decision on this and other considerations, the doctor will tell you which route to use.

Injection equipment

To give an injection, you'll need the following equipment: a syringe with needle attached, a bottle or ampule of medication, and several alcohol swabs.

To learn about the syringe, take one out of its package and compare it with the syringe in the illustration. Identify all the parts, and check the needle length. For a subcutaneous injection, it will be less than 1 inch (2.5 centimeters) long. For an intramuscular injection, it will be between 1 and 3 inches (2.5 and 7.6 centimers) long.

Parts of a syringe

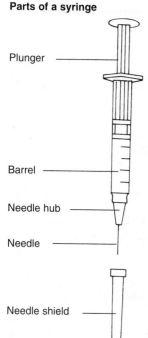

Plunger

Barrel

Needle hub

Needle

Needle shield

Safe disposal of the syringe and needle

Always dispose of used syringes and needles as follows:
• Never recap the needle.
• Place the syringe with the needle attached into a container such as a coffee can (with lid) or plastic milk container.
• Mark the container as "Biohazard."
• Place the container in a safe place, out of a child's reach.
• Once you've filled the container, seal it with tape and label it "Sharp Objects." Check with your local trash collector about how to discard the container.

Check the medication

Every time you get ready to give an injection, examine the bottle or ampule of medication first. To make sure the medication's safe to use, ask yourself these questions:
• How does the medication look? If it's normally clear but looks cloudy when you examine it, check with the doctor or pharmacist before injecting it. He may tell you to discard it. (*Note:* Some medications, such as NPH insulin, are normally cloudy.)
• Has the expiration date on the medication passed? Check the label and, if so, discard the medication. Contact the pharmacist or doctor for a new supply of medication.
• Now, check the medication's label again. Are the correct

names on it—the patient's name and the name of the pre-scribing doctor? Is the name of the medication exactly the same as what the doctor said he would prescribe? Unless your answer to all these questions is yes, don't give the injection. Instead, call the doctor (or the pharmacist or home care nurse) and follow his or her instructions.

If you're giving more than one medication by injection or another person in your household is also receiving medication this way, always double-check all label information before giving an injection.

Keep injection records

If you're giving a series of injections, you need to keep records that you and the doctor can refer to. For subcutaneous injections, expect to make a site rotation pattern for alternating injection sites.

For both subcutaneous and intramuscular injections, you'll also need a calendar record. Use a conventional calendar, with a month for each page. As you begin each month, write at the top of the new page the type of medication you'll be injecting. Then every time you give an injection, record the time and the site (for example, "6 a.m., left thigh") in the appropriate day box on the calendar. If the amount or strength of medication you inject can vary, record this information for each injection as well.

Reducing injection discomfort

For most people, getting an injection hurts. But you can do several things to lessen the pain when you give someone in your care—or yourself—an injection.

If the person's anxious or afraid, prepare him for the injection by stressing that the medication is important to his recovery.

You can also apply ice to the area for 10 to 15 minutes before the injection to numb the site.

If the person's a child, let him make some of the decisions (such as which arm will get the injection).

He'll probably ask if it'll hurt, or he'll be tense and fearful because he knows it'll hurt. Be honest: "Yes, it will hurt—but it will be over quickly." Then give the injection as quickly as possible.

If the child cries, comfort him and let him know that crying is OK.

Offer to put an adhesive strip over the injection site; if the strip is decorated or brightly colored, you can pretend with him that it's a badge he's earned for his bravery. This gesture will also help calm any fear he may have that blood will leak out. (If he doesn't mention this, don't bring up the subject.)

Preparing to give an injection

The 6 steps below provide all the specific information you need for giving an injection.

1 Remember, always wash your hands thoroughly before you handle the medication or give an injection. Then gather the equipment you'll need: the medication (and a gauze pad if the medication comes in a glass ampule), a syringe with needle attached, and several alcohol swabs.

2 Examine the medication to be sure that it looks the way it should and that all the label information is correct. If you have any doubts, call the doctor, pharmacist, or home care nurse and follow his or her instructions.

Swabbing the stopper of an open bottle

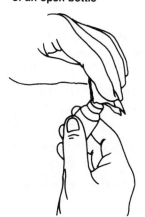

Snapping off the top of a glass ampule

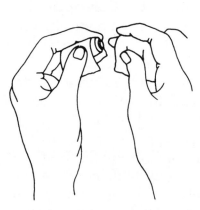

3 The medication will be either in a bottle with a metal pull-tab top or in a glass ampule.

Open a bottle by pulling back on the tab, exposing the rubber stopper; swab the stopper with alcohol before you handle the syringe.

Open a glass ampule by grasping the top with a gauze pad and snapping it off.

4 Unwrap the syringe and remove the needle shield. If the medication is in a bottle, pull back on the plunger of the syringe until you've drawn air into the barrel in an amount equal to the amount of medication you'll inject. Then inject this air into the bottle, through the rubber stopper, without withdrawing the needle. This procedure will make drawing up the medication easier. How? By preventing a vacuum from forming in the bottle.

Injecting air   **Drawing up the medication**

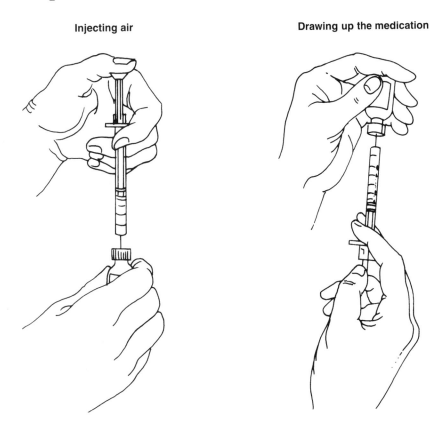

If the medication is in a glass ampule, this procedure isn't necessary.

Draw the medication into the syringe by pulling back on the plunger, measuring the correct amount by checking the markings on the side of the syringe as it fills. Draw up only the amount of medication the doctor has ordered, and then withdraw the needle from the bottle or ampule.

Now, check for air bubbles. Hold the syringe with the needle pointing up, and tap the syringe lightly so that the bubbles rise to its top. Then push out the air, and, if necessary, draw up more medication to obtain the correct amount.

Hold the syringe with the needle pointing up and pull back on the plunger a little bit more. This will cause a tiny air bubble to form inside the syringe; when you inject the medication, this bubble will help clear the needle and seal the medication into the subcutaneous tissue.

Replace the needle shield.

5 Select an appropriate injection site. Be as accurate as possible when you locate that site, making sure that it is free of lumps and skin depressions.

For frequent injections, change the site each time to minimize such injection problems as injecting in the same site too often or using a site that's still tender from a previous injection.

This discussion of sites, called "site rotation patterns," assumes that you're giving a series of injections, one per day. If you're giving two per day, alternate injection areas (such as the right thigh in the morning, left thigh in the afternoon), and make two site rotation patterns, one for each area. If you're giving three or more injections per day, just use the number of injections you're giving as your guide to the appropriate number of injection sites and site rotation patterns. For more details, see "Rotating injection sites," later in this chapter.

Wiping in an outward-moving pattern

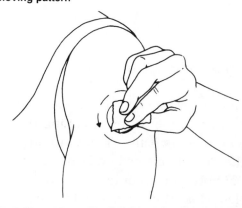

Cleaning the injection site

6 Clean the injection site with one of the alcohol swabs. Begin at the center of the site, wiping the swab continuously outward in a circular pattern. That way, you move any dirt particles away from the site.

Allow the swabbed skin to dry completely—this should take only 5 to 10 seconds—before you inject the medication. If you don't do this, the injection may push alcohol into the skin and cause burning pain.

Giving a subcutaneous injection

1 Remove the needle shield. Then firmly grasp the skin at the site. This elevates the subcutaneous tissue and helps prevent the needle from entering the wrong skin layer.

2 With your other hand, position the syringe and needle at a 45-degree angle so that the beveled (angled) part of the needle tip is facing upward.

Needle inserted at a 45-degree angle

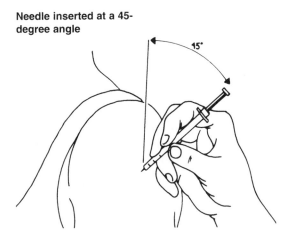

3 Holding the syringe and needle at a 45-degree angle to the skin, insert the needle in one quick motion. Don't hesitate. With your other hand, immediately release your grasp on the skin.

4 Holding the syringe firmly in place, pull back slightly on the plunger.
   If blood appears in the syringe, the needle isn't positioned properly. Take the needle out quickly, and press an alcohol swab over the site. Discard everything and begin again. If no blood appears in the syringe, you can begin injecting the medication.

5 Using your other hand to hold the needle steady, depress the syringe plunger slowly, maintaining the 45-degree angle. *Warning:* Never inject rapidly because this puts pressure on tissues and causes pain.

6 When you've injected all the medication, place an alcohol swab over the needle and the injection site and withdraw the needle at the same angle as you inserted it, applying pressure with the swab. The pressure will help seal the punctured tissue and prevent medication from seeping out.

7 Use an alcohol swab to massage the site; this will help distribute the medication and promote its absorption into the skin. *Warning:* Don't do this if you're injecting insulin or heparin.

8 Record the injection. On your calendar record, write the details of the injection. Discard the needle and syringe.

Injecting insulin

If you're diabetic and need insulin injections, you probably already have received detailed instructions on how to give yourself an injection. The instructions given here can't replace a health care professional's guidance; use them only to reinforce what he or she has taught you.

To inject insulin, follow the general instructions for giving a subcutaneous injection.

• Be sure you vary injection sites, using one or more site rotation patterns as appropriate.

• Double-check that all the label information is correct. This is important if two or more persons in your household are taking different types or dosages of insulin.

1 If you keep your insulin in the refrigerator, remove it. Then warm and mix it by rolling the vial between your palms—*Don't* shake it.

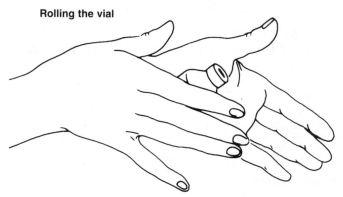

Rolling the vial

2 When you draw up the correct amount of insulin into the syringe, check for air bubbles. If you see any, tap the syringe lightly so they will rise to its top. Push out the extra air.

If necessary, draw up more insulin to obtain the correct dose.

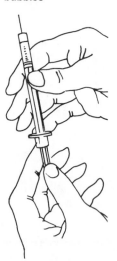

Checking for air bubbles

3 Grasp the injection site between your thumb and forefinger. Quickly plunge the syringe needle into the skin at a 90-degree angle, and insert it up to its hub.

Don't massage the site after withdrawing the needle; do apply pressure with an alcohol swab.

Grasping the injection site

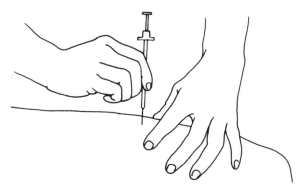

Injecting the medication

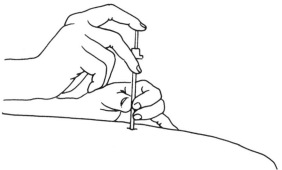

Mixing insulins in a syringe

If the doctor has prescribed regular and either intermediate or long-acting insulin to control your diabetes, you can avoid giving yourself separate injections by mixing the two types of insulin in a syringe and injecting them together. Here's what to do.

1 Wash your hands. Then prepare the mixture in a clean area. Make sure you have alcohol swabs, both types of insulin, and the proper syringe for your prescribed insulin concentration. Then mix the contents of the intermediate or long-acting insulin by rolling it gently between your palms.

Injecting air into the vial

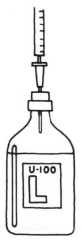

2 Using an alcohol swab, clean the rubber stopper on the vial of intermediate or long-acting insulin. Then draw air into the syringe by pulling the plunger back to the prescribed number of insulin units. Insert the needle into the top of the vial. Make sure the point doesn't touch the insulin (see illustration). Now, push in the plunger, and remove the needle from the vial.

3 Next, clean the rubber stopper on the regular insulin vial with an alcohol swab. Then pull back the plunger on the syringe to the prescribed number of insulin units, insert the needle into the top of the vial, and inject air into the vial. With the needle still in the vial, turn the vial upside down and withdraw the prescribed dose of regular insulin.

Withdrawing regular insulin

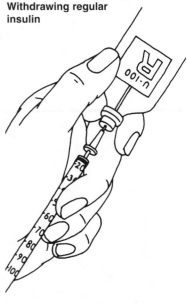

4 Clean the top of the intermediate or long-acting insulin vial. Then insert the needle into it without pushing the plunger down. Invert the vial and withdraw the prescribed number of units for the total dose. (For example, if you have 10 units of regular insulin in the syringe and you need 20 units of intermediate or long-acting insulin, pull back the plunger to 30 units.)

Never change the order in which you mix insulins, and always inject the insulin immediately to prevent loss of potency.

Rotating injection sites

Whether you administer your insulin by needle or by an insulin pump, you need to rotate the injection sites.

Why rotate sites?

Rotating the site for injecting insulin reduces injury to the skin and underlying fatty tissue. It prevents a buildup of scar tissue and swelling and lumps.

It can also minimize a slow insulin absorption rate. This can result from repeated injections in one spot, which can cause fibrous tissue growth and decreased blood supply in that area.

Site rotation can also offset changes that exercise causes in insulin absorption. Exercise increases blood flow to the body part being exercised, thereby increasing the insulin absorption rate. So don't inject yourself in an area about to be exercised. (For example, don't inject yourself in the thigh before you go walking or bike riding.)

Where can I inject insulin?

You can inject insulin into these areas:
• the outer part of both upper arms
• your right and left mid-torso, just above and below your waist (except for a 2-inch (5-centimeter] circle around your navel)
• your right and left back below the waist, just behind your hip bone

Injection sites

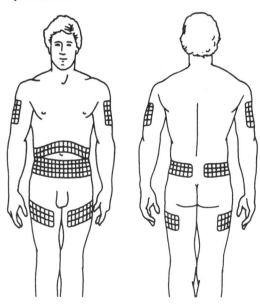

• the front and outsides of both thighs, from 4 inches [10 centimeters] below the top of your thigh to 4 inches above your knee.

Keep in mind that different parts of the body absorb insulin at different rates. The stomach area absorbs insulin best, then the upper arm, and last the thighs. Use the following approach:
• Inject into the same body area for 1 to 2 weeks, depending on the number of injections you need daily. For example, if you need four injections a day, use one area for only about 5 days.
• Cover the entire area within an injection site, but don't inject into the same spot.

• Don't inject into spots where you can't easily grasp fatty tissue.

• Have a family member give you injections in hard-to-reach areas.

• Check with the doctor if a site becomes especially painful or if swelling or lumps appear.

Injecting heparin

Wash your hands and clean the injection site. Refer to the diagram below as you choose an area on your stomach between the iliac crests.

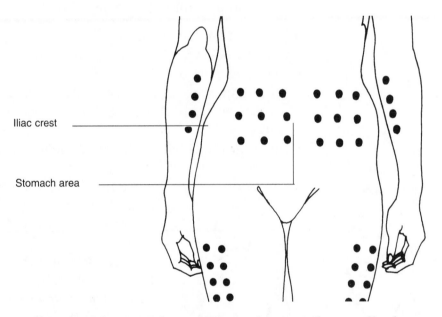

Iliac crest

Stomach area

Now, pinch your skin gently and insert the needle deep into the underlying fat layer. Slowly inject the drug. Don't check for blood backflow. Leave the needle in place for 10 seconds before you withdraw it. Don't massage or rub the area. Change the injection site each time you take this medicine.

Ensuring the right dose

Inject heparin exactly when the doctor directs. If you miss a dose, take it as soon as possible. If it's almost time for the next dose, forget the missed dose and don't double the next one. Instead, go back to your regular schedule.

Giving an intramuscular injection

Use these instructions to review how to give an intramuscular injection.

Locating injection sites

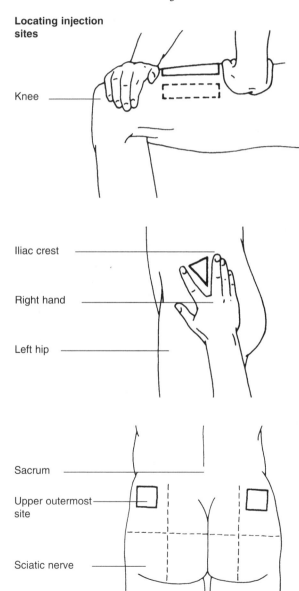

Knee

Iliac crest

Right hand

Left hip

Sacrum

Upper outermost site

Sciatic nerve

Selecting the injection site

Choose the injection site. You can use the thigh, hip, buttock, or upper arm. Avoid using the upper arm because the muscle there is small and close to the brachial nerve.

Thigh

To find the target, place one hand on the person's knee and the other hand at his groin. Use the area marked by solid lines, as shown in the illustration at left, for adult injections. Use the area marked by dotted lines for injections for infants and children.

Hip

To find this site, place your right hand on the person's left hip (or place your left hand on the person's right hip). Then spread your index and middle fingers to form a V. Your midxdle finger should be on the highest point of the pelvis, known as the iliac crest. The triangular area shown in the illustration is the injection site.

Buttock

Imagine lines dividing each buttock into four equal parts. Give the injection in the upper outermost area near the iliac crest, as shown. Don't give it in the sciatic nerve area.

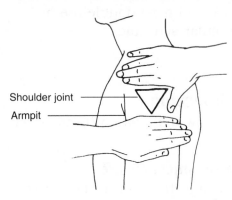

Shoulder joint

Armpit

Upper arm

Locate the injection site by placing one hand at the top of the person's shoulder and extending your thumb down his upper arm. Place the other hand at armpit level, as shown. The triangular space shown between the hands is the injection area.

If a series of injections is necessary, rotate the sites. To reduce pain and improve drug absorption, don't use the same site twice in a row.

Giving the injection

Follow the steps shown under "Preparing to give an injection." Then continue with these steps:

1 Remove the needle shield. Now, with one hand, stretch the skin taut around the injection site. This makes inserting the needle easier and helps disperse the medication after the injection.

With your other hand, hold the syringe and needle at a 90-degree angle to the injection site. Then insert the needle with a quick thrust.

Holding the needle at a 90-degree angle

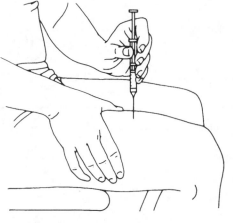

2 Holding the syringe firmly in place, remove the hand stretching your skin and use it to pull back slightly on the plunger. If blood appears in the syringe, you've entered a blood vessel. Take the needle out and press an alcohol swab over the site. Then discard everything and start again. If no blood appears, inject the medication slowly, keeping the syringe and needle at a 90-degree angle. Never push the plunger forcefully.

3 When you've injected all the medication, press an alcohol swab around the needle and injection site, and withdraw the needle at the same angle as you inserted it.

Using a circular motion, extending from the center outward, massage the site with the alcohol swab to help distribute the medication and promote its absorption.

4 Dispose of the used syringe and needle properly.

9 I.V. Therapy

Understanding essential measures

Taking care of a person with an intravenous (I.V.) line is a complex procedure. You must be particularly careful about washing your hands whenever you touch the equipment or are working with the I.V. insertion site.

You'll also need to keep the work area clean. Develop the habit of wiping down the surface with alcohol before working with the solutions or tubing.

Also, whenever working with the I.V. site, you should wear gloves if you have an infection on your hands or the person you're caring for has a blood disease that you could contract—for example, hepatitis. This precaution is important because the I.V. site is a potential place where germs can enter the person's bloodstream and, conversely, where germs can exit and infect you.

Warning: Carefully dispose of needles, tubing, and solution containers. You'll need a special container for sharp items, and anything you dispose of should be marked "Medical Waste."

Caring for an intermittent infusion device

To care for an intermittent infusion device, also called a heparin lock, you'll need to check the dressing and the area around the insertion site daily. Do this before administering a solution or medication or flushing the device, explained below.

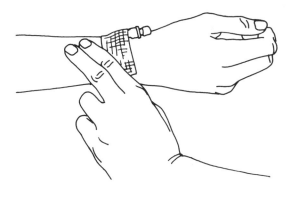

Intermittent infusion device covered by dressing

Check for redness and swelling, and ask the person if the area is tender. If any of these symptoms are present, contact the home health care nurse. The infusion device may have to be replaced.

If the dressing covering the device becomes wet, cover it with another gauze dressing and notify the home health care nurse. The home health care nurse will probably change the dressing as needed.

Flushing an intermittent infusion device

You may be asked to flush the intermittent infusion device after the person has received medication or an I.V. solution or as part of maintenance to keep the device in good working order. Depending on the doctor's or home health care agency's policy, you'll be flushing with a low-dose heparin or normal saline solution.

1 Gather the supplies: flush solution and an alcohol sponge.

2 With one hand, stabilize the device by holding it below the rubber cap. Try to keep the device steady because the less a catheter is moved in a vein, the longer the device will last.

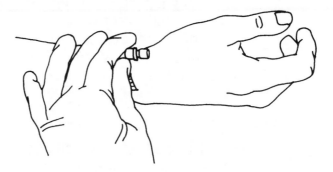

3 Using your other hand, clean the cap with an alcohol sponge.

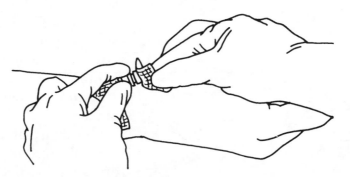

4 Next, insert the needle attached to the syringe containing the flush solution into the rubber cap on the infusion device. Pull back slowly on the plunger, and watch for blood return in the syringe.

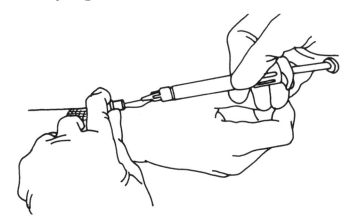

5 If you see blood return, slowly and steadily inject the flush solution. If you feel resistance or the person complains of discomfort, stop immediately.

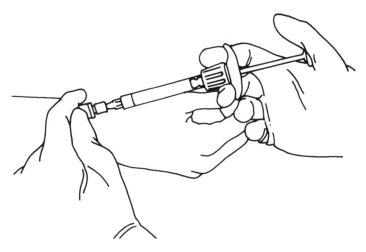

6 Remove the needle and syringe that contained the flush solution, and dispose of them properly.

Preparing for an infusion

Remember to wash your hands thoroughly and clean the work area. This helps prevent contamination, which can cause an infection.

1 You'll need the prescribed I.V. solution, an administration set (tubing), an I.V. pole, and alcohol sponges.

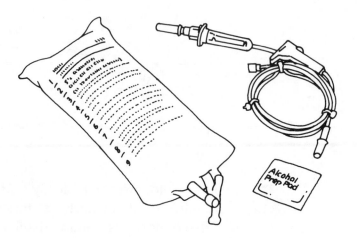

2 Carefully read the label on the solution container, and make sure you have the correct solution.

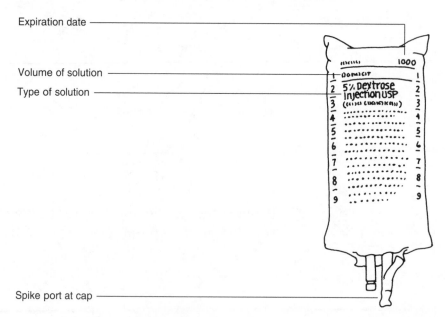

Expiration date

Volume of solution

Type of solution

Spike port at cap

3 Closely inspect the container. Hold a glass container up to the light and rotate it. Keep in mind that cracks and chips in glass will reflect the light.

If you're using a plastic bag, squeeze it to check for leaks.

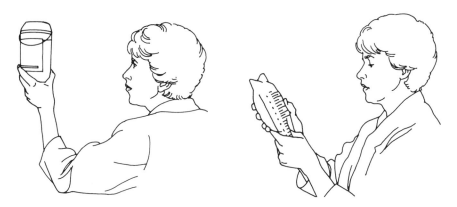

Also check the solution for particles, discoloration, and cloudiness. If you see any of these defects, notify the I.V. solution supplier and the home health care nurse. Don't administer the solution until they tell you that it's safe to use.

Preparing the I.V. bottle or bag

1 Unwrap the tubing and close the clamp below the drip chamber. "Spike" the solution container by pushing the pointed end of the tubing (the spike) into the container. If you're using an I.V. bottle with a rubber stopper, remove the

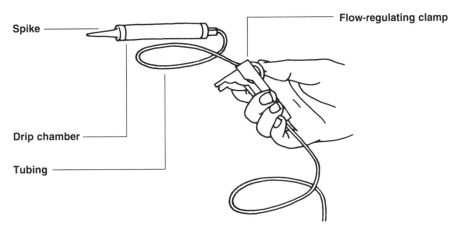

Spike

Flow-regulating clamp

Drip chamber

Tubing

Spiking the bottle

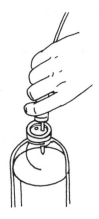

protective metal cap. Place the bottle on a stable surface, and wipe the stopper with an alcohol swab.

Next, remove the protective cap from the spike on the end of the tubing, which should have a vent. Then, holding the bottle steady, push the spike into the rubber stopper far enough so that you can see the spike through the bottle. Don't touch the spike or the stopper with your hands.

2 If you're using an I.V. bottle with a vent, remove the protective metal cap and latex diaphragm. Place the bottle on a stable surface, and wipe the stopper with an alcohol sponge. Remove the plastic cap from the spike on the end of the tubing, and push the spike through the larger hole in the entry port. The smaller hole is an air vent. Be careful not to touch the spike with your hands.

If you're using an I.V. bag without a grip port, hang the bag first. Then remove the protective cap from the entry port by pulling the cap to the right, and wipe the port with an alcohol sponge. Remove the protective cap from the spike. Hold the base of the entry port in one hand without squeezing the bag, and quickly insert the spike with the other hand.

| **Tubing with a vent** | **Bottle with a vent** | **Bag without a grip port** | **Bag with a grip port** |

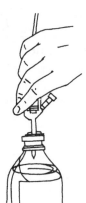 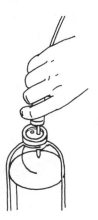 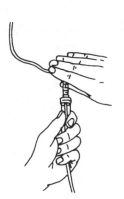 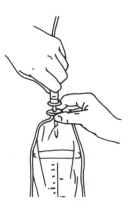

If you're using an I.V. bag with a grip port, spike the bag before hanging it.

Then gently squeeze the drip chamber, allowing it to fill about halfway. Make sure the tubing is clamped.

Squeezing the drip chamber

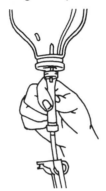

3 If the tubing contains a filter, release the clamp to allow solution to flow into the filter. Fill the filter according to the manufacturer's directions. Then reclamp the tubing.

4 Next, remove the protective cap from the end of the tubing and place the cap on a clean towel. (Don't touch the inside of the cap.) Holding the end of the tubing over (but not touching) a wastebasket or cup, release the clamp. Leave the clamp open until the solution flows through the entire length of the tubing, forcing out all air. When the solution begins to drip out, reclamp the tubing. This is known as priming the I.V. tubing.

5 Check the filter and tubing for air bubbles. If you find any, gently tap the tubing until the bubbles rise into the container.

Tapping the tubing

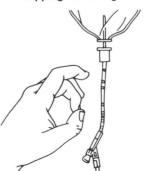

6 Once the tubing's clamped and clear of air, replace the protective cap and hang the tubing on the I.V. pole.

Hanging tubing on I.V. pole

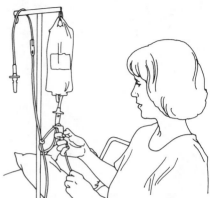

Giving the solution

1 Place the I.V. pole close to the person you're caring for.

2 Using an alcohol sponge, wipe the cap of the heparin lock that has been placed by the home health care nurse, and hang the solution container with the primed tubing on the I.V. pole.

Wiping the cap

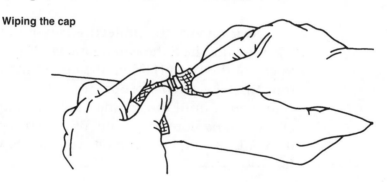

3 Remove the protective cap from the I.V. tubing, and carefully attach a needle.

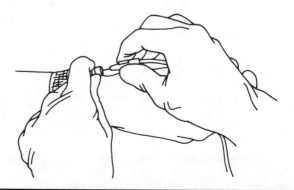

4 Remove the needle cap, and insert the needle into the rubber end of the intermittent infusion device. Watch for a backflow of blood into the tubing, confirming that the I.V. device is properly placed.

Adjusting the flow rate

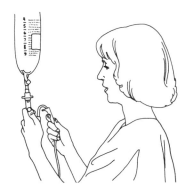

5 Adjust the flow rate of the solution. The doctor orders the amount of fluid the person is to receive in a specified time. The home health care nurse will tell you the flow rate in drops per minute that you will need to maintain to comply with the doctor's orders. To count the drops per minute, hold a watch with a second hand next to the drip chamber, and count the number of drops in 60 seconds. Use the roller clamp to adjust the flow. Push the roller up to increase the flow and down to reduce the flow.

Discontinuing the infusion

1 After all the solution has run in, close the roller clamp. Then grasp the needle hub, and pull it out of the intermittent infusion device.

2 Carefully remove the needle from the end of the tubing. Take special care not to stick yourself, and dispose of the needle in the proper container. Next, dispose of the empty solution container and tubing.

Hand positions for removing the needle

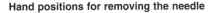
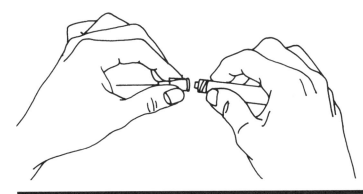

3 Now, record the amount of fluid the person received on the intake- and output-record.

Caring for a central venous catheter

To keep a central venous catheter trouble-free, you must flush the catheter and change the dressing regularly.

Flushing the catheter

Flush the catheter at least once a day to prevent blood clots from forming in it.

1 Gather the following equipment: a bottle of heparin-lock flush solution, a disposable syringe with needle, two alcohol or povidone-iodine swabs, several 4-inch by 4-inch (10.2-centimeter by 10.2-centimeter) gauze pads, and tape.

2 Wash and dry your hands. Then open the bottle of heparin-lock flush solution, and wipe the bottle top with an alcohol or a povidone-iodine swab. Don't touch the top after you've cleaned it.

3 Pick up the syringe, remove the needle guard, and pull back the syringe plunger. Then insert the needle into the flush solution bottle top, and push down on the plunger. Turn the bottle upside down, and pull back on the syringe plunger to fill the syringe with solution. Remove the needle from the bottle, and put the bottle aside. Replace the needle guard.

Filling the syringe with solution

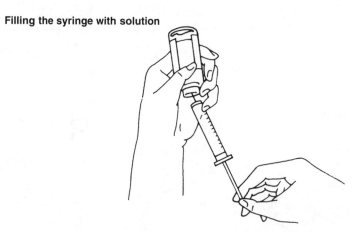

4 Remove and discard the gauze pad protecting the end of the catheter. Using a clean alcohol or povidone-iodine swab, wipe the end of the catheter. When the end is dry, remove the catheter's clamp. After removing the needle guard, insert the needle into the catheter.

Inserting the needle

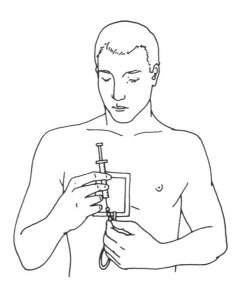

Push down on the syringe plunger to inject the flush solution into the catheter. Replace the clamp after you withdraw the needle. Wrap the catheter end in a sterile gauze pad, and tape it on top of the dressing.

Changing the dressing

Change the dressing over the catheter every other day or whenever it becomes wet or dirty. When you change the dressing, carefully check the skin around the catheter. Call the doctor at once if you see any sign of infection, such as redness, swelling, or pus. Also call him if a fever or pain develops.

Cleaning the skin using a circular motion

1 To change the dressing, obtain a dressing change kit or assemble the supplies recommended by the nurse or doctor. Then wash your hands, and remove the soiled dressing. Wash your hands again. (If suggested by the doctor, you may want to put on sterile gloves to avoid possible contamination.)

Clean the skin around the catheter with an

alcohol swab, beginning near the catheter and working outward in a circular motion. Repeat the procedure, using a povidone-iodine swab.

2 Squeeze some povidone-iodine ointment onto a sterile gauze pad. Put the pad over the catheter exit site. Cover it with a dry sterile gauze pad.

Squeezing ointment onto gauze

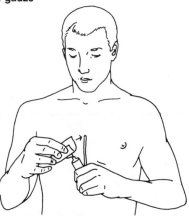

3 Apply an adhesive bandage over both gauze pads so that the bandage edges stick to your skin. For extra security, tape the bandage edges to your skin. Now, wrap the catheter end in a sterile gauze pad, and tape it on top of the bandage.

Applying bandage to skin

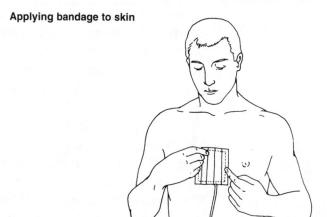

Giving total parenteral nutrition

Use the guidelines below to review your instructions for giving total parenteral nutrition (TPN) to the person in your care. They'll help you give TPN correctly and confidently.

Preparing the feeding solution

Begin by removing the feeding solution from the refrigerator 1 hour before you'll use it. This will allow time for the solution to warm to room temperature. Then follow these steps.

1 Always read the container's label to make sure you have the right solution. And always check the solution's preparation and expiration dates. Don't use a solution that was prepared more than 1 week ago, and never use a solution whose expiration date has passed. If the solutions are numbered, make sure to use them in sequence.

2 Inspect the container. Holding it to the light, look for cracks, leaks, or breaks. Also note whether the solution is discolored or cloudy. If you notice anything wrong, discard the solution and use another container. Make sure to tell the supplier that you're short one solution container. Once you've taken a container of solution from the refrigerator, use it within 24 hours or discard it.

3 Clean your work area with an alcohol-soaked swab. Let the surface air-dry. Then set out the following equipment: the solution container, tubing, alcohol and antimicrobial swabs, needles and syringes, containers of saline solution and heparin solution, tape, scissors, and materials for a dressing change (if necessary).

   Wash your hands thoroughly with soap and water, and spike and prime the solution container (see *Preparing the I.V. bottle or bag* earlier in this chapter).

Setting up the pump

1 Make sure the pump is working correctly. Following the manufacturer's instructions, turn the control to ON to check the power, displays, alarms, and battery. If you have any problems, call the supplier immediately for a replacement pump.

2 Set the pump controls. As directed, set the flow rate, the amount to be infused, and the time the infusion will take. Thread the tubing through the pump, according to the manufacturer's directions. When it's in place, check to make sure it isn't pinched or kinked.

3 Now, do a trial run. Here's how to proceed.
• Remove the tubing's protective cap.
• Hold the tubing over—but not touching—a wastebasket or cup.
• Start the pump.

The solution should flow freely and smoothly from the end of the tubing. If it doesn't, recheck the threading (the tubing can get pinched if it's not threaded exactly right). When the solution is flowing correctly, stop the pump and reclamp and recap the tubing.

Giving the solution

First, remove the tape and gauze pad that secure the catheter cap to the person's dressing. Now you're ready to infuse the solution.

1 Thoroughly clean the tubing-catheter connection. This will help to prevent infection.
• If a threaded screw lock connects the tubing and the catheter, remove the protective cap from the end of the catheter and set it aside on a sterile towel. Don't touch the inside of the cap. Wipe the junction

Using an antimicrobial swab

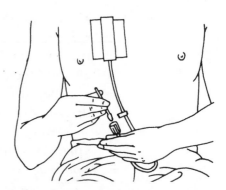

between the catheter tip and the catheter's protective cap with an alcohol swab and an antimicrobial swab.
• If a needle connects the tubing and the catheter, the catheter will have an injection cap on the end (a rubber covering you can use for several injections). Clean the cap with an alcohol swab and an antimicrobial swab.

Screwing the tubing into the catheter

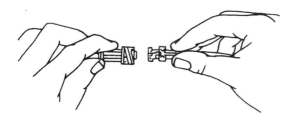

Piercing the cap

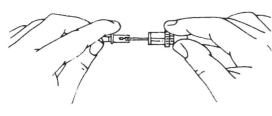

Taping the connections

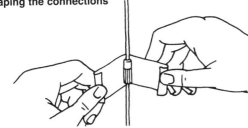

2 If a threaded screw lock connects the tubing and the catheter, remove the protective caps from both the tubing and the catheter. Screw the end of the tubing into the catheter. Don't touch the ends of the tubing or the catheter with your hands.

If a needle connects the catheter and the tubing, attach a needle to the end of the tubing, and remove the needle's protective shield.

Release the clamp on the tubing to let a little of the solution drip out. This primes the needle and forces out any air.

3 Now, without touching the injection cap or the needle, pierce the cap on the end of the catheter. Make sure the needle is all the way in and flush against the cap to make a connection.

4 For security, tape the connections (both the screw lock and the needle). Fold the ends of the sticky side of the tape together to form tabs. This makes the tape easier to remove later.

5 To start the infusion, release the catheter clamp. You've already set the pump for the prescribed rate, so check one last time for air bubbles, kinks, and twists. Now, start the pump.

Finishing the infusion

Here's what to do when you hear the signal that means the infusion has ended.

1 Stop the pump, and turn off the power. Wash your hands with soap and water, and clean your work area again with alcohol.

2 Clamp the catheter. Remember to clamp it in a different place each time to avoid weakening any one section.

3 Carefully remove the tape that secures the connection between the catheter and the tubing.

4 Disconnect the tubing according to the kind of connection.
• If you have a screw lock connection, first clamp the catheter, and then unscrew the connection. Next, clamp the tubing so that the solution doesn't drip, and replace the catheter's protective cap.
• If a needle connects the catheter and the tubing, pull the needle out of the injection cap and clamp the catheter. Carefully put the protective shield over the needle, and remove the needle from the end of the tube. Dispose of the needle properly. Clamp the end of the tubing so that the solution doesn't drip out. Record the amount of solution the person received on the fluid intake-and-output record.

Flushing the catheter and cleaning up

After the infusion, you'll flush the catheter with saline solution to remove any remaining feeding solution. Then you'll flush it with heparin to prevent blood clots from forming in the catheter. Use the following steps for flushing a Hickman catheter with saline solution. Repeat the steps for flushing with heparin. If you're using another type of catheter, follow the nurse's or doctor's orders.

Wiping the top of the vial

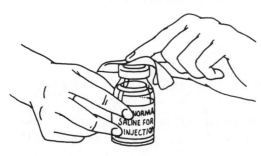

1 Assemble the equipment: a vial of saline solution and a vial of heparin solution, disposable syringes with plastic needle shields or syringes prefilled with saline and heparin solutions, two povidone-iodine sponges, a 4-inch by 4-inch (10.2-centimeter by 10.2-centimeter) gauze pad, and tape.

Wash your hands. If necessary, remove the protective cap on the saline solution vial. Then wipe the top of the vial with a povidone-iodine sponge. Don't touch the top after you've cleaned it.

2 Remove the needle shield, and pull back the plunger until the top of its rubber stopper meets the prescribed dosage line on the syringe. Then insert the needle into the vial top and push down on the plunger. This forces air into the vial and makes it easier to remove the solution.

3 Turn the vial and syringe upside down, and pull back on the plunger to fill the syringe with solution. Remove the needle from the vial, and replace the needle shield. Set the syringe down within reach.

Preparing the syringe   **Filling the syringe**

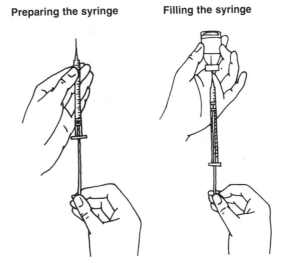

4 Remove and discard the gauze pad protecting the catheter cap. Using a clean povidone-iodine sponge, wipe the top of the catheter cap and let it air-dry. Don't let anything touch the cap after you've cleaned it.

Inserting the needle into the cap

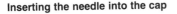

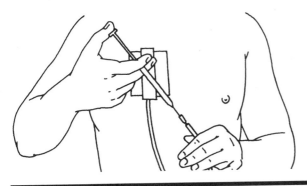

5 Remove the catheter clamp. Then remove the needle shield, and insert the needle into the cap.

Don't puncture the catheter with the needle. Slowly and steadily press the syringe plunger until you've injected all the prescribed solution into the catheter. Never use force to inject the solution. Replace the clamp, withdraw the needle from the cap, and properly dispose of the needle and syringe.

6 Tear four strips of tape. Then fold the new sterile gauze pad around the cap. Lay the wrapped catheter cap on the dressing over the catheter exit site. Use the four strips of tape to secure the pad to the dressing. To keep the catheter cap from slipping out the bottom, pinch a strip of tape around it.

Applying tape strips

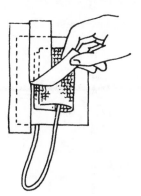

Pinching the tape

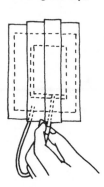

7 Make sure to discard all the equipment that's disposable (tubing, tape, sterile towels, solution container, swabs, needles, and syringes). Also make sure the pump's plugged in so that the batteries stay fully charged.

Caring for an implanted port

Here are some guidelines for flushing and injecting medication into an implanted port.

Flushing the port

To keep an implanted port trouble-free, flush the port according to the doctor's instructions (usually monthly). Check with the doctor if the person develops a fever or if you observe redness, pain, swelling, or pus at the port site.

1 Gather the following equipment: a 10-milliliter syringe with needle, a bottle of heparin (if you don't have a prefilled syringe), a special needle (called a Huber needle), one or two alcohol swabs, and one or two povidone-iodine swabs. Wash your hands. Open the bottle of heparin, and wipe the top with an alcohol or a povidone-iodine swab. Don't touch the top after you've cleaned it.

2 Remove the needle cover from the syringe needle, and pull back the syringe plunger, permitting air to enter the syringe. Pull back on the plunger until the amount of air in the syringe equals the amount of solution that you'll withdraw from the heparin bottle.

Then insert the needle into the heparin bottle top, and push down on the plunger. Turn the bottle upside down, and pull back on the syringe plunger to fill the syringe with the correct amount of solution. Now, remove the needle from the bottle and put the bottle aside. Be sure to replace the needle cover until you've prepared the injection site.

Change the needle on the heparin flush syringe to the Huber needle.

3 Locate the port by feeling for the small bump on the person's skin. (The site is over a bony area, usually on the upper chest.)

Feeling for the port

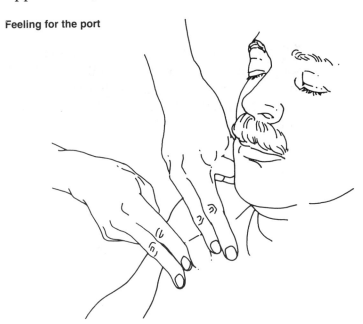

4 Clean the injection site first with an alcohol swab (allow the site to air-dry) and then with a povidone-iodine swab. Hold the port between two fingers. Push the Huber needle firmly through the skin and port septum until it hits the bottom of the port's chamber. Be sure to insert the needle at a 90-degree angle.

Pushing through the skin

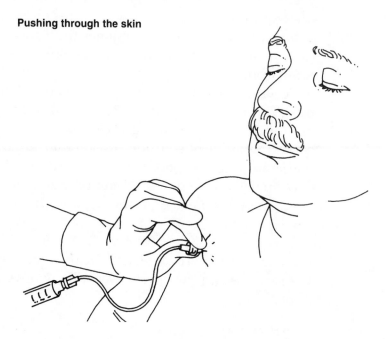

5 Then attach extension tubing. Now, push down on the syringe plunger, which will inject the heparin solution into the port. You'll normally feel a small amount of resistance. Notify the doctor immediately if the solution won't flow into the port.

6 Remove the needle. To keep the solution from flowing back into the syringe when you remove the needle, continue to push down slowly on the syringe plunger as you withdraw the needle.

Injecting medication into the port

1 Gather the needed equipment: an extension set with a special needle (Huber needle), a clamp, a 10-milliliter syringe filled with saline solution, a syringe containing the prescribed medication, a sterile needle filled with heparin flush solution, a povidone-iodine swab, and two alcohol swabs.

2 Wash and dry your hands. Attach the 10-milliliter syringe filled with saline solution to the end of the extension set. Gently push on the plunger of the syringe until the extension tubing and needle are filled with solution and all the air has been forced out. Flick the tubing of the extension set to make sure all the air has been removed.

3 Locate the port by feeling for the small bump on the person's skin. Hold the port between two fingers. Clean the site with an alcohol swab and then with a povidone-iodine swab.

4 Push the Huber needle firmly through the skin and port septum until it hits the bottom of the port's chamber. Be sure to insert the needle at a 90-degree angle.

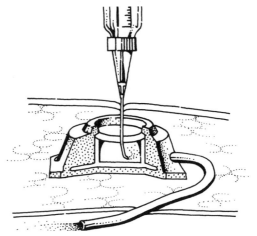

5 Check for a backflow of blood by pulling back on the syringe that's attached to the extension set.

6 Flush the port with 5 milliliters of saline solution by pushing down on the plunger of the syringe with the saline solution. Clamp the extension set, and remove the saline-filled syringe.

7 Connect the medication-filled syringe to the extension set. Open the clamp, and inject the medication, as ordered by the doctor. Check the skin around the needle for swelling and tenderness. If you note these signs, stop the injection and call the doctor.

8 When the injection is complete, clamp the extension set and remove the medication syringe.

9 Attach the saline-filled syringe to the extension set. Then open the clamp, and flush the port again with 5 milliliters of saline solution by pushing down on the plunger of the syringe. Remember to flush the port after each medication interaction. Clamp the extension set, and remove the syringe. Put a protective cap on the end of the extension set. Tape the needle in place, and apply a gauze dressing.

10   Incontinence

Learning about incontinence

If you accidentally leak urine or stool from time to time, then you've experienced incontinence—the involuntary release of urine or stool. This intensely private problem is no doubt embarrassing and uncomfortable for anyone who has it. When severe, incontinence may even discourage a person from socializing with family and friends.

Many causes of incontinence can be treated, so the person may be able to regain control. If not, the person can learn to cope with incontinence and return to a satisfying and secure lifestyle.

Bladder incontinence

The urge to urinate normally occurs when the bladder collects enough urine to stretch its smooth-muscle walls, sending a message up the spinal cord to the brain. In young adults, this occurs when the bladder's about half full. But as a person grows older, bladder capacity decreases and the urge to urinate may not occur until the bladder's almost full. To complicate matters, the urge to urinate then may occur with little warning. So a person who has been ill or has difficulty walking or undressing may not have time to get to a toilet before incontinence occurs.

Besides aging, many other causes—such as pressure, muscle weakness, urinary tract or nervous system disorders, medication, and psychological problems—may contribute to incontinence.

Bladder incontinence may be temporary or permanent, involving large volumes of urine or just dribbling. Types of incontinence include stress, overflow, urge, and complete. In stress incontinence, sudden physical strain, such as a cough, a sneeze, or an abrupt movement—causes intermittent leaking of urine. Overflow incontinence is a dribble that results when urine spills from an overly full bladder. An inability to suppress a sudden urge to urinate characterizes urge incontinence. In complete incontinence, the bladder can't retain any urine, resulting in constant leaking.

Structures of the urinary system

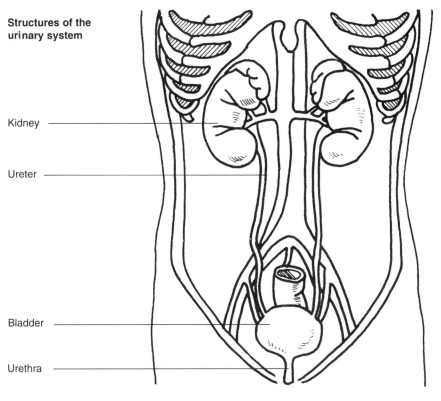

Kidney

Ureter

Bladder

Urethra

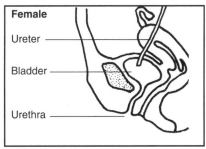

Female

Ureter

Bladder

Urethra

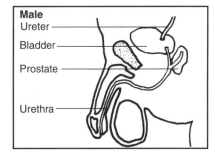

Male

Ureter

Bladder

Prostate

Urethra

Bowel incontinence

Like bladder incontinence, the inability to control the bowels—bowel incontinence—can make a person feel miserable and socially outcast. To understand why bowel incontinence occurs and how to control it, you need to remember know how the body normally digests food.

Digestion begins when you chew and swallow food. At that point, gravity and peristalsis take over, moving food through the gastrointestinal (GI) tract.

Peristalsis—a series of wavelike contractions—pushes food

through the GI tract to the rectum. It's triggered by accumulating food that distends the GI tract. Increased peristalsis gives the GI tract less time to absorb fluid. The result is liquid bowel waste—either diarrhea or a loose bowel movement. The opposite occurs when peristalsis is inadequate. The GI tract absorbs more fluid, making bowel waste very solid and difficult to pass (constipation), which may lead to fecal impaction.

Among the causes of bowel incontinence are fecal impaction (liquid bowel waste leaks around the blockage and oozes from the rectum); nervous system disorders or damage to nerve pathways that control bowel movements, as in head injury; disease of the intestines, rectum, or anus; infections, such as intestinal flu and food poisoning; not enough bulk and fluid in the diet; changes in peristalsis and loss of internal sphincter muscle tone (or strength); long-term dependence on laxatives; psychological stress; and the effects of surgery.

Retraining the bladder

You can help the person you're caring for "retrain" his bladder—and correct or manage incontinence—by reestablishing a normal urination pattern.

First, keep a careful record of the person's fluid intake and urination pattern. Then schedule urination at regular intervals and gradually increase the time between urinations. The person's goal will be to urinate no more than once every 3 to 4 hours.

Step 1: Keeping a record

Do accidental urinations follow a pattern? You'll know at a glance by recording fluid intake, how the person urinated (intentionally or by accident), and why you think an accident occurred. Keep a chart like the one shown here throughout the retraining program. Also keep the training chart that follows. Record exact times and amounts. Make notations.

After a few days, your chart will show when

Date 10/17		
Time	Fluid intake	Urinated in toilet
6 to 8am	small glass of orange juice	✓
8 to 10am	2 cups of coffee	

the person is most likely to become incontinent—for example, after meals or during the night. Your chart will also help the doctor evaluate progress and adjust treatment, if necessary.

Step 2: Scheduling urination

Schedule the person for specific times to urinate. He should practice this technique at home, where he's relaxed and close to the bathroom. He can start by urinating every 2 hours, whether or not he feels the need. If he has to urinate sooner, he can practice "holding" it by relaxing, concentrating, and taking three slow, deep breaths until the urge decreases or goes away.

He should wait 5 minutes, and then go to the bathroom and urinate—even if the urge has passed. Otherwise, the next urge may be strong and difficult to control.

If the person has an accident before the 5 minutes are up, shorten the next waiting time to 3 minutes. After a week of training, if waiting 5 minutes is easy, increase the waiting time to 10 minutes.

Using the method above, gradually increase the interval between urinations. Strive for 3- or 4-hour intervals. Caution the person against being discouraged. if he does have an accident.

Tips for success

• Photocopy and use the training chart on the next page to record daily times of fluid intake and outflow.
• Set an alarm clock to remind the person when to use the toilet.
• Make sure the person can reach the bathroom or portable toilet easily.
• Urge him to walk to the bathroom slowly.
• He should always urinate just before bedtime.
• He should drink 8 to 10 eight-ounce glasses (about 2 liters) of fluid every day. This helps to prevent urinary tract infection and constipation, which also can cause incontinence. To prevent nighttime accidents, he should drink most fluids before 6 p.m.

Remember to count foods that are mostly liquid (such as ice cream, soup, and gelatin) as fluids.

TRAINING CHART

Date   Name

Time	Fluid intake	Urinated in toilet	Small or large accident	Reason for accident if known
6 to 8 a.m.				
8 to 10 a.m.				
10 a.m. to noon				
12 to 2 p.m.				
2 to 4 p.m.				
4 to 6 p.m.				
6 to 8 p.m.				
8 to 10 p.m.				
10 p.m. to midnight				
12 to 2 a.m.				
2 to 4 a.m.				
4 to 6 a.m.				

Exercising your pelvic muscles

Exercising your pelvic muscles every day can make them stronger and help to prevent incontinence. The following exercises, called Kegel exercises (named for their inventor), are easy to learn and simple to do.

If you have stress incontinence, try to do these exercises just before a sneeze or a cough. Also try to do a few exercises before you lift something heavy or cumbersome.

By exercising faithfully and correctly, you'll notice an improvement in about 4 weeks. In 3 months, you'll notice an even greater improvement. Here's how to do the exercises.

Finding the right muscle

The muscle you want to strengthen is called the pubococcygeal (PC) muscle. It controls the flow of urine. You can find this muscle in two ways:
• by voluntarily stopping a stream of urine
• by pulling in on your rectal muscle as you would to retain gas.

Once you've mastered these motions, you've mastered the exercises.

Practicing the exercises

Strengthen and tone your PC muscle by performing one of the two motions described above. Hold the muscle tight, working up to 10 seconds. Then relax the muscle for 10 seconds. Do 15 exercises in the morning, 15 in the afternoon, and 20 at night. Or exercise for about 10 minutes three times a day.

Where and when to exercise

You can do Kegel exercises almost anywhere and at any time. Most people sit in a chair or lie on a bed to do them. You can also do them standing up.

How can you remember to do these exercises? One way is to combine them with an activity you do regularly. For example, if you spend a lot of time in the car, do an exercise at every red light. Or exercise while standing in line at the grocery store or at the newsstand, while waiting for the bus or train, and especially while urinating.

Avoiding mistakes

Take time to think about which muscles you're using. If you find yourself using your abdominal, leg, or buttocks muscles, you're not performing the exercises correctly.

Here's an easy way to check yourself: Place one hand on your abdomen while you perform the exercise. Can you feel your abdomen move? If you can, you're using the wrong muscles. Or if your abdomen or back hurts after exercising, you're probably trying too hard or using abdominal or back muscles that you shouldn't be using.

If you get a headache after exercising, be careful not to tense your chest muscles or hold your breath.

Remember: These exercises should feel mild and easy—not strenuous.

Using a condom catheter

Here are some guidelines for wearing a condom catheter temporarily for urinary incontinence. This catheter fits over the penis and connects to a drainage bag that straps on one leg. You'll need to empty and clean the bag about twice a day.

Follow these steps for applying the catheter, connecting the drainage bag, removing the catheter and bag, and solving problems.

1 Wash your hands. Then gather your equipment: correct-sized condom catheter, double-sided elastic stomal tape, leg drainage bag with tubing, clamp, manicure scissors, soap, washcloth, towel, and protective ointment.

2 Trim the hairs on the shaft and at the base of the penis. That way they won't stick to the stomal tape you'll use. Before each catheter change, wash, rinse, and dry the penis. To protect the skin from urine, coat the penis with protective oint-

Leg strap

Tubing

Double-sided tape

Leg drainage bag

Condom catheter

Connector tip

Leg strap

Drainage port

ment and let the ointment dry (it'll feel sticky).

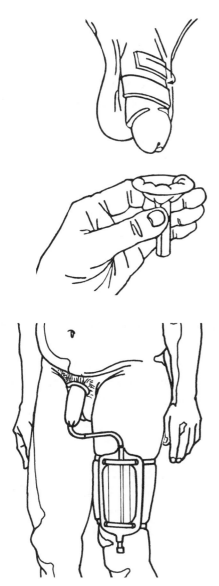

3 Now, remove the backing from both sides of the stomal tape. Place the side marked "skin side" against the penis. Starting at the penis base, spiral the tape.

Caution: Don't let the edges of the tape overlap. Don't stretch the tape or you'll wind it too tightly. And never wrap the tape in a circle around the penis—it may interfere with circulation.

4 Tightly roll the condom sheath (balloon-like part) to the edge of the connector tip. Now, place the catheter sheath on the end of the penis, leaving about $\frac{1}{2}$ inch (1.3 centimeters) of space between the tip of the penis and the connector tip.

Gently stretch the penis as you unroll the condom. When the condom is unrolled, gently press it against the penis so that it sticks to the tape.

5 Connect one end of the tubing to the connector tip and the other end to the drainage bag. Strap the drainage bag to the thigh. You can put on boxer shorts over the catheter. (Knit briefs may kink the tubing.)

6 To remove the drainage bag, clamp the tube closed. Release the leg straps, and disconnect the extension tubing at the top of the bag. Remove the condom catheter and the tape by rolling them forward.

Special instructions

• If the tape doesn't stick to the skin, make sure the penis as well as the protective ointment is completely dry.

• If the tape pulls away from the skin, you may need to apply more ointment. Also make sure the tape is snug (but not tight).

• If urine leaks when the person is wearing the catheter, squeeze the sheath to get a better seal.

• If the catheter sheath wrinkles in contact with the tape, the sheath may be too large. If so, select a smaller-sized sheath.

• Empty the drainage bag every 3 to 4 hours. Never let it fill to the top.

• Wash the drainage bag twice a day with soap and water. Rinse it with a solution of one part vinegar and seven parts water.

• Don't use the same drainage bag longer than 1 month.

• Use only ointments and adhesives prescribed by the doctor. Don't wash with povidone iodine—this can irritate skin.

• Remember to change the condom catheter every 24 hours. Make sure to thoroughly wash and dry the penis between changes.

• Check the penis every 2 hours for swelling or unusual color. If it feels uncomfortable or doesn't look normal, take off the condom catheter and call the doctor.

• Call the doctor if the person feels pain or burning when he urinates, has the urge to urinate very frequently, the urine has an unpleasant odor, or if you see blood or pus in the urine.

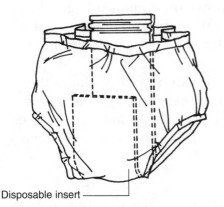

Disposable insert

Using incontinence briefs

Plastic incontinence briefs are available with either disposable or reusable liner pads. Disposable briefs, such as Depends, are also available. Used for moderate urine flow, these briefs can keep the person dry and comfortable. For intermittent dribbling, a sanitary pad designed for menstrual flow may be adequate.

When these briefs are worn, be sure to:

• frequently check the brief and change it when it's wet or soiled.

• wash the perineum (the area between the thighs) each time you change a pad, and gently dry it. Then apply a protective ointment to guard against skin irritation from contact with urine.

- continually check for signs of skin irritation.
- wash the reusable briefs and pads daily or as needed.

Bowel retraining

If the doctor recommends bowel retraining to control bowel
incontinence, here's what to do.

Establishing an individual pattern

Set a specific time for the person to have a bowel movement,
such as once a day or once every other day after breakfast or
another meal. Just remember that a daily bowel movement
isn't necessary. Every 3 days may be normal.

Adjusting the diet

To adjust diet, give the person plenty of fluids—2 to 3 quarts
(about 2.8 liters) each day. Also add high-fiber foods to the
diet. For example, serve more raw fruits and vegetables and
whole-grain breads and cereals. High-fiber foods, like the
ones listed below, can help relieve constipation and may also
help prevent intestinal cancer.

Fruit	**Vegetables**	**Whole-grain breads and cereals**
Apples	Avocado	Whole wheat bread
Apricots	Baked beans	Bran cereal
Cantaloupe	Bean sprouts	Shreddedwheat
Dates	Broccoli	Oatmeal
Figs	Brussels sprouts	Puffed wheat
Honeydew	Cabbage	
Oranges	Carrots	
Peaches	Corn	
Pears	Green beans	
Strawberries	Lima beans	
Watermelon	Peas	
	Potatoes	
Nuts	Sauerkraut	
Almonds	Squash	
Peanuts	Sweet Potatoes	
Pecans	Turnips	

Tips for success

• If necessary to ensure regularity, the doctor may order a suppository—either glycerin or bisacodyl—to be inserted about 30 minutes before the time of the scheduled bowel movement. Or if the person hasn't had a bowel movement for several days, the doctor may order an enema. *Important:* Be sure the person avoids the routine use of laxatives like suppositories and enemas because he can become dependent on them.

• Have the person use the toilet or a portable commode—not a bedpan—if possible. That way he can assume a sitting position, instead of a more recumbent position. The sitting position is more natural and lets gravity help the muscles that control a bowel movement. Respect his privacy, and encourage him to try to relax.

• Caution the person against being discouraged if accidents occur. They're normal and don't represent a failure. If needed, he can wear incontinence briefs for protection.

• Help the person take regular walks, if the doctor approves. Even walking around the room, sitting in a chair, and walking to the bathroom help stimulate peristalsis.

Performing bowel stimulation

Manual bowel stimulation is an important part of a bowel retraining program. It's done about 30 minutes after inserting a glycerin or bisacodyl (Dulcolax) suppository.

Although you may feel hesitant at first about performing this procedure, you'll feel more comfortable once you learn how. If the doctor orders bowel stimulation, follow these steps.

1 Wash your hands with soap and water and dry them, using a clean terry towel or a paper towel. Then gather the equipment you'll need: a disposable glove, water-soluble lubricant, and a towel or linen-saver pad.

2 Place the towel or linen-saver pad on your bed.

3 Put a disposable glove on your right hand (or on your left hand if you're left-handed), and lubricate your gloved index finger with a water-soluble lubricant.

4 Then lie on your left side on the towel or pad, keeping your left leg straight and your right knee drawn up toward your chest.

Note: If you're left-handed, reverse these instructions by lying on your right side with your right leg straight and your left knee drawn up.

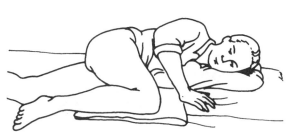

5 Insert the index finger ½ inch (1.3 to 2.5 centimers) to 1 inch into your rectum. Rotate it to stimulate the bowel.

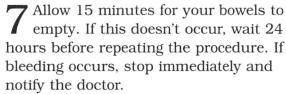

6 Then, if possible, use the toilet—not a bedpan. That way you'll be able to assume a sitting position. This position lets gravity help the muscles that control a bowel movement.

7 Allow 15 minutes for your bowels to empty. If this doesn't occur, wait 24 hours before repeating the procedure. If bleeding occurs, stop immediately and notify the doctor.

8 After the procedure, remove the glove and discard it. Then wash your hands with soap and water and dry them.

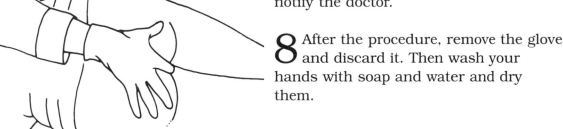

11 Pressure Ulcers

How pressure ulcers develop

Although they're called pressure ulcers (or sometimes bed-sores) and most commonly occur in older adults who are confined to bed, anyone, at any age, can develop these painful skin ulcers. They can occur on any part of a person's body and usually occur from prolonged sitting or lying in one position. This puts pressure on the skin, especially over bony areas. Being confined to bed is only one such situation. For example, a cast or splint can pinch skin and cause an ulcer, and a bedridden person in a wheelchair or an arm chair is subject to ulcer-producing pressure on his buttocks and heels.

The outermost layer of skin, the layer you see and feel, is called the epidermis. Beneath it lies the dermis, the skin layer that contains nerve receptors, blood vessels, hair follicles, and sweat and oil glands. Together the epidermis and dermis act as a waterproof membrane to protect the body against infection, prevent loss of fluids, and control temperature. So these two skin layers are essential to survival. Without them, normal body functions could not continue.

Beneath the epidermis and dermis lies a layer of fatty subcutaneous tissue that protects the underlying muscle and bone.

Each of the billions of skin cells—like all body cells—receives life-sustaining oxygen and nutrients from circulating blood. When blood vessels in the skin are compressed or stretched, skin cells don't receive nourishment and, therefore, they die. When skin cells die, they produce irritating toxins that prevent new skin formation.

The result is an opening in the skin. This opening most commonly is called a bedsore, although the nurse or doctor may call it a pressure ulcer. Whatever you call it, it's painful, slow to heal, and quick to become infected. Any of the following factors, or a combination of them, can cause pressure ulcers.

• Direct pressure from body weight pressing skin against a surface long enough to slow or stop blood flow in the area. If the surface is hard, and particularly if pressure occurs over a thin-skinned bony area, chances are good that a bedsore will develop.

• Shearing force from pulling or stretching skin to the point where blood supply to the area is interrupted. A person who's bedridden, for instance, may develop ulcers from slowly sliding downward from a sitting position.

• Friction from dragging skin across a rough surface. Example: A person pulling across rough or wrinkled sheets may irritate his skin and cause an ulcer to develop. Special equipment, such as a body brace or traction device, can also create ulcers by producing friction.

• Chemical irritation from contact with urine- or sweat-soaked sheets or clothing or from lying or sitting in urine or feces.

Other factors that contribute to the development of pressure ulcers include poor health, poor nutrition, poor circulation, diabetes, skin dryness, and paralysis or extreme muscle weakness.

Pressure ulcer sites
The labels in each of the following four common body positions identify specific locations where pressure ulcers are likely to develop if the conditions cited above exist.

Side-lying position

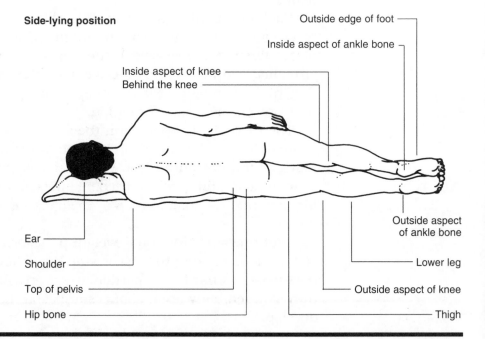

Outside edge of foot

Inside aspect of ankle bone

Inside aspect of knee
Behind the knee

Outside aspect of ankle bone

Ear

Shoulder

Top of pelvis

Lower leg

Outside aspect of knee

Hip bone

Thigh

Prone position (lying on stomach)

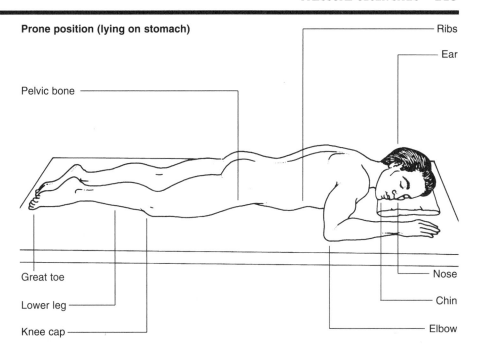

Ribs

Ear

Pelvic bone

Great toe

Lower leg

Knee cap

Nose

Chin

Elbow

Supine position (lying on the back)

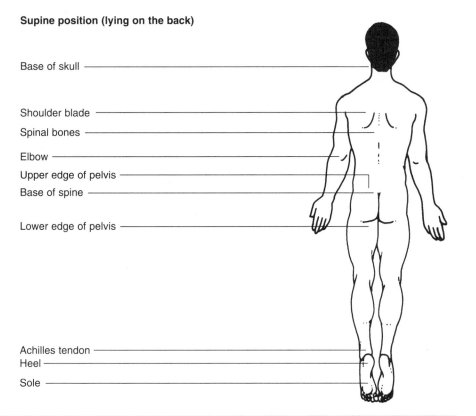

Base of skull

Shoulder blade

Spinal bones

Elbow

Upper edge of pelvis

Base of spine

Lower edge of pelvis

Achilles tendon

Heel

Sole

Sitting position

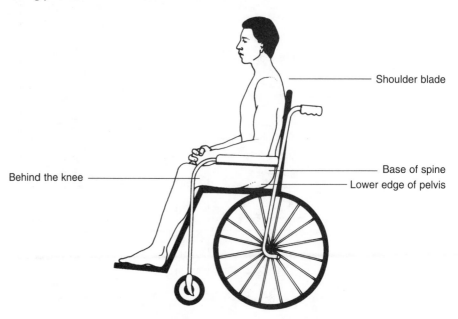

Shoulder blade

Base of spine

Lower edge of pelvis

Behind the knee

Inspect the skin for dry or irritated patches and for superficial breaks. A reddened area over a bony prominence or a pale area that remains pale even after you've massaged it and changed position may be a pressure ulcer in an early stage.

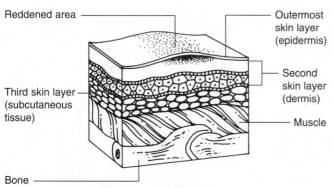

Reddened area

Outermost skin layer (epidermis)

Second skin layer (dermis)

Third skin layer (subcutaneous tissue)

Muscle

Bone

Identifying the stages of pressure ulcers

Four stages of pressure ulcers are characterized by changes in the skin. Inspect the skin of the person you're caring for daily for changes, and contact the doctor immediately if you spot a new ulcer or enlargement or signs of infection in an existing ulcer.

Stage 1

The skin stays red for 5 minutes after pressure is removed, and an abrasion or brush burn may develop. (Very dark or

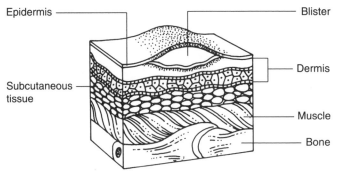

Epidermis — Blister

Subcutaneous tissue — Dermis

— Muscle

— Bone

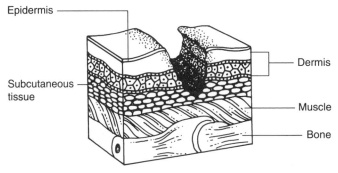

Epidermis —

Subcutaneous tissue — Dermis

— Muscle

— Bone

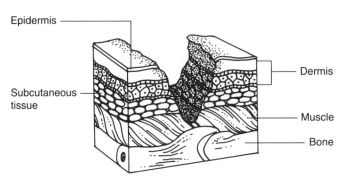

Epidermis —

Subcutaneous tissue — Dermis

— Muscle

— Bone

black skin may look purple.) The skin also feels warm and firm. The ulcer usually is reversible at this stage if pressure is relieved.

Stage 2
Breaks appear in the skin, and discoloration may occur. The ulcer has penetrated the skin's fat layer. It is painful and may be visibly swollen. If pressure is relieved, the ulcer may heal in 1 to 2 weeks.

Stage 3
A hole develops, and foul-smelling yellow or green fluid oozes from it. A black, leathery crust or eschar may form at the ulcer's edges and, eventually, at the center and may extend into the muscle. The ulcer isn't painful, but healing may take months.

Stage 4
The ulcer can destroy tissue from the skin to the bone. You'll notice foul-smelling drainage and deep tunnels that extend from the ulcer. It make take months or even a year for the ulcer to heal.

Using a pressure ulcer record sheet
Use the following chart to remind you to check the skin daily for pressure ulcers. They may develop at spots where bones are prominent and close to the skin, such as at the elbow, shoulder, hip, knee, or ankle.

Every day mark the block for each body site with N

(normal), R (red), or M (moist). If you think that an ulcer is developing, contact the doctor.

Also use this chart to keep track of the treatments and prevention techniques you're using, including skin care, exercise, and diet.

Pressure ulcer record

Name

Date												

Skin Inspection

Back of head												
Left side of head												
Right side of head												
Rim of left ear												
Rim of right ear												
Left shoulder												
Right shoulder												
Left elbow												
Right elbow												
Left side of middle back												
Right side of middle back												
Left hip												
Right hip												
Front of left knee												
Front of right knee												
Inner left knee												
Inner right knee												
Outer left knee												
Outer right knee												

Pressure ulcer record *continued*

Date													

Skin Inspection — *continued*

Inner left ankle													
Inner right ankle													
Outer left ankle													
Outer right ankle													
Left heel													
Right heel													
Tailbone area													

Skin Care

Pressure relief device used (Yes, No)													
Skin massage with lotion (Yes, No)													
Treatment as ordered (Yes, No)													

Exercise

Number of times out of bed													
Number of times turned while in bed													
Range-of-motion exercises performed (Yes, No)													

Diet (for each meal, indicate the percentage of food served that was actually eaten—100%, 75%, 50%, less than 50%)

Breakfast													
Lunch													
Dinner													

Caring for the skin

Follow these basic guidelines to keep the skin of the person you're caring for healthy.

• Keep the skin clean and dry at all times, and make sure only dry clothing and bed linens touch the skin.

• Don't use harsh alkali soaps, alcohol-based products such as witch hazel and astringents, tincture of benzoin, or hexachlorophene. (Be sure to read product labels to find out if a product contains these irritants.)

• Massage the person's skin regularly with lotion to keep it flexible and less likely to crack.

• Encourage activity and exercises to increase blood circulation to the hands and feet.

• Keep sheets and other bed linen dry and wrinkle-free.

• If the person is overweight, dry the skin inside fat folds by directing a hand-held hair dryer over the area while you hold the skin folds apart.

Special devices are available that help to relieve pressure and promote healthy skin in people who are bedridden (see "Pressure-relief devices," in Chapter 6, Hospital Beds).

Using a turning schedule

When the person in your care must stay in bed, proper positioning and frequent turning help to prevent and treat pressure ulcers. Frequent turning relieves skin pressure and irritation, promotes comfort, and stimulates blood circulation (For more information about how to reposition a person in bed, see also Chapter 5, Comfort Measures.)

If he can, the person should turn himself. But if he can't, he'll need your help.

Turning schedule

As ordered, turn and reposition the person every 2 hours, first on one side and then on his back, stomach, and other side.

Adjust the schedule for comfortable positioning to coincide with the person's activities, such as positioning him on his back when he eats.

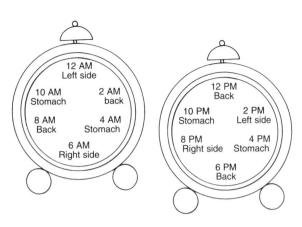

12 AM
Left side

10 AM
Stomach

2 AM
back

8 AM
Back

4 AM
Stomach

6 AM
Right side

12 PM
Back

10 PM
Stomach

2 PM
Left side

8 PM
Right side

4 PM
Stomach

6 PM
Back

Use two clocks, as shown here, to remind you which position to use.

Changing your position in a wheelchair

Sitting for a long time in a wheelchair can cause pressure uclers. By shifting your weight and doing push-ups, you can relieve pressure on the contact points and prevent pressure ulcers.

Shifting your weight

A wheelchair is much more confining than a bed, so you have fewer options for changing your position. But you should try (or ask your caregiver) to shift your weight from buttock to buttock at least once every hour. When you shift your weight to one buttock, hold the position for 1 minute and then shift to the other buttock and hold for 1 minute.

Doing push-ups

If you can move your arms, try these wheelchair push-ups. Grip the arms of the chair and push down hard with your hands and arms to try to raise your upper body off the seat. If you can, use this same technique to shift your weight.

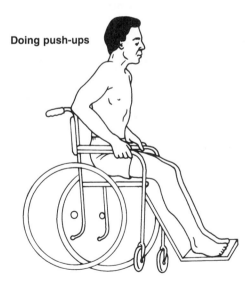

Doing push-ups

Treating pressure ulcers

Depending on the stage of the ulcer, the doctor will order specific treatment. Stage 1 treatments prevent skin breakdown and improve circulation. Stage 2 treatments, used with stage 1 treatments, prevent further skin damage. Those at stages 3 and 4 treat and prevent infection and remove dead tissue.

Stage 1 treatments
Lubricants
Lubricants increase tissue pliability and stimulate blood circulation. Massage the lotion *gently* over the affected area. Vigorous massage can further damage skin.
Clear plastic dressings (transparent film dressing)
This type of dressing adheres to the skin, protecting it against friction. Permeable to moisture vapor, it allows oxygen to enter but keeps germs and water out. If you have trouble securing the dressing in a moist area, dry the area first with a hair dryer, set on low.
Gelatin-type wafers
These wafers promote healing and protect the skin.
Whirlpool baths
Besides cleaning the skin, whirlpool baths stimulate blood circulation. Don't use a whirlpool bath too frequently because it may dry the skin.

Stage 2 treatments
Normal saline solution or water
Normal saline solution or water cleans the ulcer and prevents infection. Clean the ulcer gently to avoid further skin damage.
Hydrogen peroxide
A 25% solution of hydrogen peroxide cleans the ulcer, removes debris, and prevents infection. Follow this cleaning with a saline rinse.

Stages 3 and 4 treatments
Hydrogen peroxide
A 50% solution of hydrogen peroxide cleans the ulcer, acts as an antibacterial agent, and brings dead tissue to the surface. Follow cleaning with a normal saline rinse.
Povidone iodine
A 50% solution of povidone iodine cleans the ulcer and fights infection. Don't use this treatment if the patient is allergic to iodine.
Granular absorbent dressing
This treatment draws drainage from the ulcer. Apply the powder form directly to the ulcer. Don't use this treatment on a healing ulcer because it may damage new tissue.

Gel-like absorbent

This dressing liquefies on contact with drainage, which helps draw exudate from the ulcer.

Enzymatic ointment

Enzymatic ointment breaks down dead tissue to aid drainage.

Healing gel or ointment

This treatment encourages new cell formation.

Sodium chloride–impregnated dressing

This treatment and dressing clean deep or infected ulcers by drawing drainage, debris, and bacteria from the ulcer, while maintaining a moist environment that promotes healing. Secure this dressing with hypoallergenic tape.

Gauze dressings

Gauze adheres to dead tissue, removing it along with the old dressing. Avoid nonstick dressings because they won't adhere to and remove dead tissue.

Wet-to-dry dressings

When making a wet-to-dry dressing, soak gauze in a normal saline solution or an antiseptic solution. As the dressing dries, it adheres to the ulcer. When the dressing is removed, debris comes with it. (For specific information about appropriate dressings, see Chapter 12, Dressings and Bandages.)

Other therapies include concentrated oxygen treatments to promote wound healing.

12 Dressings and Bandages

Learning about dressings and bandages

If the person you're caring for has a wound, you'll need to know about the uses and types of dressings. A dressing may be used to:

- control bleeding
- absorb wound drainage
- protect the wound from germs
- keep wound germs from spreading
- protect the wound from further damage.

Three major types of dressing are used:

- standard gauze pad, which commonly comes in four sizes: 2 inches by 2 inches, 2 inches by 3 inches, 4 inches by 4 inches, and 4 inches by 8 inches (5 centimeters by 5 centimeters to 10.2 centimeters by 20.3 centimeters)
- nonadhering gauze pad, which comes in the same sizes as the standard pad but is coated on one side with a shiny material that prevents it from sticking to wounds
- thick surgical dressing, which can absorb more than the other dressing types because it's larger and has more bulk. It's usually used with the smaller pads.

The doctor or nurse will tell you which type of dressing pad to use, how often to change it, and what to use to hold it in place: tape made of adhesive, elastic, paper, or clear plastic; Montgomery straps; or bandages and binders.

Before you change a dressing, review these special precautions.

- Dressings (or other supplies) that are stored, applied, or discarded carelessly are potential sources of infection. That's why you need to take every precaution to keep the dressing materials as well as the wound germ-free.
- Before you open or use sterile supplies, check the packaging for holes, tears, and punctures. If you see any, discard the package and select a new one—and give it the same check.
- Check the expiration date on all supplies and equipment. If the expiration date on an item has passed, don't use the item.
- Before every dressing change, wash your hands with soap and water or an antimicrobial cleaning agent and dry them with a fresh paper towel.
- Put on sterile gloves before touching a dressing that has

drainage on it.
• Place all soiled dressings and disposable equipment in a plastic bag. Then discard the bag.
• Whenever possible, use single-use containers of solution and ointment.

Cleaning a wound and applying a dry, sterile dressing

Follow this step-by-step guide to cleaning, treating, and dressing a wound.

Assemble the equipment

Gather the equipment: dressings (gauze pads or transparent adhesive dressings are most common), scissors, hypoallergenic tape, a cleaning solution (such as peroxide or povidone-iodine solution), antibacterial ointment (if ordered), two bowls in which to pour the cleaning solution, gloves (sterile and clean), disposable plastic bags, and baby oil.

Have the new dressing ready before you remove the old one. Cut strips of hypoallergenic tape in advance, too. Pour boiling water into the bowls to sterilize them, and then discard the water. Then pour sterile water into one bowl and the cleaning solution into the other bowl.

Position the person so that you can reach the bowl easily.

Remove the old dressing

Wash your hands thoroughly. Carefully remove the tape from the person's skin. If this is painful, moisten the tape with baby oil before you attempt to remove it. If the skin under the tape is inflamed, don't apply the new tape there. Remove the old dressing, but don't touch any part of it that touched the wound (if the dressing is wet with drainage, put on clean gloves before removing it). Write down the amount and color of any drainage on the dressing (estimate the amount of drainage based on something familiar—for example, drainage the size of a quarter).

Fold the dressing's edges together, place it (and gloves, if worn) in a disposable bag, and close the bag.

Check the wound

Inspect the wound for—signs of infection, swelling, redness, and drainage, including pus. Is the wound healing?

Does the wound appear to be infected, healing, or unchanged since the last dressing change? Write down what you see. Do this every time you change the dressing. Don't touch the wound.

Put on sterile gloves

Remove all hand jewelry and wash your hands thoroughly before touching the sterile gloves. Start with the glove for the hand you use most often. Grasp its cuff with your thumb and forefinger, and lift it from its wrapper. Be careful to touch only the inside of the glove (to keep the outside surface sterile). Now, slip it on.

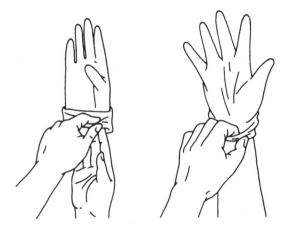

Pick up the second glove by slipping your gloved fingers under its cuff, touching the outside (sterile side) of the glove.

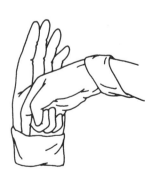

Pull on the second glove.

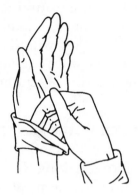

Clean the wound

Saturate a gauze pad with the prescribed cleaning solution. Now, lightly scrub both the wound and the area around it.

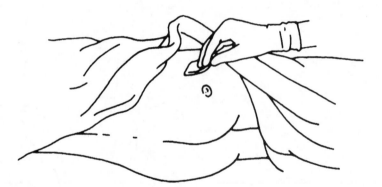

Place a catch basin under the wound, and saturate a second gauze pad with sterile water. Wring it out over the wound.

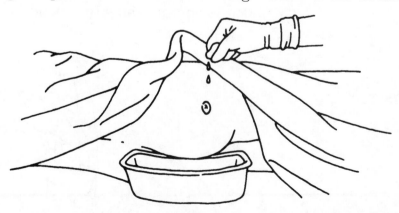

Use another gauze pad to gently blot dry the wound and the skin around it. Discard all pads in a disposable bag.

Put on the new dressing

If you're applying a gauze dressing, be careful not to touch any area of it that will touch the wound. If the doctor has ordered it, squeeze antibacterial ointment onto the dressing before applying it. Tape the dressing securely in place.

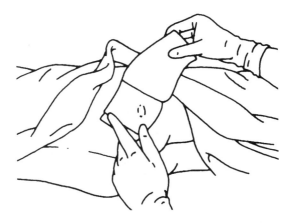

Dress the wound with a drain

1 If the wound has a drain, take two gauze pads and cut halfway through them. Place one of the cut pads around the drainage tube. Place the other cut pad around the drainage tube from the other direction, so that the pads overlap and surround the tube.

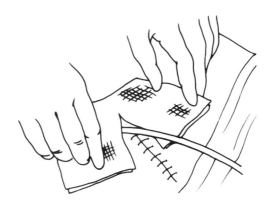

2 Layer more gauze dressing pads around the drain to collect the drainage, cover the wound with gauze or a surgical dressing, and tape in place.

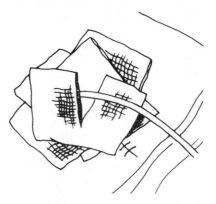

3 If you're applying a transparent adhesive dressing, take the packet it comes in and remove part of the protective paper. Then use your thumb to press that part of the dressing onto the skin near the wound. Peel the remainder of the paper off the dressing, and smooth it over the wound and the surrounding skin.

Press down all four sides of the dressing to prevent leakage.

After you've finished applying the dressing, remove your gloves, discard them in a disposable bag, seal the bag, and wash your hands thoroughly.

Protecting the bed

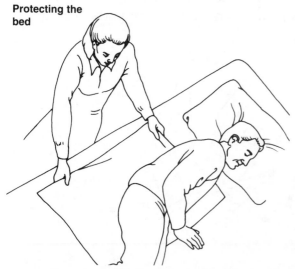

Changing a wet dressing

The doctor may instruct you to wet the dressing before applying it (this type of dressing is also called a compress). Use the same procedure as for applying a dry, sterile dressing with the following added steps.

1 If the person's in bed, protect the sheets with towels or a plastic bag before you start changing the dressing.

2 Soak the new dressing for a few minutes in a bowl filled with sterile water or the medicated solution the doctor has ordered. Lukewarm water that's been boiled for 5 minutes to make it sterile and then cooled is most commonly used. If you use this method to soak the pads, make the bowl germ-free, too. To do this, wash and rinse the bowl well and then immerse it in boiling water for 5 minutes.

Securing the dressing

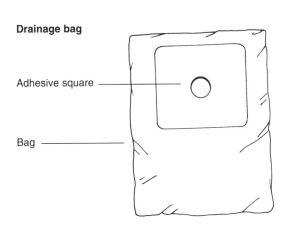

3 After applying the dressing, cover it with a surgical dressing to keep the person's clothes and bedding dry. Then secure it with tape or Montgomery straps (see *Using Montgomery Straps* later in this chapter).

Using a drainage bag

The doctor may instruct you to apply a drainage bag or pouch to a wound that's producing a large amount of drainage. The bag collects the excess drainage.

Drainage bag

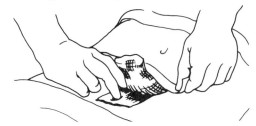

Adhesive square

Bag

1 You'll need just two items:
• a drainage bag (you'll probably use a temporary colostomy bag) that has an attached adhesive square for applying it to the person's skin
• a supply of skin-barrier (protective) solution that you'll brush, wipe, or spray around the drain to protect the skin under the adhesive square.

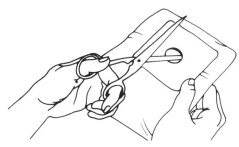

2 If the adhesive square on the bag isn't already cut to fit, you'll need to measure the wound and cut an opening in the adhesive square. *Note:* Make the opening no more than $\frac{1}{8}$ inch (3 millimeters) larger than the wound. Otherwise, the seal will be too loose.

3 Apply the skin barrier to the skin around the wound. Don't apply it directly to the wound.

4 Peel off the adhesive square's cover. Center the square over the wound, and then apply it and the bag in the centered position.

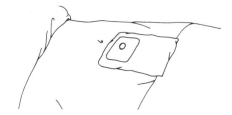

Applying a wet-to-dry dressing

Wet-to-dry dressings can help relieve flare-ups of dermatitis; soothe inflammation, itching, and burning; remove crusting and scales from dry lesions; and help dry up oozing lesions.

What's more, using these dressings may prevent such complications as bacterial and fungal infections. You can apply the dressings in four steps. Here's how.

1 Moisten a piece of gauze or a soft, clean cloth with warm tap water, normal saline solution, or Burow's solution. Squeeze out the excess moisture. Don't squeeze the gauze or cloth completely dry; it should still make a squishy sound when gently squeezed.

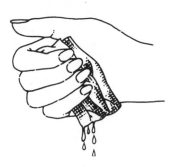

2 Apply the wet dressing to the affected area, making sure you cover all of it.

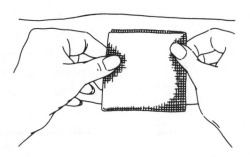

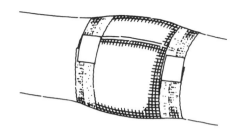

3 Cover the wet dressing with a dry dressing. Hold the dry dressing in place with dry roller gauze or pin a towel to hold the dressing in place. Allow the dressing to air-dry.

4 Remove the dressing without remoistening it. Repeat the entire procedure, changing the dressing material every 24 hours or more as ordered by the doctor.

Applying a special wound-cleaning agent

Follow these steps to apply a special wound-cleaning agent.

1 You'll need several 4-inch by 4-inch (10.2-centimeter by 10.2-centimeter) sterile gauze pads, a 5-inch by 9-inch (12.7-centimeter by 22.9-centimeter) sterile dressing, hypoallergenic tape, linen-saver pads, an irrigation syringe, irrigating solution (usually sterile water) and a container to pour it into, a container to catch irrigation runoff, a wound-cleaning agent (beads or paste) prepared as directed, sterile disposable gloves, and a disposable bag.

2 Remove the old dressing, and check it for drainage. Then fold its sides together with the soiled side in, and discard it in the disposable bag. Carefully inspect the wound for signs of infection: redness, swelling, or yellowish-white drainage. Don't touch the wound. Write down a description of the wound, including the color and amount of any drainage.

3 Pour the irrigating solution into its container, and wash your hands. Draw about 1 ounce (30 milliliters) of the solution into a bulb syringe or a large syringe with a plunger.
After placing the irrigation-runoff container against the skin below the base of the wound, hold the irrigation syringe with its tip about 2 inches (5 centimeters) from the wound and squirt all the solution into the wound. Be sure to remove all the old paste and debris from the wound; if necessary, irrigate the wound again. Don't touch the wound with the syringe tip or the syringe will become contaminated and un-

Irrigating the wound

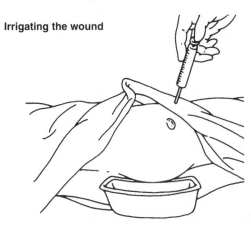

usable for future dressing changes.

Put on the sterile gloves. Then wrap a sterile gauze pad around your finger and gently pat dry the area around the wound. Leave the wound moist to stimulate the action of the beads or paste. Then discard the pad in the disposable bag.

4 If you're using wound-cleaning paste, apply it with a sterile gauze pad into the wound—at least $\frac{1}{4}$ inch (6 millimeters) deep. If you're using wound-cleaning beads, pour the beads into the wound at least $\frac{1}{4}$ inch (6 millimeters) deep.

Cover the wound with a sterile dressing. Tape down the dressing on all four sides. Finally, remove the sterile gloves, discard them in the disposable bag, and wash your hands thoroughly.

Check every 8 hours to see if the wound-cleaning agent has changed color. If it has, remove the beads or paste by irrigating again. If it hasn't, change the beads or paste every 12 hours.

Using Montgomery straps

If the person in your care has sensitive skin that's irritated by the tape used to apply dressings or if he has a large dressing that requires frequent changing, you may want to make one or more Montgomery straps to use in place of tape. Although making the straps takes a little time, you'll find that they make dressing changes easier for you and less painful for the person you're caring for.

1 You'll need to gather:
• 2-inch (5-centimeter) wide nonallergenic tape
• twill tape (available at most fabric stores)
• scissors
• skin-barrier protective solution.

Cutting a small hole in the tape

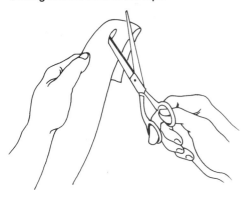

Applying tabbed strips

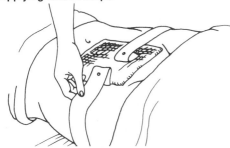

Running twill tape through the tabs

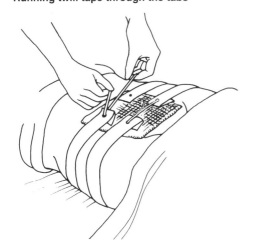

2 Cut a strip of nonallergenic tape at least 4 inches (10.2 centimeters) longer than you'd normally need to tape down the dressing.

3 Fold one end of the tape back on itself, sticky sides together, to form about a 2-inch (5-centimeter) tab.

Cut a small hole in the center of the tab. Then make at least three more of these tabbed strips of tape.

4 Apply the dressing to the wound. Then use the skin-barrier wipes or solution on the skin around the dressing where you'll be applying the tabbed adhesive strips.

5 Apply one of the tabbed strips to the skin so that the tabbed part falls almost halfway across the dressing.

Now, apply another tabbed strip to the skin so that the tabbed part is about 1 inch (2.5 centimeters) away from the tab of the strip you've already applied.

6 Next, cut a piece of twill tape long enough to double back through the holes of both tabs.

Run the twill tape through the tabs, and tie the ends of the twill tape together. This is the Montgomery strap. Now, when you have to change the dressing, you can simply untie the tabbed strips. You don't have to use tape.

Make and apply as many Montgomery straps as you need. Replace the tabbed strips when they become soiled or loose.

Using bandages

If the person in your care needs a bandage, you'll need to know more about their uses and types.

A bandage may be used for one or more of the following reasons:
- to keep a dressing or splint in place
- to limit motion
- to apply pressure
- to provide support.

Many types of bandage are used. Some have names that describe their appearance or what they're made of, such as the elastic and gauze bandages shown below. Other bandages take their names from their shapes, such as the triangular bandage, the straight binder, and the many-tailed binder.

Some bandages, such as adhesive strips, combine a dressing with the bandage.

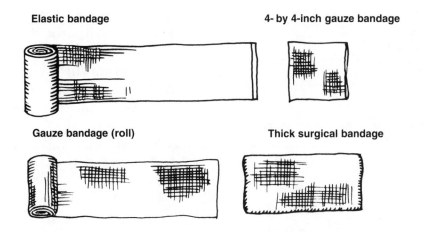

Elastic bandage

4- by 4-inch gauze bandage

Gauze bandage (roll)

Thick surgical bandage

Applying a gauze bandage

Gauze bandage is made of lightweight woven cotton in such a way that it stretches and molds to the shape of the body. It's also called roller gauze or woven gauze.

Gauze bandage usually comes in rolls 1 inch to 3 inches

Beginning the wrap

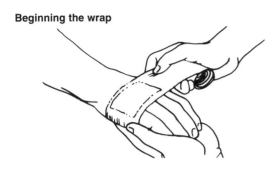

Making figure-eight turns

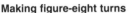

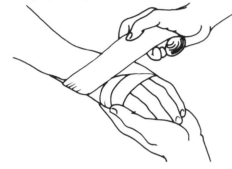

Making circle turns

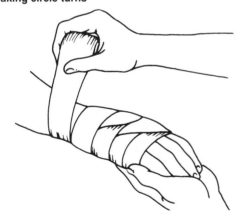

(2.5 centimeters to 7.6 centimeters) wide. Although the procedure shown here applies a gauze bandage to the hand, you can wrap any part of the body the same way. The width of the gauze bandage you use depends on the size, condition, and location of the wound as well as the amount of drainage present.

1 With one hand, hold the loose end of the gauze roll just below the person's knuckles. With your other hand, pass the roll around the hand twice to secure the bandage.

2 Angle the bandage to begin making a figure-eight turn. Then pass the roll under the wrist and back up toward the fingers to complete the figure-eight turn. Repeat until the wrist is covered.

3 Finish wrapping the hand by passing the roll around the wrist and circling up the forearm several times. Finally, secure the end of the bandage with adhesive tape.

Applying an elastic bandage

An elastic bandage compresses the tissues around a sprain or strain to help prevent swelling and provide support. The directions below explain how to wrap an elastic bandage around an ankle. You can modify them for wrapping your knee, wrist, elbow, or hand.

1 With one hand, hold the loose end of the elastic bandage on the top of your foot between your instep and toes. With the other hand, wrap the bandage twice around your foot, gradually moving toward your ankle. Make sure to overlap the bandage in a spiral manner.

Overlapping the bandage

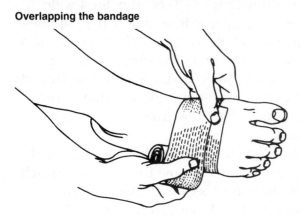

2 After wrapping your foot twice, move your hand to support your heel. Use your other hand to wrap the bandage in a figure-eight manner, leaving the heel uncovered.

To do this, angle the bandage up, cross it over the foot, and pass it behind the ankle. Next, angle the bandage down, cross it over the top of the foot, and pass it under the foot to complete the figure-eight turn. Do this step twice.

3 Now, circle the bandage around your calf, moving toward your knee. Overlap the elastic as you wrap. Stop just below the knee. Don't wrap downward. Secure the end of the bandage with a metal clip or adhesive tape.

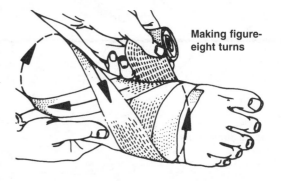

Making figure-eight turns

Comfort and safety tips

Aim for a snug—not tight—fit. Never wrap the bandage so tightly

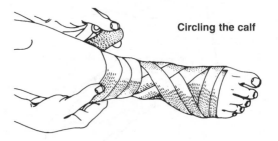

Circling the calf

that it restricts or cuts off your circulation. If you're stretching the bandage material, chances are you're wrapping it too tightly.

Promote circulation by removing and rewrapping the bandage at least twice daily.

Remove the bandage immediately if you experience numbness or tingling. When these symptoms disappear, you can reapply the bandage. If the numbness or tingling doesn't subside, call the doctor.

Applying a sling

The doctor wants the person you're caring for to wear a sling (also called a triangular bandage) temporarily to support and rest his sore shoulder. Ask the doctor when and how often the person can remove the sling. Follow these directions to help the person put on the sling.

1 A sling looks like a triangular scarf. Place the triangle's center point at the elbow of the affected arm. The longest side of the triangle should be parallel to the person's body.

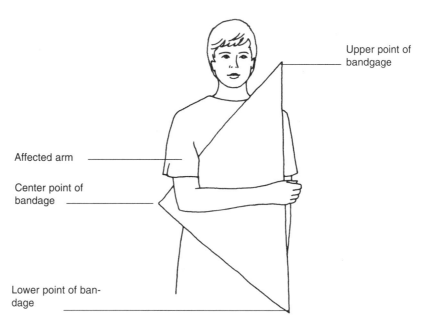

Upper point of bandgage

Affected arm

Center point of bandage

Lower point of bandage

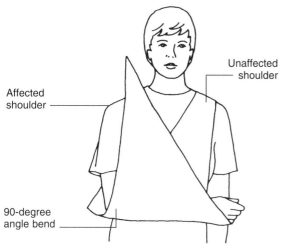

Affected shoulder

Unaffected shoulder

90-degree angle bend

2 Drape the upper point over the unaffected shoulder. Help the person bend the elbow of his affected arm at a 90-degree angle, with his thumb pointing up. Place the lower point of the triangle over the affected shoulder, enclosing the forearm in the sling.

3 Now, knot the two ends of the sling loosely around his neck. Always position the knot to the side—never in the back of his neck. To keep the knot securely in place and to prevent skin irritation, place the sling outside his collar or insert a gauze pad under the knot.

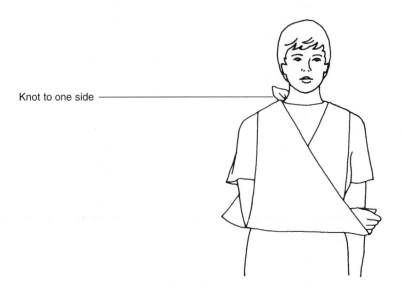

Knot to one side

4 If the knot is uncomfortable, pin each point to the opposite side. Make sure that the edge of the sling extends to the first joint of the little finger. This holds the wrist in line with the arm to prevent wrist damage. Now, use a safety pin to fasten the overflap at the elbow to the sling fabric. This will keep the sling from falling off.

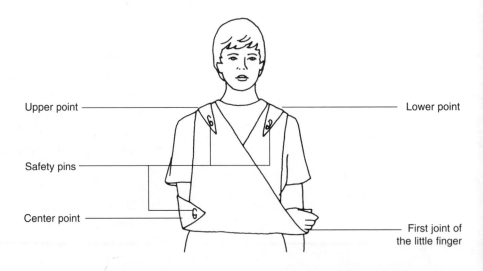

Upper point

Lower point

Safety pins

Center point

First joint of the little finger

Applying an abdominal binder

The abdominal binder (also called a straight binder) is a rectangular bandage about 12 inches wide (30.5 centimeters) and long enough to wrap around a person's stomach with a few inches to spare. It's used to provide chest, abdomen, or groin support after surgery or to keep a dressing in place. A straight binder may also be used as a replacement for tape if the person's skin is too sensitive for taping.

1 Place the binder around the person's stomach. Make sure the binder's ends overlap for a secure fit.

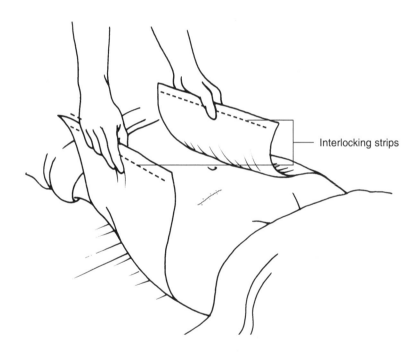

Interlocking strips

2 To secure the binder, start at the lower edge and work upward, pressing the interlocking strips together. Then check the binder to make sure it's not too tight. You can tell that the snugness is right when you can fit one finger between the top of the binder and the person's skin.

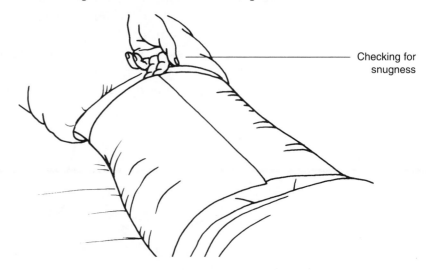

Checking for snugness

When to call the doctor

If you note any of the following changes, call the doctor immediately.

• The wound begins to bleed.
• A stitch (also called a suture) breaks.
• The wound's edges appear to be separating.
• The wound begins to drain more fluid or pus than the doctor told you to expect.
• The drainage color changes and appears white or green.
• The area around the wound is red or swollen.
• The size of the wound increases.
• Pain increases at or near the wound.
• The person with the wound develops a fever.

13   Crutches and Canes

Choosing crutches

The doctor wants you to use crutches to reduce the amount of weight you put on your injured leg or foot or to avoid putting any weight on it. Using crutches helps to speed healing by taking pressure off the injured bone as you stand and walk.

Your crutches should come with rubber tips to prevent slipping and with padded underarm and hand supports to prevent injury. Also, they need to be fitted just for you. When you use the crutches, remember to support your weight on your hands, not your underarms.

Before you select a pair of crutches, put them to the test. Ask yourself these questions to determine if you've found the right ones.

Are the crutches in good condition?

Make sure that your crutches have rubber tips to prevent sliding. Also make sure they have padded underarm pieces for comfort.

Are they the right size?

Stand with your crutches, and place their tips about 6 inches (15 centimeters) from the sides of your feet. Check to see if the underarm pieces come to about 1 to $1\frac{1}{2}$ inches (roughly 2 fingerwidths or 2.5 to 3.8 centimeters) below your armpits. If the underarm pieces touch your armpits, the crutches are too long. Ask the doctor to shorten them. Remember, you should support your weight with the handgrips, not the crutch tops.

Do they cause problems?

Support yourself by distributing your weight on your hands, wrists, and arms. If you experience tingling or numbness in the side of your chest below your armpits or in your upper arms, you're probably using the crutches incorrectly—or you may need to adjust their size or fit. For either problem, notify the doctor.

Be careful to use your crutches correctly. Otherwise, they may damage the nerves in your armpits or palms.

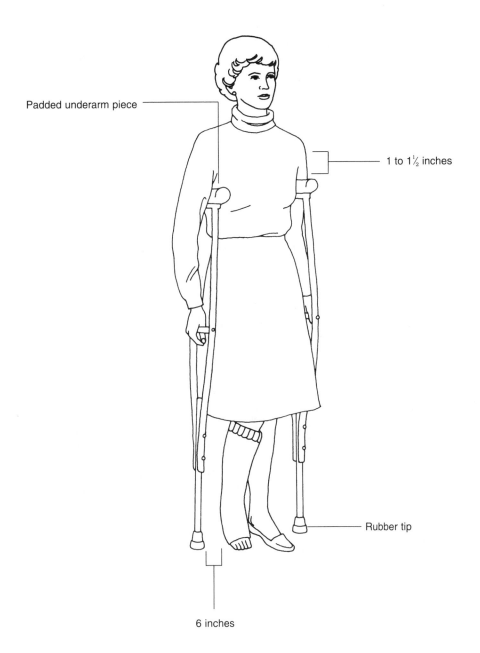

Padded underarm piece

1 to 1½ inches

Rubber tip

6 inches

Learning to walk with crutches

Learning to walk with crutches requires time and patience. You'll use one of the techniques described below.

Crutch-walking with partial weight on your injured leg

The doctor may allow you to place some of your weight on the injured leg. The diagrams below show you how to walk with crutches if your right leg is injured. The foot and crutch patterns duplicate your stance. (If your left leg is injured, place most of your weight on your right leg, and adapt the instructions.)

1 Stand straight with your shoulders relaxed and your arms slightly bent. Lean your body slightly forward, distributing your weight between the crutches and your uninjured leg. You can put some weight on your injured leg (shown as the darkened footprint).

2 Move the crutches forward. Then move your injured leg up to meet them.

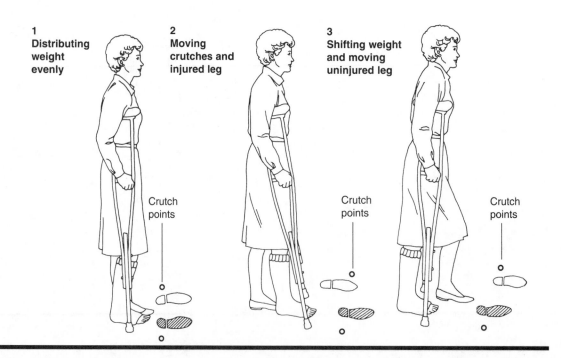

1
Distributing weight evenly

Crutch points

2
Moving crutches and injured leg

Crutch points

3
Shifting weight and moving uninjured leg

Crutch points

3 Put some weight on your injured leg as you move your uninjured leg ahead of the crutches. Repeat these steps to keep walking.

Crutch-walking with no weight on your injured leg

The step patterns below show how to walk with crutches if your left leg is injured and you can't put weight on it. (If your right leg is injured, rest your weight on your left leg, and adapt the instructions. You may want to draw the step patterns for yourself.)

1 Stand straight with all your weight on your uninjured leg. Relax your shoulders. Hold the foot of your injured leg off the floor, flexing your knee slightly.

Balancing all your weight on the crutches, position the uninjured leg's foot so that it's even with the crutch tips, slightly in front of you. Use the uninjured leg and the crutches to support your weight as you lean your body slightly forward.

2 Shift all your weight to the uninjured leg, and move the crutches forward together, swinging the injured leg along with them. Don't put any weight on your injured leg.

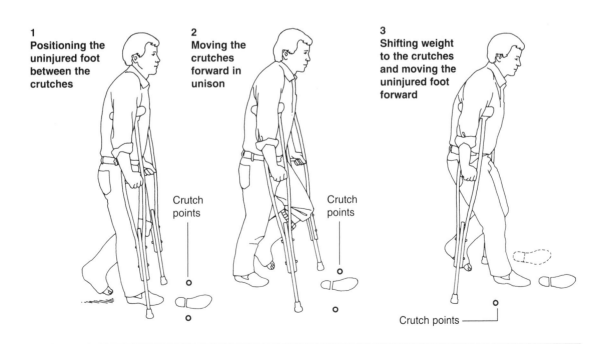

1
Positioning the uninjured foot between the crutches

Crutch points

2
Moving the crutches forward in unison

Crutch points

3
Shifting weight to the crutches and moving the uninjured foot forward

Crutch points

**Preparing to
climb stairs**

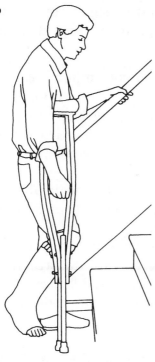

3 Now, shift all your weight back to the crutches by way of your hands and wrists, swing your uninjured leg forward, and again, place all your weight on this leg, using the crutches to keep your balance.

To keep walking, repeat steps 2 and 3.

Using crutches on stairs

Climbing stairs and getting into and out of a chair with your crutches may seem hard. Put yourself at ease, and do these maneuvers slowly at first. The following guidelines will help.

How to climb stairs

If the banister is on your left side and your right leg is injured, follow the directions below.

1 Standing at the bottom of the stairs, shift both crutches to your right hand. Then grasp the banister firmly with your left hand. Using your right hand, carefully support your weight on the crutches.

**Hopping onto
the first step**

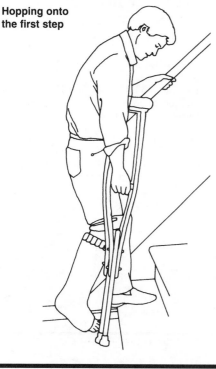

2 Next, push down on your crutches and hop onto the first step, using just your uninjured leg. Lift your injured leg as you go.

Support your weight on that leg as you continue to grasp the banister tightly. Then swing the crutches up onto the first step. Now, hop onto the second step, using your uninjured leg. Repeat this procedure, but go slowly.

To get down the stairs, reverse these maneuvers. But always advance the crutches and your injured leg first. Remember: Your strong leg goes up first and comes down last.

Getting into and out of a chair using crutches

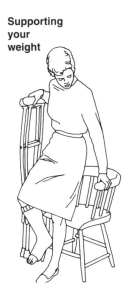

Supporting your weight

How to sit down

1 Using your crutches, walk over to the chair. Turn around, and step backward until the back of your uninjured leg touches the chair's front edge.

2 Keeping your weight on your uninjured leg, transfer both crutches to the hand on the same side as your injured leg. Support most of your weight on your crutches. Next, reach back with your other hand and grasp the chair arm.

3 Carefully sit down, making sure to keep your weight off your injured leg. Keep your crutches next to the chair.

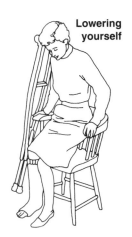

Lowering yourself

How to get up

Preparing to get up

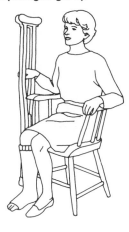

1 Move your uninjured leg backward until it touches the back of the chair's front edge. While you're still sitting, take the crutches and stand them upright.

2 Using the hand on the same side as your injured leg, hold onto the handgrips. With your other hand, hold onto the chair arm.

3 Slide forward, with your uninjured leg slightly under the
chair. Push yourself up onto your
uninjured leg. Once you're standing,
transfer a crutch to your uninjured
side. Or push yourself up while
grasping the handgrip of a crutch in
each hand.

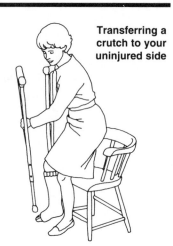

Transferring a crutch to your uninjured side

Coping with a fall

If you fall when using crutches, follow these steps to get back on your
feet safely.

1 Sit with your legs extended and your hands beside your
hips. Look around the room for a low, sturdy piece of furniture, such as a sofa. Then, inch backward toward the sofa
by pushing your hands down on the floor and lifting up your
buttocks. Slide the crutches along with you.

2 When you're next to the sofa, lean the crutches against it
and move the cushion to the side if the sofa is high. Then
reach back and place both hands on the sofa seat.

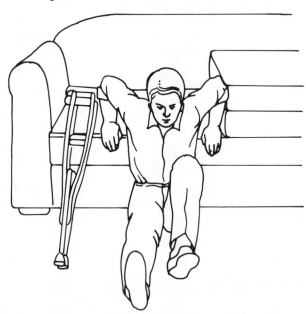

3 Next, press down on the sofa seat and lift your buttocks onto the sofa.

4 Then grasp both crutches in one hand. As you steady yourself with the crutches, raise yourself to a standing position by pushing down on the sofa with your other hand. After that, transfer one of the crutches to your other hand.

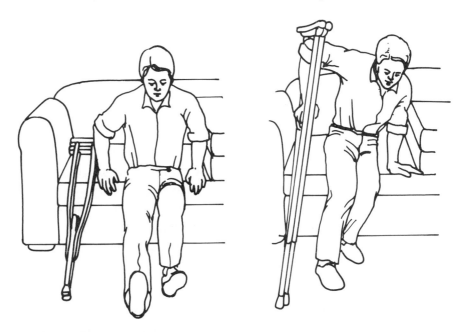

Choosing a cane

The doctor may order a cane if you have weakness on one side of your body or if you have poor balance. Either the doctor or the physical therapist will help you select the cane that's best for you.

Hold the cane in the hand opposite your weaker side, and flex your elbow at a 30-degree angle. If the cane's made of aluminum, you can adjust it by pushing in the metal button on the shaft and raising or lowering the shaft. If the cane's wooden, you or a helper can remove the rubber safety tip, saw off any excess wood, and replace the tip. Available in several types, canes can be standard, straight-handled, or broad-based.

Standard canes

The doctor may recommend a standard cane if you'll be going up and down stairs often. Made of wood or metal, a standard cane commonly comes in 34- to 42-inch (86 to 107 cm) sizes. It features a single foot and a half-circle handle. It's usually inexpensive, easy to use, and hooks onto your belt or arm when you go up or down stairs and onto the back or arm of a chair when you sit down.

Choose a cane with a wooden or plastic handle rather than a metal one. If your hand perspires, you may lose your grip on a metal handle. Besides, a metal handle may feel uncomfortable for you to hold onto in cold weather.

Straight-handled canes

The doctor will recommend a straight-handled cane if your hand is weak. Made of wood, plastic, or metal, a straight-handled cane has easy-to-hold handgrips and a rubber safety tip. If you're selecting one, make sure the handgrip isn't too thick or too thin for you to hold comfortably and that the cane is the correct height. Because this cane doesn't hook over railings or chair arms, you can place it on the floor near you when you sit down.

Broad-based canes

This lightweight metal cane has three or four prongs or legs that provide a sturdy supportive base. Its height can be adjusted, and extra-long handles and child sizes are available. A broad-based cane stands upright when not in use.

Cane bases range from narrow to wide. A narrow broad-based cane fits on the standard stair step in the normal cane position, whereas a wide broad-based cane fits on the step if you turn the cane sideways. Usually, the narrower the cane's base, the less you rely on it for support.

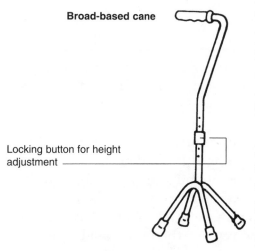

Broad-based cane

Locking button for height adjustment

Walking with a cane

You can use the following guidelines for walking with a cane if your left leg is weaker. If your right leg is weaker, start with the cane on your left side, and adapt the instructions.

Examining the cane's tip

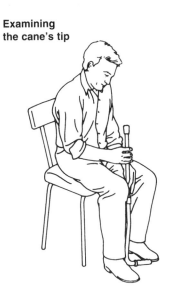

1 Be sure you're wearing nonskid, flat-soled, supportive shoes, and check that they fit securely (loose laces can be hazardous). Avoid wearing sandals or clogs because they don't support your weight properly. Next, check your cane's rubber tip to be sure it has no cracks or tears and is wearing evenly. Also, make sure the tip fits securely and evenly on the cane's end.

If possible, remove throw rugs and avoid walking on slippery, wet, or waxed floors or on gravel driveways. Also, try to walk close to a wall so that you have something to lean against if you drop your cane.

Distributing weight evenly

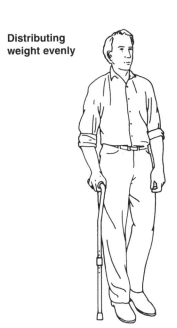

2 Now, position the cane about 4 inches (10 centimeters) to the side of your stronger leg. Distribute your weight evenly between your feet and the cane.

3 Shift your weight to your stronger leg and move the cane about 4 inches (10 centimeters) in front of you.

4 Now you're ready to move your weaker foot forward so that it's even with the cane.

5 Shift your weight to your weaker leg and the cane. Now, move your stronger leg forward, ahead of the cane. If you've done this step correctly, your heel will be slightly beyond the tip of the cane.

6 Next, move your weaker leg forward so that it's even with your stronger leg. Then move your cane in front of you about 4 inches (10 centimeters).

Repeat these steps. As you proceed, remember to keep your head erect, shoulders back, and back straight. Your abdomen should be tucked in and your knees slightly bent.

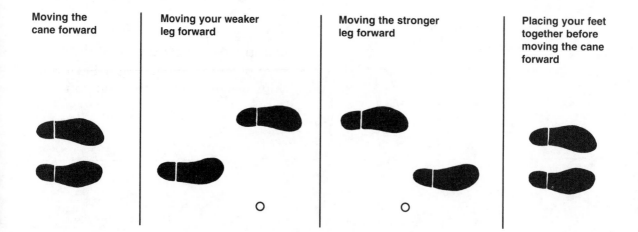

Moving the cane forward

Moving your weaker leg forward

Moving the stronger leg forward

Placing your feet together before moving the cane forward

Using a cane on stairs

With practice you'll learn to master going up and down stairs. You'll be able to go up and down facing forward if stairs have two banisters. But if they have only one, you'll have to learn to go up and down facing backward.

How to climb stairs facing forward

Stand at the bottom of the stairs with your feet about 6 inches (15 centimeters) apart. If your right side is stronger, grasp the banister with your right hand about 4 inches (10 centimeters) from the end. Transfer the cane to your left hand and hook it over your arm or under your belt. If you have a broad-based cane, place it on the step ahead of you.

Now, firmly grasp the banister as you shift your weight to your left leg. Pull yourself forward with your right hand, using the banister, as you lift your right foot to the first step.

Next, shift your weight to your right leg. Then, use the banister to pull yourself forward with your right hand as you lift your left foot to the first step. Continue this sequence until you reach the top of the stairs.

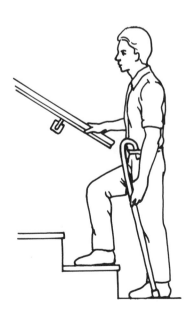

How to go down stairs facing forward

To get down the stairs, face the bottom of the stairs. If your right side is stronger, grasp the banister with your right hand. Now, lower your left foot and then your right onto each step.

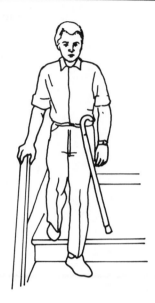

How to climb stairs facing backward

If the banister is on your weaker side (as you look up the stairs), you'll need to go up the stairs facing backward. Stand with your back to the stairs and your stronger side next to the banister. Grasp the banister and lift the foot on your stronger side to the first step. Then lift the foot on your weaker side to the first step. Repeat this sequence of steps until you reach the top of the stairs.

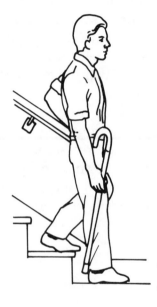

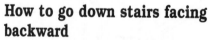

How to go down stairs facing backward

To get down the stairs if the banister is on your weaker side (as you look down the stairs), go down the stairs facing backward. Stand with your back to the stairs and your stronger side next to the banister. Grasp the banister, and lower your weak foot one step. Then lower your stronger foot one step. Repeat this sequence until you reach the bottom.

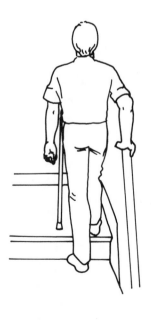

Getting into and out of a chair using a cane

After learning how to walk with a cane, you'll want to learn how to get into and out of a chair. Follow these steps if you're using a chair with armrests.

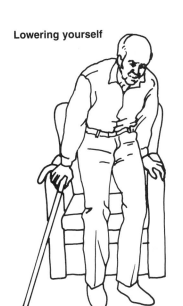

Lowering yourself

1 To sit down, steady yourself with the cane as you stand with the backs of your legs against the chair seat. Move the cane out from your side, and reach back with both hands to grasp the armrests. Supporting your weight on the armrests, lower yourself onto the seat. Hook or lean the cane on the armrest or chair back.

2 To get out of the chair, unhook the cane, and hold it in your stronger hand as you grasp the armrests. Place your stronger foot slightly forward. Lean slightly forward, and push against the armrests to raise yourself. Steady yourself by placing the cane's tip about 4 inches (10 centimeters) to the side of your stronger foot.

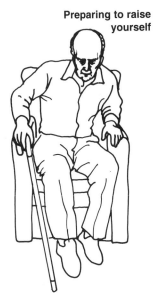

Preparing to raise yourself

Using special aids

If you're walking with crutches or a cane, the special aids described below can help save you time and effort.

Carrying devices

When using crutches or a cane, you may be able to carry lightweight objects in a canvas, vinyl, or nylon knapsack strapped to your back. Be sure your arms are strong and your balance is good before you use a knapsack. And don't try to carry heavy objects in a knapsack.

To carry small objects when using crutches, attach a 12-inch (30.5-centimeter) dog collar to the handle of the crutch you're using on your stronger side. The collar can be unbuckled and slipped through the handle on any small object you want to carry—a handbag or a portable radio, for example.

Reachers

If you want to reach an object beyond your grasp, you may be able to get it yourself by using a reacher. Reachers are available in most medical supply stores. Some have magnetized

Magnetized reacher

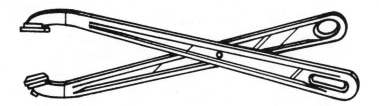

tips for picking up small metal objects, such as safety pins. Others come with hooked ends for picking up nonmetal objects like sweaters. Kitchen tongs or a bent metal clothes hanger can also serve as a reacher in some situations.

Hooked reacher

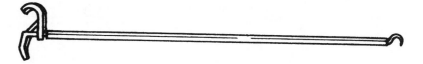

14   Exercises

Understanding exercise

If you've been ill or injured—even if you're confined to a bed or wheelchair while you recover—you need to exercise. Why? Because not exercising may result in weakened muscles; stiff, locked joints; and, possibly, impaired circulation, including dangerous blood clots.

Don't attempt any exercise without the doctor's knowledge and permission. Also, be sure the doctor tells you which of the exercises described in this chapter are safe for you.

In general, exercise maintains or increases muscle strength, improves blood circulation, assists in the elimination of waste products, and aids in the delivery of oxygen and nutrients to the body's tissues and organs. Exercise also contributes to a sense of well-being, increased relaxation, and an improved outlook on life. The following are some specific benefits:

• Exercise increases the heart's pumping action so that your heart can more easily pump blood to your legs and arms.

• Exercise helps your lungs: you breathe quicker and more often while exercising. This helps keep your lungs functioning normally. It also helps prevent infections that can occur if you don't breathe or cough deeply enough to bring up lung secretions.

• Exercise speeds up gastrointestinal (GI) motion, so it can be an important factor in preventing or relieving constipation or other GI problems.

• Exercise promotes urinary function by improving blood flow to and from the kidneys.

Limbering up your hands and feet

A gentle, daily hand and foot exercise program can help you stay limber. What's more, it promotes muscle strength and increases blood flow to your tissues. Try to set aside time to exercise every day. Then follow these instructions for gentle range-of-motion exercises.

Finger curls

Slowly curl each finger toward your palm. Begin at the top with the joint closest to your fingertip. Tip it gently toward

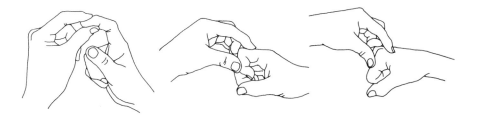

your palm.

Then fold the middle two finger joints gently and naturally into a curl.

When your fingertips are as close as possible to your palm, bend your knuckle joint.

You may exercise your fingers individually or together. If necessary, use your other hand to guide the movement. Do the exercise five times with each hand.

Finger stretches

Place your right hand on a table, with your palm facing down and your fingers and thumb touching. Now, one by one, fan your fingers to the right and "walk" them away from your thumb, as though you're playing a keyboard. Then walk your fanned fingers back toward your thumb and relax. Repeat the exercise with your left hand.

Making fists

Close your hand into a tight fist. Then slowly open it, stretching out your fingers as far as you can. Repeat this exercise 10 times with both hands.

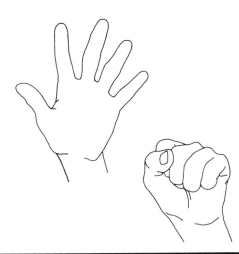

Hand presses

Place your hands together, palms touching and fingers slightly entwined (as if praying). Press the right hand backward with the left hand and then reverse and press the left hand backward with the right hand. Exert pressure at the palm, not the fingertips. Coax the hand just past the point of discomfort, unless the doctor or physical therapist tells you not to.

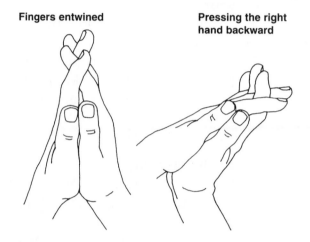

Fingers entwined   Pressing the right hand backward

Wrist looseners

Hang your hand, palm side down, over the edge of a table or arm rest. Raise your hand as far as you can using your other hand to help. Then lower your hand so that it's almost at a right angle to your wrist.

Use your other hand to complete the movement. Do this exercise five times with each wrist.

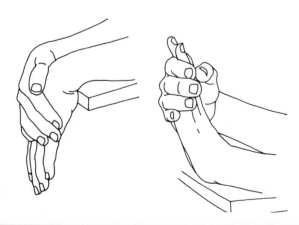

Heel and toe lifts

Sit in a chair or on the edge of a bed with both feet flat on the floor. Keep your toes on the floor and raise your heels as high as you can. Lower your heels and relax. Repeat five times.

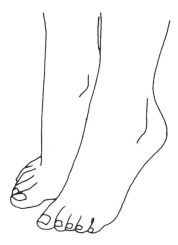

Next, keep your heels on the floor, and raise your toes as high as you can. Lower your toes and relax. Repeat five times.

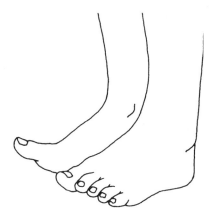

Foot rolls

Place a rolling pin under one foot. Then use your foot to roll the pin back and forth for a few minutes. Repeat with the opposite foot.

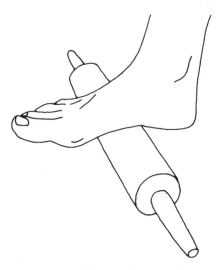

Performing active range-of-motion exercises

Review the following guidelines before you begin doing active range-of-motion exercises.

Some guidelines

Do your exercises daily to get the most benefit from them.

• Repeat each exercise three to five times or as often as the doctor recommends. (As you become stronger, he may tell you to increase your activity.)

• Impose order on your routine. If you're exercising all your major joints, begin at your neck; then work toward your toes.

• Move slowly and gently so that you don't injure yourself. If a particular exercise hurts, stop doing it. Then ask the doctor if you should keep doing that exercise.

• Take a break and rest after an exercise that's especially tiring.

• Consider spacing your exercises over the day if you prefer not doing them in a single session.

Neck exercise

Slowly tilt your head as far back as possible. Next, move it to the right, toward your shoulder.

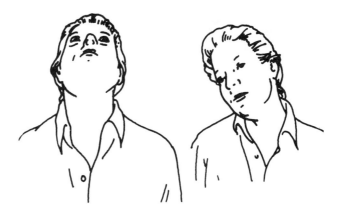

Still with your head to the right, lower your chin as far as you can toward your chest. Then move your head toward your left shoulder. Complete a full circle by moving your head back to its usual upright position.

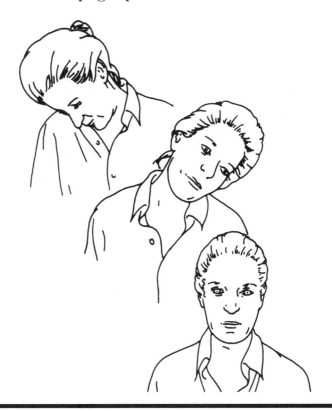

After you do the recommended number of counterclockwise circles, reverse the exercise, doing an equal number of clockwise circles.

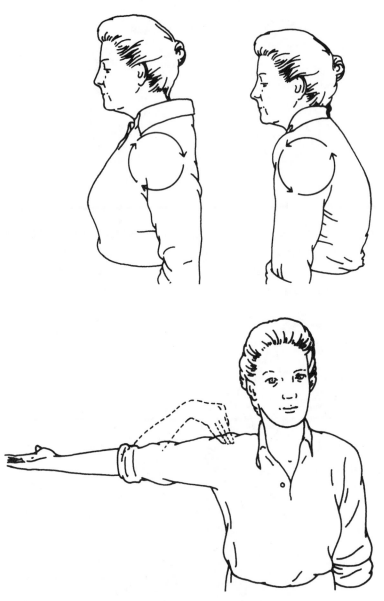

Shoulder exercise

Raise your shoulders as if you were going to shrug. Next, move them forward, down, and then up in a single circular motion.

Now move them backward, down, and then up in a single circular motion.

Continue to alternate forward and backward shoulder circles throughout the exercise.

Elbow exercise

Extend your arm straight out to your side. Open your hand, palm up, as if to catch a raindrop. Now, slowly reach back with your forearm so that you touch your shoulder with your fingers. Then slowly return your arm to its straight position. Repeat with your other arm.

Alternate your left and right arm throughout the exercise.

Wrist and hand exercise

Extend your arms, palms down and fingers straight. Keeping your palms flat, slowly raise your fingers and point them back toward you. Then slowly lower your fingers, and point them as far downward as you comfortably can.

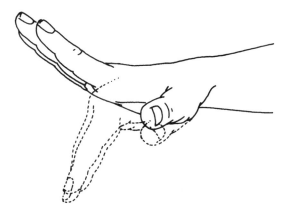

Finger exercise

Spread the fingers and thumb on each hand as far apart as possible without causing discomfort. Then bring the fingers back together into a fist.

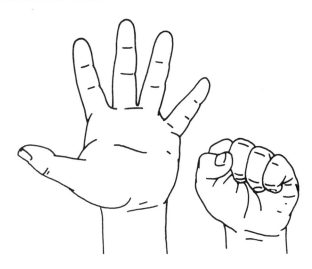

Leg and knee exercise

Lie on a bed or on the floor. Bend one leg so that the knee is straight up and the foot is flat on the bed or floor.

Now, bend the other leg, raise your foot, and slowly bring your knee as close to your chest as you can without discomfort.

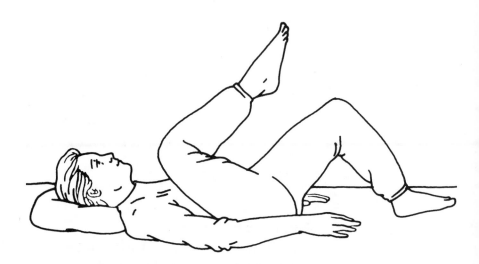

Then straighten this leg slowly while you lower it. Repeat this exercise with your other leg.

Ankle and foot exercise

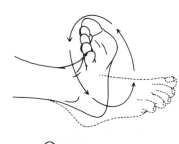

Raise one foot and point your toes away from you. Move this foot in a circular motion—first to the right and then to the left.

Point your toes back toward you. With your foot in this position, make a circle with it, first to the right and then to the left. Now do the same exercise with your other foot.

Toe exercise

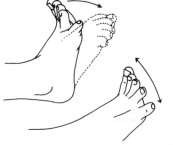

Sit in a chair or lie on a bed. Stretch your legs out in front of you with your heels resting on the floor or the bed. Slowly bend your toes down and away from you. Next, bend your toes up and back toward you. Finally, spread out your toes so that they're separated. Then squeeze them together.

Helping someone else exercise

Passive range-of-motion exercises are important if the person in your care can't exercise part of his body. Even though these exercises are called "passive," have the person help as much as possible because any movement can improve his muscle tone and strength. Be careful to support, control, and move each joint correctly as you perform the exercise. If you need to, consult a therapist, nurse, or doctor.

Repeat the exercises for the prescribed number of times.

Neck exercise

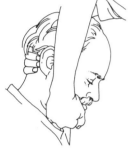

Lay the person on his back with his head flat (no pillow). With one hand, support the back of his head; with your other hand, support his chin. Extend his neck by moving his head backward so that he's looking at the ceiling. Next, bring his head forward until his chin comes as close to his chest as possible without causing discomfort. Now, turn his head first to the left and then to the right.

Shoulder exercise

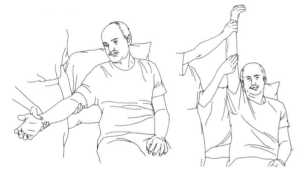

With the patient sitting or lying down, extend his arm straight out to the side with his palm facing up. Place one hand under the elbow; use your other hand to grip his wrist. Then keep his arm straight, and bring it up until it reaches his ear. Return the arm to its original position. Repeat with the other arm.

Elbow exercise

Extend the person's arm straight out to the side with his palm facing up. Grasp his wrist to keep his hand from drooping. Now, bend his arm at the elbow, and bring his hand up toward his shoulder and then return it to its original position. Repeat with the other arm.

Forearm exercise

Place the person's arms along his sides. Grasp the wrist and hand of one arm. Keeping the person's elbow on the bed, raise his hand and gently twist it so that his palm is facing up. Then twist it so that his palm is facing down. Repeat with the other arm.

Wrist exercise

Place the person's arms along his sides. Keeping his elbow on the bed, hold one arm slightly below the wrist and raise it. Grasp the hand with your other hand, lift it, and bend it gently back and forth. Then rock the hand back and forth sideways. Gently twist the hand from side to side. Do the same thing with the other hand.

Finger exercise

Place the person's arms along his sides. With one of your hands, grasp one of his but keep his wrist straight. With your other hand, gently straighten out his fingers. Now, working from his little finger to his thumb, spread apart each pair of adjoining fingers and then bring them back together. Pinch the thumb together with each of his fingers, one finger at a time. Repeat with the other hand.

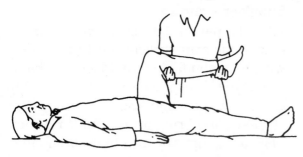

Hip and knee exercise

Straighten the person's legs flat on the bed. Place one hand under his ankle and the other under his knee. Then bend his knee toward his chest.

Bring his leg down, straighten it, and then gently move it out to the side away from his other leg. Gently move it back to the center, over and across the other leg, and then back to the center. Repeat with the other leg.

Ankle exercise

Straighten the person's legs on the bed. Place one hand under his heel and the other hand against the ball of his foot. Push the ball of his foot gently toward his head as you pull his heel down.

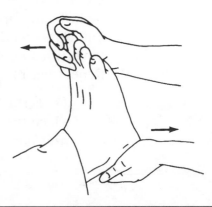

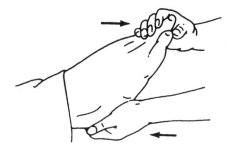

Next, pull his toes down toward the bed while you push his heel up.

Finally, straighten the foot and move it gently from side to side. Repeat with the other foot.

Foot exercise

Straighten the person's legs on the bed. Place one hand under one of his heels and the other hand under the ball of his foot. Gently twist his sole inward toward the other foot, back to the center, and then outward. Repeat this exercise with the other foot.

Toe exercises

Straighten the person's legs on the bed. Support his heel or ankle with one hand and use the other hand to curl his toes toward his sole. Straighten his toes, bend them gently back toward the top of his foot and then straighten them.

Next, working from the little toe to the big toe, spread apart each pair of adjoining toes and then bring them back together.

Repeat these exercises with the toes of the other foot.

Performing isometric exercises

To perform isometric exercises correctly, you'll exercise against resistive force to increase the muscle-strengthening effect of the exercises. Remember to repeat each exercise as many times (typically three) as the doctor directs. Then review the following tips.

Some guidelines

In isometric exercise, you don't move your joints; instead, you contract your muscles against the resistance of a stationary object, such as a bed, a wall, or another body part. If you press your palms together (pushing with one, resisting with the other) until you feel a tightness in your chest and upper arm muscles, you're doing a basic isometric exercise.

You don't have to be in any special position for most isometric exercises, so you can do them anytime, anywhere. Hold each contraction for 3 to 5 seconds. Repeat the entire series at least five times a day.

For the first week, don't contract your muscles fully; this will give them a chance to get used to the exercises. After that, contract them fully.

Neck exercises

Place the heel of your right hand above your right ear. Without moving your head, neck, or arm, push your head toward your hand. Then repeat this exercise with your left hand above your left ear.

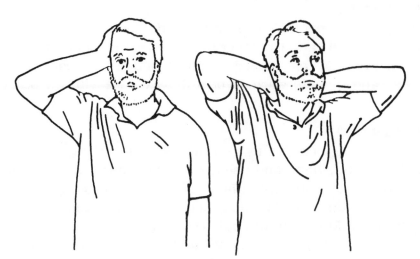

Clasp your fingers behind your head. Without moving your neck or hands, push your head back against your hands.

Shoulder and chest exercise

Hold your right arm straight down at your side. Grasp your right wrist with your left hand. Then try to shrug your right shoulder, but prevent this by keeping a firm grip on your right wrist.

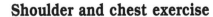

Do the same exercise with your left arm and left shoulder.

Arm exercise

Bend your elbow at a 90-degree angle. Turn your right palm up, and place your left fist in it. Then try to bend your right arm upward while you resist this force with your left fist.

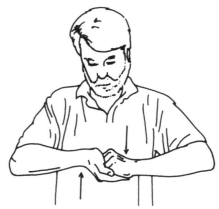

Repeat this exercise with your left arm and right fist.

Abdominal exercise

Begin by sitting on the floor or on a bed with your legs out in front of you. Then bend forward, and place your hands palm down on the midfront of your thighs. Try to bend further forward, but resist this movement by pressing your palms against your thighs.

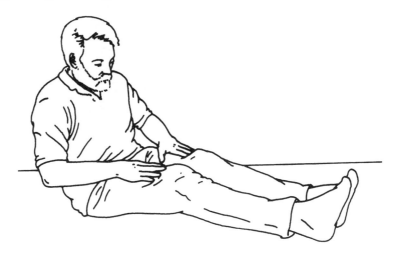

Buttocks exercise

While standing, squeeze your inner thighs and buttocks together as tightly as possible. If you're doing this exercise in bed, place a pillow between your knees to make the exercise more effective.

Thigh exercise

For leg support, sit on the floor or on a bed. With your legs completely straight, vigorously tighten the muscles above your knees so that your kneecaps move upward.

Calf exercise

While sitting up in bed, bend down and grasp your toes. Then pull gently backward, and hold this position briefly.

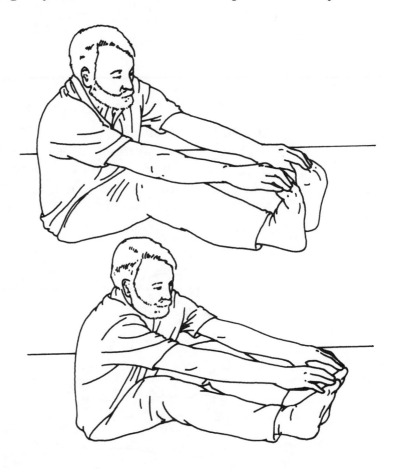

Still touching your toes, push them forward and down as far as possible, and hold this position briefly.

Performing back-strengthening exercises

The doctor may have prescribed special exercises to strengthen your back and help relieve your lower back pain. (They're called Williams flexion and McKenzie extension exercises.) Perform only the exercises the doctor has recommended. If you do the others, you could aggravate your back condition, causing more pain.

If the doctor approves, do each exercise 10 times every day. After 2 weeks, increase the number of times you do each exercise every day by 10 until you're doing each exercise 30 times every day. Then cut back to 30 times every other day.

Head and shoulder lift

Lie on your back with your knees bent, feet flat on the floor, and arms folded across your chest. Lift your head and shoulders off the floor. Do not elevate your head and chest more than 45 degrees. Hold for a count of 5 and then relax back to the floor.

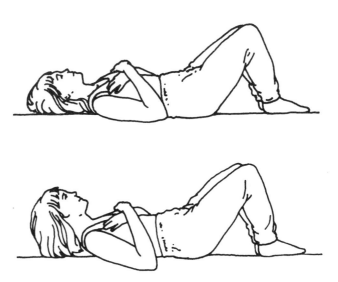

Pelvic tilt while lying on your back

The pelvic tilt is the basic starting point for most back exercises. Lie on your back with your knees bent and feet flat on the floor. Pull in your stomach, and pinch your buttocks together to flatten your lower back to the floor. Hold for a count of 5 and then relax.

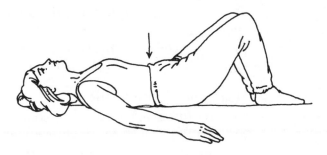

Foot flex and leg lift

Lie on your back with your knees bent and feet flat on the floor. Straighten one knee without moving your thighs. Then bend (flex) the foot of the straight leg toward your head.

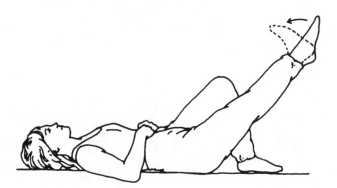

Next, lift your straight leg as far as you can, keeping the knee straight and the foot flexed toward your head.

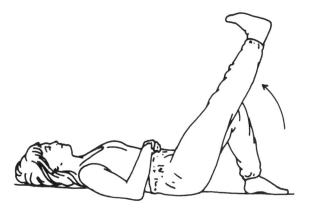

Hold for a count of 5, lower the straight leg, relax your foot, and bend your knee until your foot is flat on the floor. Perform the exercise with the other leg.

Foot flex and bent leg lift

Lie on your back with one knee bent so that your foot is flat on the floor. Hold the other leg firmly to your chest with your hands under the knee. First, bend (flex) your elevated foot toward your head.

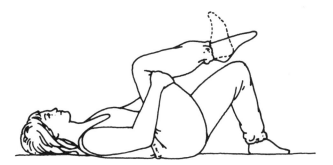

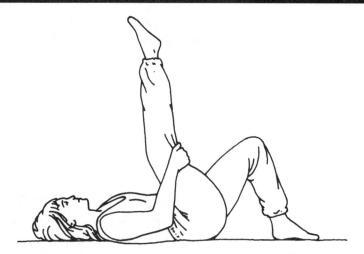

Then straighten that leg, keeping your thigh close to your chest. Hold for a count of 5 and then relax to the starting position. Do the same exercise with the other leg.

Leg stretches

Hold the ends of a towel in each hand, place your foot against the middle of the towel, and extend your leg to stretch out your hamstring muscles. Then do the same stretching exercise with your other leg.

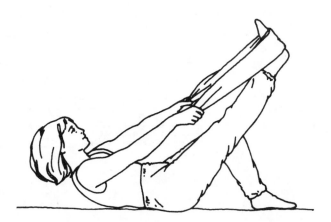

Pelvic tilt while lying on your stomach

Lie on your stomach with your hands at your sides and tighten your buttocks as hard as you can. Hold for a count of 5 and then relax.

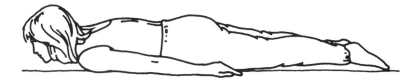

Shoulder blade squeeze with head and chest lift

Lie on your stomach with your arms at your sides and palms facing down. Squeeze your shoulder blades together, and raise your head and chest as far as you can. Hold for a count of 5 and then relax.

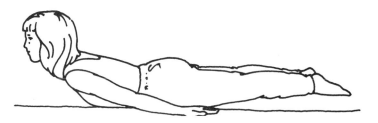

Single leg lift

Lie on your stomach with your arms at your sides and your palms facing down. Keep your legs straight and slowly lift one leg off the floor as far as possible. Don't hold the position. Return your leg slowly to the floor, and perform the exercise with the other leg.

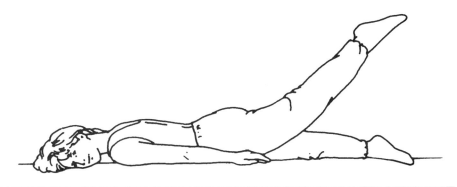

Double leg lift

Lie on your stomach with your arms at your sides and your palms facing down. Keep your legs straight, and raise both of them off the floor together as far as possible. Don't hold the position. Return your legs slowly to the floor.

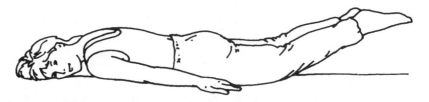

Alternate arm and leg lift

Lie on your stomach with your arms extended past your head and your palms facing down. Raise one arm and the opposite leg from the floor as high as possible without bending either. Don't hold the position. Return your arm and leg slowly to the floor. Perform the exercise with the other arm and leg.

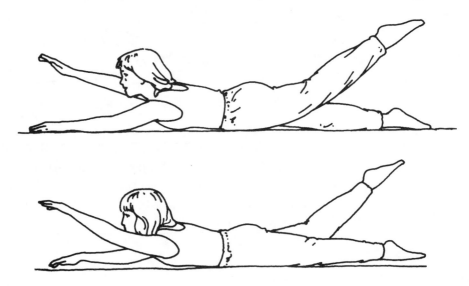

15 Walkers and Wheelchairs

Importance of mobility

When illness or injury strikes, your ability to move around (mobility) can be limited or lost. To increase your mobility, the doctor has ordered a walker or wheelchair for you. A walker provides the stability and balance you need to walk safely. Or, if you're unable to walk, a wheelchair supports your weight while you propel yourself where you want to go.

A walker or a wheelchair helps you move around independently. But these devices also have another important benefit: They give your body a chance to keep moving. And that's important because moving your muscles and joints keeps them from becoming weak and stiff. Mobility also keeps your body's fluids—blood and mucus, for example—from collecting so that you can avoid complications such as phlebitis and pneumonia. What's more, mobility helps keep your skin free from pressure ulcers, which develop when you sit or lie down for long periods without changing your position. In a nutshell, you need to keep moving, even if you don't always feel like it.

Before you use a walker or a wheelchair

Before you can use a walker or a wheelchair safely and comfortably, you'll need to take certain steps. These include adapting your home and learning how to use a walker or wheelchair safely.

Adapting your home

You don't have to spend a lot of money to adapt your home. In fact, some of the ideas listed here cost little or nothing and will greatly increase your safety and comfort. If you'll be using a wheelchair permanently, you may want to consider remodeling certain areas of your home—the kitchen, for example, to make counters and cabinets accessible. If you don't think you can afford adapting your home, talk to the doctor or nurse. He or she can refer you to the hospital's social service department or to another agency that can discuss financial help.

Kitchen

• Remove area rugs from the floor. Also, make sure the floors are kept dry and don't have excess wax.

• If you have unused storage space, such as below the sink, make use of this area for supplies. Consider lowering the countertops.

• Make sure the stove's controls, a telephone, and a fire extinguisher are within easy reach.

• Angle a mirror over the cooking surface.

• Hang adapters on a pegboard within easy reach.

Living room

• Remove thick carpeting or area rugs. A hardwood floor or low-pile carpet provides better stability and ease of movement.

• Put a raised cushion on your easy chair.

• Make sure you have easy access to a telephone and a table.

• Arrange furniture along the walls for more moving space.

Bedroom

• Remove thick carpeting or area rugs, as in your living room.

• Use a hospital-type bed with side rails and attached trapeze, if necessary.

• Keep a commode chair in the room.

• Place the telephone on an overbed table for easy access.

• Keep a fire extinguisher handy.

Bathroom

• Have safety rails or grab bars installed around the toilet and bathtub.

• Get an elevated toilet seat and a tub seat.

• Have nonslip strips installed in the bathtub.

• Use a hand-held shower head.

Other areas

• Have handrails installed along walls.

• Consider obtaining an electric chair lift to take you up and down stairs. Also consider installing a ramp alongside or in place of steps outside your home.

• Make sure smoke and heat detectors are installed on each floor.

• Have narrow doorways enlarged.

Using your walker or wheelchair safely

Follow these important and practical tips:

Safety tips for using a walker

• Be sure you wear shoes that fit well—tennis shoes or tied oxfords with rubber soles are good choices. Avoid shoes that slide off your feet (such as slippers). Also avoid shoes with high heels or slippery soles.

• To safely carry small items, attach a lightweight basket or bag to the walker's metal frame with snaps, self-sticking strips, or hooks. If you have good arm strength and balance, you may prefer to carry lightweight items in a knapsack on your back.

• Make sure the surface you're walking on is clean, flat, dry, and well-lighted.

• When you're walking, remember to look ahead rather than at your feet.

• Each time you use your walker, stand for a few minutes with the walker to get your balance. Remember: Feeling a little dizzy at first is normal. If your dizziness is severe or doesn't go away, sit down and call for help.

Safety tips for using a wheelchair

• Remember to lock the wheelchair's brakes before transferring yourself into it from your bed or car—or moving from it.

• To avoid developing pressure ulcers from prolonged sitting in the wheelchair, practice wheelchair push-ups: Press down on the armrests with your hands as you lift your buttocks off the seat. If you can't do push-ups, try shifting your weight

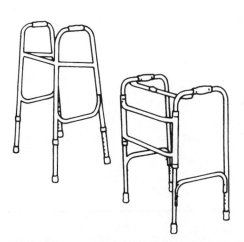

from one side to the other. To keep pressure ulcers from forming on your arms, partially fill two small hot water bottles with water and place them on the armrests. This will cushion your arms and help reduce pressure.

• Never lean forward in the wheelchair if you can't place both feet flat on the floor or if you have poor arm strength or a displaced center of gravity (because of a leg cast, for example).

Learning about walkers

Two types of walkers are available: stationary and reciprocal. Which one the doctor will

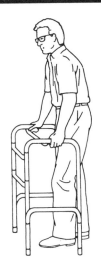

order for you depends on how much muscle strength you have and how well you can keep your balance when you stand or walk.

Stationary walker

Usually lightweight, inexpensive, and stable, a stationary walker consists of an adjustable metal frame with handgrips and four legs. Most stationary walkers have no movable parts, but some models have small front wheels and others fold for travel and easy storage.

The doctor may order a stationary walker for you if your arms are strong but you have general muscle or leg weakness or only a minor balance problem. He may also order it if you have a broken hip, leg, or foot.

Reciprocal walker

A reciprocal walker consists of a metal frame with handgrips, four legs, and a hinge mechanism that allows one side to be advanced ahead of the other. Its height usually is adjustable from 27 to 37 inches (68 to 94 centimeters), and some models fold for travel and storage.

This type of walker is recommended for people with decreased arm strength and balance. It's also recommended for people with arthritis and Parkinson's disease.

Using a three-point gait

If the doctor has recommended that you use a three-point gait with your walker, follow these steps.

Moving your weaker leg

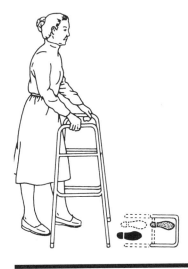

Place the walker slightly in front of you. Distribute most of your weight between your stronger leg (the right leg in the picture) and the walker, but try to support some weight on your weaker leg as well. Now, shift all your weight to the stronger leg while you lift and advance the weaker leg and the walker as far as 8 inches (20 centimeters). (The foot and walker patterns duplicate your stance.)

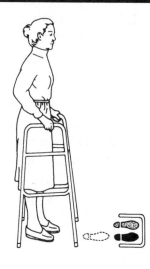

Moving your stronger leg

Next, shift your weight to the weaker leg and the walker while you move the stronger leg as far as 8 inches (20 centimeters) forward.

Repeat these steps, moving first the walker and the weaker leg and then the stronger leg. Never attempt to put all your weight on the weaker leg.

Using a two-point gait with swing through

If you can't put any weight on one leg but have normal use of your arms, upper body, and other leg, the doctor may recommend that you use the two-point gait with swing through with your stationary walker. Follow these steps.

Shifting your weight

Stand with the walker in front of and partially around you. Then distribute your weight evenly between the walker and your stronger leg. Hold your weaker leg off the floor. Now, simultaneously shift your weight to the stronger leg as you lift and advance the walker about 8 inches (20 centimeters).

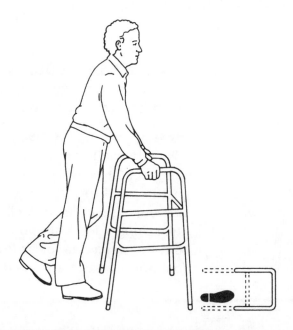

Moving forward

Swing the stronger leg about 8 inches (20 centimeters) forward while you support your weight on the walker. Repeat these steps, moving first the walker and then the stronger leg. Remember, don't put any weight on the weaker leg.

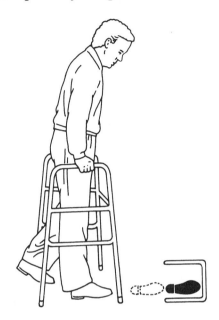

Using a four-point gait

If you can't support your full weight on either leg, the doctor may recommend that you use a four-point gait with your reciprocal walker. These steps explain how.

Moving your left foot forward

Stand with the walker in front of and partially around you. Distribute your weight evenly between the walker and both legs. Then move the right side of the walker forward. Now, move your left foot forward.

Distributing weight evenly

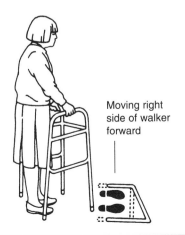

Moving right side of walker forward

Moving left foot forward

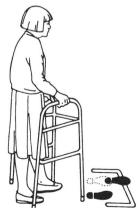

Moving your right foot forward

Next, move the left side of the walker forward. Then move your right foot forward to complete the four-point gait. Repeat the procedure to continue walking.

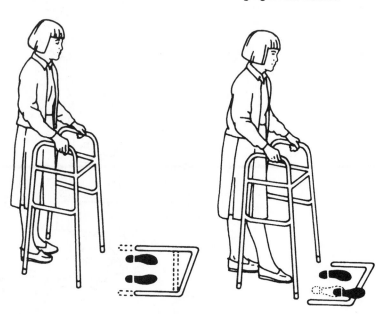

Moving left side of walker forward   **Moving right foot forward**

Using a two-point gait

If you can't support your full weight on your legs but your arms are strong and your muscle coordination is good, the doctor may recommend a two-point gait for you. Follow these steps for using this gait with a reciprocal walker.

Positioning the walker

Stand with the walker in front of and partially around you. Keep your weight evenly distributed between the walker and both legs. The foot and walker patterns duplicate your stance.

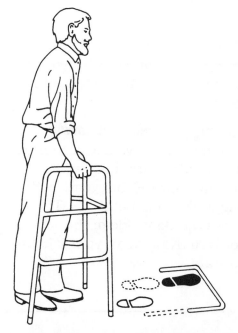

Moving forward

Simultaneously advance the walker's right side and your left foot. Next, advance the walker's left side and your right foot. Continue in this manner.

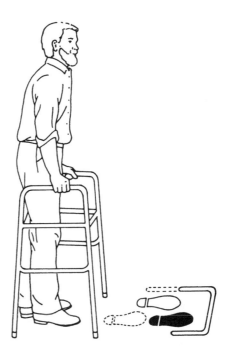

Sitting down in a chair

To use your walker to help you sit, follow these steps.

Shifting your weight

Stand with the back of your stronger leg against the front of the chair, your weaker leg slightly off the floor, and the walker directly in front of you. Now, grasp the armrest with the hand on the weaker side. Then shift your weight to the stronger leg and to the hand grasping the armrest. Next, grasp the other armrest with your free hand.

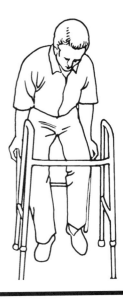

Lowering yourself

Lower yourself into the chair and slide backward. After you're seated, place the walker beside the chair.

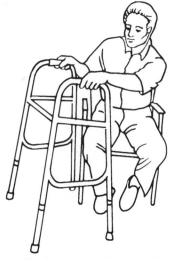

Getting up from a chair

Follow these two steps to rise from a chair and position yourself upright with your walker.

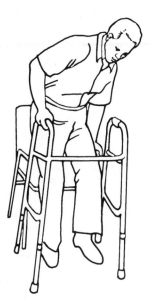

Pushing upward

Move the walker in front of you, and slide forward in the chair. Place the back of your stronger leg against the seat. Then advance your weaker leg. Now, placing both hands on the armrests, push yourself to a standing position. Support your weight with the stronger leg and the opposite hand. Then grasp the walker's handgrip with your free hand.

Securing your grip

Grasp the free handgrip with your other hand. Now, distribute your weight evenly between your hands and your stronger leg. Take a moment to get your balance.

Coping with a fall while using a walker

If you fall while using a walker, call for help. If no help is available, use the following method to help yourself up.

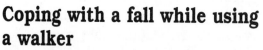

1 Look around the room for a low, sturdy piece of furniture, such as a coffee table. Inch backward toward the table by pushing your hands down on the floor and lifting your buttocks. As you do this, pull the walker with you, using one hand.

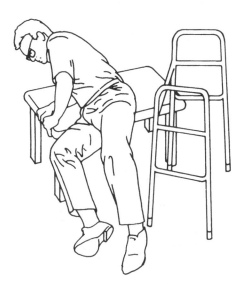

2 When you get to the table, position the walker near it. Then reach back and place both hands on the table top. Next, press down on the table top and lift your buttocks onto the table.

3 Place the walker in front of you, and raise yourself to a standing position by pushing your hands down on the handgrips.

Remember: You may feel a little dizzy when you first stand up. Take a moment to gain your balance before walking. If the dizziness doesn't go away or if it seems excessive, lower yourself back onto the table and call for help. Or you may want to sit a while before attempting to stand again.

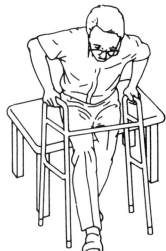

Learning about wheelchairs

Two types of wheelchair are available: standard, which is suitable for most people, and motorized, which is recommended for people who have severe arm and hand weakness.

Choosing a wheelchair that meets your needs

Both standard and motorized wheelchairs offer optional features that modify the handrims, brakes, armrests, and legrests. These features can be combined in various ways to meet your special needs. For example, if you have arm or hand weakness, you may want a wheelchair with hand projections on the handrims. Hand projections allow you to grasp the handrims more firmly.

A wheelchair can be custom-made for your particular needs, but it will cost more than a ready-made model. Your wheelchair should also be the right size, with a seat low enough so that your feet touch the floor but high enough so that you can move easily from the chair to a bed or car.

Standard wheelchair   **Motorized wheelchair**

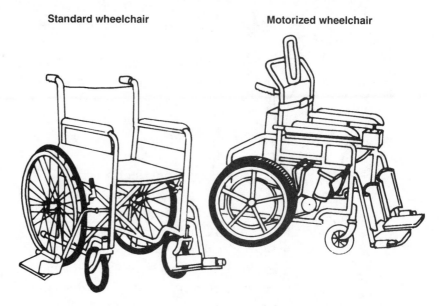

Your condition and prognosis—whether your condition might worsen or improve—also affect the type of wheelchair you'll need. For example, if you have progressive muscular dystrophy, you eventually may have upper-body weakness. A wheelchair with a semi-reclining back or a higher backrest will provide the support and comfort you'll need.

When choosing wheelchair features, consider the method you'll use to transfer from your bed or car to your wheelchair. A wheelchair with removable or swing-away legrests is recommended for most transfers. One with removable arms may be a good choice if you'll use a sitting transfer. You can read more about transfer methods beginning on the next page.

Finally, consider your home environment and lifestyle. For

example, if you spend a lot of time outdoors, you may want to order a wheelchair with pneumatic tires. These tires will help you maneuver the chair on soft or uneven ground. The doctor, nurse, or physical therapist can offer more suggestions for choosing the best wheelchair for you.

How a motorized wheelchair works

Most motorized wheelchairs are battery-powered. The battery pack is located at the back of the chair, near the floor. The batteries must be recharged every night to make sure they have enough power for the next day's use.

Motorized wheelchairs operate in different ways—for example, by a toggle switch, a mouthpiece, or a chin control. A wheelchair with a toggle switch is hand-controlled—you push the switch in the direction you want to move. A wheelchair with a mouthpiece control allows you to propel the wheelchair without using your hands. The mouthpiece control attaches to a tube connected to the motor. You direct the wheelchair by blowing into the mouthpiece. (For example, two short puffs may make the chair steer to the left.) A wheelchair with a chin control may also be used if you have reduced hand strength. The chin lever attaches to an arm that's connected to the battery cable. You use your chin to push the lever in the direction you want to move.

Learning about transfers

You'll need to learn how to get from your bed to your wheelchair and from your wheelchair into a car. If someone's helping you do these transfers, you may want to wear a transfer

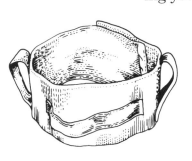

belt—a nylon, canvas, or leather strap about 3 feet (1 meter) long with handles on the sides and back. When the belt's attached to your waist, your helper can grip the handles to assist you.

Types of transfer

You can move from your bed to your wheelchair by performing a standing, sitting, backward-, or forward-sitting transfer. You can also use a transfer board. To return to your bed from the wheelchair, reverse the procedures outlined on the next few pages.

You can move from your wheelchair to a car by yourself using the sitting transfer. Or, if a family member or friend can help you, the two of you can use the stand-pivot transfer method.

Performing a standing transfer

1 Sit at the edge of the bed with your shoes on and your feet flat on the floor. Make sure the wheelchair's right side is parallel to the left side of the bed. Lock the chair's wheels and move the legrests out of the way.

Raising yourself from the bed

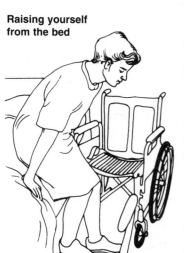

2 Put your stronger foot slightly in front of your weaker foot. Then place your hands, palms down, on the bed, next to your hips. Now, lean forward slightly. Push your hands down on the bed to lift yourself to a standing position.

3 Use the hand on your stronger side to grasp the wheelchair's armrest that's farthest from you.

Grasping the wheelchair

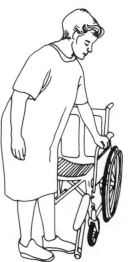

4 Pivot, or step, to your stronger side as you grasp the wheelchair's other armrest with your other hand. Position yourself directly in front of the wheelchair's seat. The backs of your legs should be touching the edge of the seat.

Support your weight with your hands as you lower yourself into the chair. Then replace the legrests and position yourself comfortably in the chair.

Performing a sitting transfer

1 Sit at the edge of the bed with your shoes on and your feet flat on the floor. The wheelchair's right side should be parallel to the left side of the bed. Lock the chair's wheels.

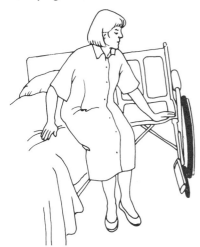

Grasping the wheelchair

2 Remove the chair's right armrest and hang it from the side of the chair. Then remove the right legrest or move it to the side. Next, place your left hand, palm down, on the wheelchair's seat. Place your right hand, also palm down, next to your right hip.

3 Push down with your right hand to lift your buttocks off the bed. Then shift your weight to your left hand as you slowly move yourself into the wheelchair's seat. Reattach the right armrest and legrest, and position yourself comfortably in the chair.

Performing a backward-sitting transfer

1 Remove the wheelchair's legrests or swing them aside. Position the front of the wheelchair as close as possible to the side of the bed. Lock the chair's wheels. The wheelchair seat should be facing the side of the bed. Make sure you're sitting in bed with your legs extended.

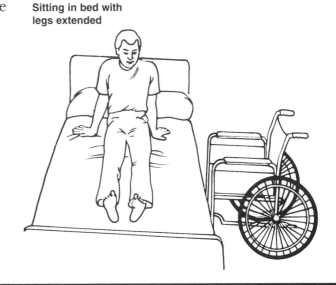

Sitting in bed with legs extended

Moving backward to the side of the bed

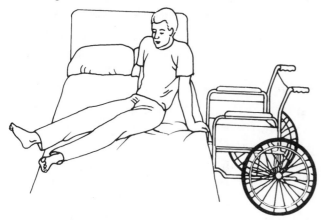

2 Next, lean slightly forward. Pushing your hands against the mattress, lift your buttocks slightly off the bed. Keeping your legs extended across the bed, inch backward to the side of the bed—close to the wheelchair. Stop when your back is in front of the wheelchair.

Lifting into the chair

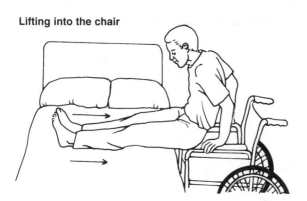

3 Now, firmly grasp the armrests of the wheelchair and gradually lift your buttocks onto the seat. Unlock the chair's wheels, and push yourself away from the bed. Position yourself comfortably in the wheelchair.

Performing a forward-sitting transfer

1 To get back into bed, position the wheelchair seat so that it's facing the bed. Lift your legs off the legrests, and then swing the legrests out of the way. Now, raise your legs onto the bed as you position the chair as close as possible to the bed. Lock the chair's wheels.

Raising your legs onto the bed

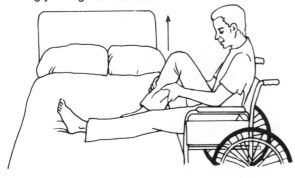

2 Next, grasp the armrests of the wheelchair, and lift your buttocks slightly off the seat. Keeping your legs extended across the bed, inch forward to the middle of the bed.

Using a transfer board

You can use a transfer board to help you perform a sitting transfer. Here's how you can move from your wheelchair to a bed using this device. *Important:* Make sure the bed and the wheelchair seat are about the same height before you attempt the transfer.

1 Move the wheelchair alongside the bed and lock the chair's wheels. Remove the legrests and the armrest closest to the bed.

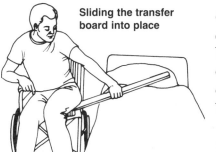
Sliding the transfer board into place

2 Shift your weight to the buttock that's farthest from the bed, and slide one end of the transfer board under your buttocks and upper thighs. Then extend the other end of the board onto the bed.

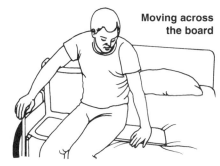
Moving across the board

3 Grasp the remaining armrest and place your other hand on the transfer board. Lift your buttocks, and inch your way across the board toward the bed.

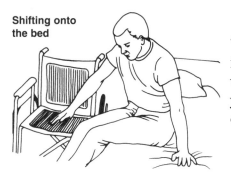
Shifting onto the bed

4 Place one hand on the bed and the other on the transfer board. Now, shift your weight toward the bed so that you can pull the transfer board out from under you.

Moving from your wheelchair into a car

You can use a sitting transfer to move from your wheelchair into a car. Or you can have a family member or friend help you, using the stand-pivot transfer method. Consider using a transfer belt to assist with the transfer. Follow these steps for a stand-pivot transfer.

1 Park the car on a level surface close to the door of the building. Make sure there's enough room for the wheelchair on the right side of the car. Next, open the car's front passenger door as far as possible.

2 Move the person in the wheelchair over to the car, and move the wheelchair's left armrest and both legrests out of the way. Then position the left side of the wheelchair next to the car seat. Lock the chair's wheels.

Moving the wheelchair

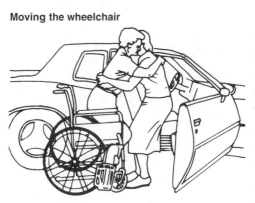

3 Now, move close to the person, and place your knees against his legs. Squat slightly and slide your arms under his arms. Then lock your arms around his waist, and help him to a standing position. Remember to support his knees with yours throughout the transfer.

Pivoting

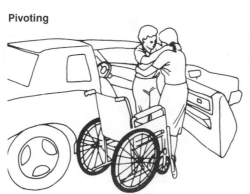

4 Now, pivot toward the car seat. Stop turning when the person's standing directly in front of the open door.

Lowering the person

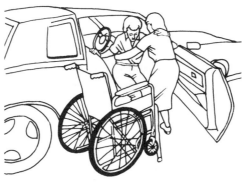

5 Next, slowly lower the person onto the car seat so that he's sitting with his legs dangling outside the car.

6 Put your hands under the person's knees, and raise his legs into the car. Ask him to help you, if possible, by guiding him with his arms. Make sure he's properly positioned on the car seat, and remove the transfer belt (if you've used one). Finally, fasten the seat belt and close the door.

Positioning the person in the car

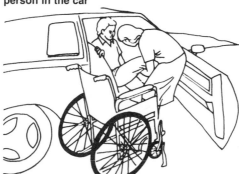

Coping with a fall from a wheelchair

If you fall from your wheelchair, follow this procedure to return to it.

1 Look around the room for a low, sturdy piece of furniture (for example, a coffee table) that you can use for support. Next, place your hands, palms down, beside your hips. Push down with your hands and lift your buttocks off the floor. As you do this, inch your way toward the wheelchair and grasp the armrest.

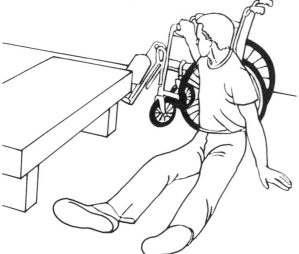

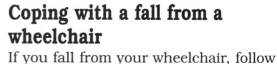

2 Unlock the wheelchair's brakes, if necessary. Then inch your way over to the coffee table, pushing or pulling the wheelchair with you.

When you reach the table, position the wheelchair so that the front of the seat is facing the table. Lock the chair's brakes, and move the legrests aside.

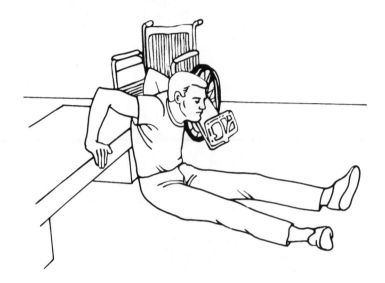

3 Position yourself with your back toward the table. Then reach back and place both hands on the table. Push down and lift your buttocks off the floor onto the table. Then slide back on the table so that you're as close as possible to the front of the wheelchair.

4 Reach back and place your hands on the wheelchair seat. Push down with both hands and lift yourself onto the seat. Then slide back into the seat and position yourself properly.

16   Oxygen Therapy

Using oxygen effectively

Oxygen is important because it provides the body's cells with the fuel they need to function. Normally, the lungs take in fresh air loaded with oxygen and let out stale air filled with carbon dioxide. When you breathe in (see the illustration), air enters your upper airway and moves through a series of tubes called a bronchial tree. At the end of these tubes, or bronchioles, are grape-like clusters of air sacs called alveoli. The alveoli have thin walls that expand to take air in and contract to let it out. Oxygen passes through these thin walls into the bloodstream by way of small blood vessels called capillaries, which surround the alveoli.

After oxygen enters the bloodstream, the blood carries it to cells in all parts of the body. In the same cells, carbon dioxide is produced as a waste product. It travels back to the lungs and is eliminated each time you breathe out.

Sometimes, a person needs more oxygen than he can get by just breathing. A doctor may prescribe oxygen if:
• a person's lungs aren't delivering enough oxygen to his blood vessels—for example, in lung disease
• a person's red blood cells aren't carrying enough oxygen to his body's cells—for example, in severe anemia
• a person's heart isn't beating as strongly as it should—for example, in heart disease.

If a doctor thinks a person needs more oxygen, the person should follow instructions carefully because without enough oxygen, a person breathes harder and faster to try to get the oxygen he needs. This makes his heart and lungs work harder to get their job done.

When the body's tissues don't get enough oxygen, a condition called hypoxia results. This can make a person feel confused, restless, and less alert than usual. It can also make him

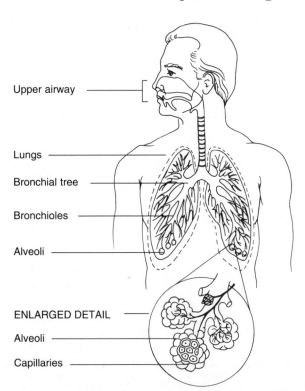

Upper airway

Lungs

Bronchial tree

Bronchioles

Alveoli

ENLARGED DETAIL

Alveoli

Capillaries

short of breath and cause his heart to beat faster and have an irregular rhythm. Unless hypoxia improves, it will damage a person's brain, heart, kidneys, and lungs. Breathing in extra oxygen, as the doctor orders, can keep this from happening.

Learning about home oxygen systems

To relieve shortness of breath, the doctor has ordered oxygen therapy for you or the person you're caring for to use at home. Your first job is to become familiar with the oxygen delivery equipment.

Oxygen options

The oxygen will be provided in a liquid oxygen container, an oxygen tank, or an oxygen concentrator.

Liquid oxygen is stored at very cold temperatures in insulated containers. When released, it's warmed up to breathe as oxygen gas. Most stationary liquid oxygen units have a contents indicator that shows the amount of oxygen in the unit, a flow selector that controls the oxygen flow rate, a humidifier bottle that connects to a humidifier adapter, and a filling connector that attaches to a matching connector on the portable unit.

An oxygen tank stores oxygen gas under pressure. Attached to the tank is a pressure gauge that shows how much oxygen is left in the tank, a flow meter that shows the flow rate, and a humidifier bottle.

Stationary liquid oxygen unit

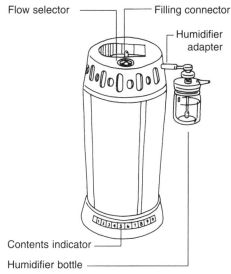

Flow selector — Filling connector

Humidifier adapter

Contents indicator —

Humidifier bottle —

Oxygen tank

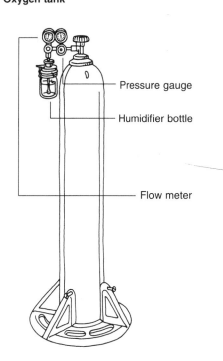

Pressure gauge

Humidifier bottle

Flow meter

Oxygen concentrator

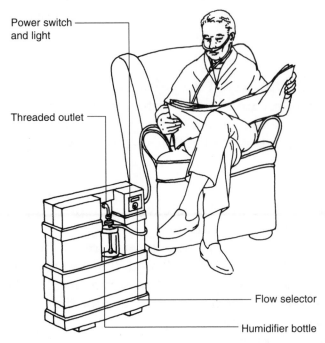

Power switch and light

Threaded outlet

Flow selector

Humidifier bottle

The oxygen concentrator removes nitrogen and other components of room air and then concentrates the remaining oxygen and stores it.

Oxygen concentrators are available in different models and sizes, but most have the following operating parts: a power switch and light, a flow selector that regulates the oxygen flow rate, an alarm buzzer that warns of power interruptions, and a humidifier bottle that attaches to a threaded outlet.

Obtaining equipment

When you obtain your home oxygen system from the medical equipment supplier, you'll learn how to set it up, check for problems, and clean it.

Your system will include a humidifier to warm and add moisture to the prescribed oxygen and a nasal cannula or face mask through which you'll breathe the oxygen. Keep a record of the prescribed flow rate, and have your supplier's phone number handy in case of problems.

Also, get a backup system suitable to use in an emergency.

General guidelines

When using an oxygen tank, an oxygen concentrator, or liquid oxygen, be sure to follow these important guidelines.

• Check the water level in the humidifier bottle often. If it's near or below the refill line, pour out any remaining water and refill it with sterile or distilled water.

• If the inside of your nose feels dry, apply a water-soluble lubricant like K-Y Jelly.

• If you'll need a new supply of oxygen, order it 2 to 3 days in advance or when the gauge reads one-quarter full.

• Maintain the oxygen flow at the prescribed rate. If you're not sure whether oxygen is flowing, check the tubing for kinks, blockages, or disconnection. Then make sure the system is turned on. If you're still unsure, invert the nasal cannula in a glass of water. If bubbles appear, oxygen is flowing through the system. Shake off extra water before reinserting the cannula.

Safely tips

• Oxygen is highly combustible. Alert your local fire department that oxygen is in the house, and keep an all-purpose fire extinguisher on hand.

• If a fire does occur, turn off the oxygen immediately and leave the house.

• Don't smoke—and don't allow others to smoke—near the oxygen system. Keep the system away from heat and open flames, such as a gas stove.

• Don't run oxygen tubing under clothing, bed covers, furniture, or carpets.

• Keep the oxygen system upright. Make sure the oxygen's turned off when it's not in use.

Using an oxygen tank or liquid oxygen

If you're using an oxygen tank or liquid oxygen, follow these important guidelines.

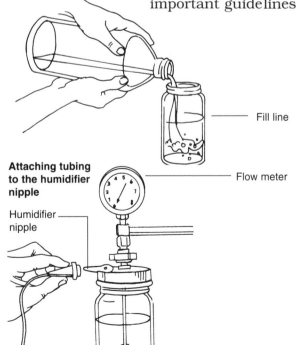

Filling the humidifer bottle with water

Fill line

Attaching tubing to the humidifier nipple

Flow meter

Humidifier nipple

Oxygen tubing

1 Check the water level in the humidifier bottle. If it's below the correct level, refill the bottle with sterile or distilled water or replace it with a prefilled bottle.

2 Attach one end of the oxygen tubing to your breathing device. Attach the other end to the humidifier nipple.

If you're using an oxygen tank, before setting the flow rate, open the tank by turning the valve at the top counterclockwise until the needle on the pressure gauge moves. If you're using a liquid oxygen system, set the flow rate to turn on the oxygen.

Flow meter with dial gauge   **Flow meter with tube scale**

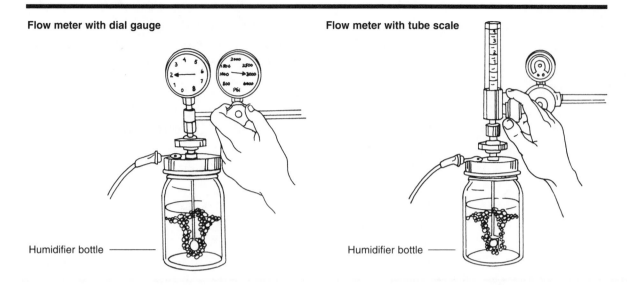

Humidifier bottle ————   Humidifier bottle ————

3 Next, set the flow rate using the appropriate method for your device. Either turn the dial to the correct number or turn the dial until the metal ball rises to the correct level on the scale. Wait for the gauge needle to reach the correct level. Never increase the flow rate on your equipment without the doctor's permission.

4 Put on your breathing device following the guidelines in "Using an oxygen cannula or mask," later in this chapter.

Using an oxygen concentrator

1 Before you plug in the unit, check the air inlet filter to make sure it's clean and in place. If it's dirty, take it out and wash it in mild soap and water. Then rinse it, pat it dry, and replace it.

2 Some oxygen concentrators have a battery-powered alert buzzer that has to be checked before you use the system. To check the alert buzzer, push the power switch. If the buzzer doesn't sound, use a different oxygen source and contact your supplier. If it does sound, push the power switch again to turn it off.

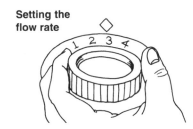

Setting the flow rate

3 Now, set the flow selector to the prescribed rate by turning the dial to the correct number. Or if your flow meter is a tube scale, turn the dial until the metal ball in the scale rises to the correct level. *Important:* Don't change the flow rate without the doctor's permission.

4 Check the water level in the humidifier bottle. If it's below the correct level, refill the bottle with sterile or distilled water or replace it with a prefilled bottle.

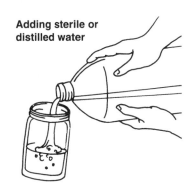

Adding sterile or distilled water

5 Attach one end of the oxygen tubing to your breathing device. Attach the other end to the humidifier nipple.

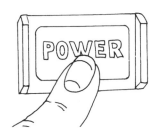

6 Plug the power cord into a grounded electrical outlet, and push the power switch to turn on the unit. The green power light should come on and the alert buzzer should sound for 60 seconds. After the alert buzzer goes off, put on the breathing device and begin breathing the oxygen.

Safety tips

To use an oxygen concentrator safely, follow these tips:
• Never operate the oxygen concentrator without a filter or with a dirty filter. Clean the filter at least twice each week.
• Don't use an extension cord with the concentrator, and don't plug the concentrator into an outlet that has other appliances plugged into it.
• Turn off the unit, use a backup oxygen source, and call the supplier if:
—the alert buzzer doesn't come on when you push the power switch
—the power light goes out and the alert buzzer sounds while you're using the oxygen concentrator
—the alert buzzer sounds even though the power supply isn't

interrupted. (If the power supply is interrupted, turn off the unit and use a different oxygen source until the power comes on again.)

Using an oxygen cannula or mask

If the doctor has prescribed a nasal cannula or an oxygen face mask so that you can breathe in extra oxygen, follow these steps for using your breathing device.

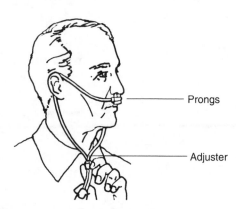

Prongs

Adjuster

Positioning a nasal cannula

If you're using a nasal cannula, insert the two prongs in your nostrils. Make sure the prongs face upward and follow the curve of your nostrils.

Also make sure the flat surface of the tab rests above your upper lip. Position the tubing for the nasal cannula behind each ear, and adjust it below your chin for a comfortable fit.

Elastic strap

Positioning an oxygen mask

If you're using an oxygen mask, place the mask over your face. Position the elastic strap over your head so that it rests above your ears and the mask fits snugly against your face.

Preventing skin irritation

To keep the cannula or mask strap from irritating your skin, pad it with 2-inch (5-centimeter) square gauze pads, placing them against your cheeks and behind your ears.

Every 2 hours, check for reddened areas around your nose

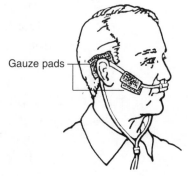

Gauze pads

and ears. If you see redness, rub the area gently and then wash your face and dry it well. Call the doctor if the redness persists.

You may moisten your lips and nose with a water-soluble lubricating jelly (such as K-Y Jelly), but take care not to get any in the cannula or mask.

Every 8 hours, remove the cannula or mask and wipe it clean with a wet cloth.

Using portable oxygen equipment

Special equipment may offer you greater freedom of movement while you're breathing extra oxygen. For instance, a portable liquid oxygen unit or portable oxygen tank will allow you to move around freely and leave your home. A wheeled carrier or extension tubing for your regular equipment will extend your range of movement inside your home.

Use these guidelines, along with specific manufacturer's instructions, to operate portable oxygen equipment.

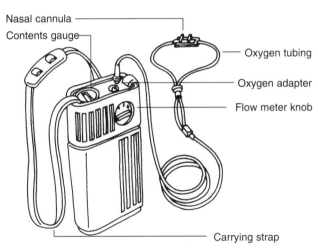

Portable liquid oxygen unit

Nasal cannula
Contents gauge
Oxygen tubing
Oxygen adapter
Flow meter knob
Carrying strap

Checking your oxygen supply

A portable liquid oxygen unit has a built-in scale that indicates the oxygen level each time you hold the unit by its carrying strap. Check the oxygen level often, and refill the unit when necessary. Your supplier will give you specific instructions for your model.

A portable oxygen tank has a contents gauge, a flow meter, and a knob to turn on the oxygen. To check the tank, turn the knob until you see the needle on the flow meter move. Then turn the knob off.

Attaching the tubing

Connect one end of the oxygen tubing to the nasal cannula or mask. Then connect the other end to the oxygen adapter on the liquid oxygen unit or the oxygen tank. Make sure the tubing connects securely and isn't kinked.

Setting the flow rate

Now, turn the flow meter knob to deliver oxygen at the prescribed rate. You should feel oxygen flowing from the prongs of the cannula or from the mask. If you don't feel oxygen flowing, briefly turn up the flow rate.

Then turn the knob back to the prescribed level. Make sure the knob on a liquid oxygen unit clicks into position or oxygen will not flow.

Carrying the portable tank

Slip the carrying strap over your shoulder, and adjust it for a comfortable fit. Try carrying the tank on each side of your body to determine which way is most comfortable. Now, put on the nasal cannula or mask and begin breathing oxygen.

When to call the doctor

You may not be getting enough oxygen if you have these signs: difficult or irregular breathing, restlessness, anxiety, tiredness or drowsiness, blue fingernail beds or lips, confusion, inability to concentrate.

You may be getting too much oxygen if you notice these signs: headache, slurred speech, sleepiness or difficulty waking up, shallow or slow breathing.

If these signs develops, call the doctor immediately. Above all, never change the oxygen flow rate without checking first with the doctor.

Troubleshooting tips

Your home oxygen system may not always work the way it should. Here are some common problems and how to cope with them. If the solutions listed here don't correct the problem, call your supplier immediately.

Diagnosing problems

PROBLEM	LIKELY CAUSE	WHAT TO DO
Oxygen isn't flowing freely through the breathing device.	• Faulty oxygen tubing	• Disconnect oxygen tubing and check for kinks or obstruction. Replace with new tubing, if needed.
	• Humidifier dirty or plugged	• Remove humidifier from oxygen supply. If the bottle is reusable, throw away any remaining water and refill the bottle with sterile or distilled water. If the bottle is disposable, replace it with a prefilled bottle.
Alert buzzer on oxygen concentrator sounds.	• Unit not plugged in securely • No power at wall outlet • Electrical power failure	• Check plug at electrical outlet. • Check fuse or circuit breaker in house. • Use backup oxygen tank until power is restored.
Oxygen hisses and empties too fast.	• Tank leaking oxygen	• Call your supplier immediately. Open windows in room. Extinguish all flames, including pilot lights.

17 Suctioning

Learning about suctioning

A healthy person clears his mouth and windpipe naturally and with little effort. But some people have difficulty swallowing or coughing, and they need help. That's the role of suctioning. It clears the mouth and windpipe of mucus, which improves a person's ability to breathe, talk, and eat and decreases the likelihood of his getting a lung infection.

Suctioning the mouth and the back of the mouth is called oropharyngeal suctioning. Suctioning the back of the nose is called nasopharyngeal suctioning. And suctioning the trachea, or windpipe, is called tracheal suctioning. (For guidelines on suctioning the trachea, see Chapter 18, Tracheostomy Care.)

You should suction a person whenever he has trouble breathing, coughing up secretions, or swallowing saliva. If the person has built up secretions in the back of his mouth or in his nose or trachea, his breathing will be labored or raspy. You may even hear a gurgling sound as he breathes. This problem usually can be prevented by suctioning the person as many times a day as the doctor orders. Sometimes, the person will need more frequent suctioning to breathe easier. In such a case, suction him as necessary. But notify the doctor if you have to suction more than once every 2 hours because you can harm the person by suctioning too frequently.

Using suctioning equipment

To perform suctioning, you'll need a portable suction machine, a disposable glove, water and a water container, and a suction catheter.

Note: Some people feel comfortable suctioning themselves. If you've been trained to do this, you'll also need a mirror to help you work.

Portable suction machine

A portable suction machine creates the air pressure you need to suction mucus and other secretions from the mouth, nose, and trachea. Most suction machines come with a regulator dial that allows you to set the suction pressure ordered by the doctor. After you turn on the machine and set the regulator dial, the needle on the pressure gauge will move, indicating the amount of suction pressure. The secretions drain through a length of connection tubing into a collection bottle that comes with the machine.

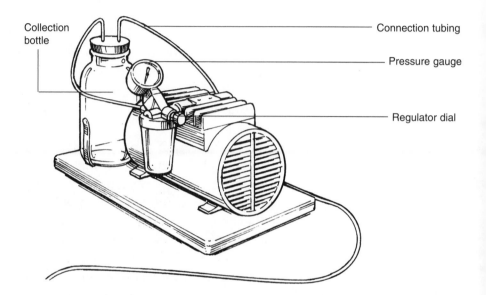

Disposable glove

If you're suctioning yourself, it isn't necessary for you to wear a disposable glove unless you have a respiratory tract infection. If you're suctioning someone else, use a glove.

Water and a water container

Use the water to test the suction pressure and to moisten the tip of the suction catheter for easier insertion. The doctor may tell you to use sterile (germ-free) water. If he does, you can sterilize normal tap water by boiling it for 5 minutes. As the water cools, put a lid on the pot so that the water stays germ-free. You can keep a supply of sterile water in a glass jar that has been sterilized by boiling. (You can also buy sterile water.)

Suction catheter

The suction catheter is the tubing that's put into the person's mouth, nose, or trachea. Inserting the catheter stimulates the urge to cough so that secretions can be suctioned.

Suction catheters are disposable or reusable. A disposable suction catheter has a knob with a hole, called a control valve. By placing your finger over the control valve when the suction machine is on, you can control suction pressure. A reusable suction catheter doesn't have a control valve. If you're using a reusable catheter, you'll also need a Y-connector, which serves the same function as the control valve on the disposable catheter. You'll insert the Y-connector between the connection tubing and the suction catheter.

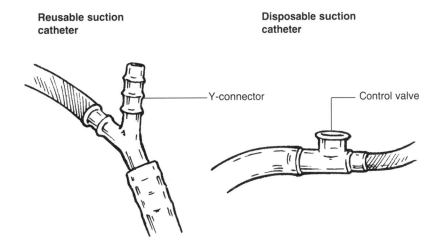

Reusable suction catheter

Disposable suction catheter

Y-connector

Control valve

Promoting deep breathing and coughing

Before you suction a person, give him a chance to fill his lungs with oxygen by breathing deeply. Deep breathing will help him cough up secretions so that they can be suctioned. It will also help him relax so that suctioning will be easier.

Between suctioning, remind the person to cough. Coughing helps loosen secretions. If he can learn to cough effectively, eventually he won't need to be suctioned. But coughing can be painful if the person is very ill or has injured his ribs. To lessen the pain, show him how to hold (splint) his ribs when he coughs. Using the following steps, teach him how to breathe deeply and cough effectively.

Deep breathing

Have the person sit up straight and inhale deeply from the bottom of his stomach, below where the diaphragm begins. Then tell him to let his stomach swell out as he slowly pulls in air. This expands and lifts the diaphragm.

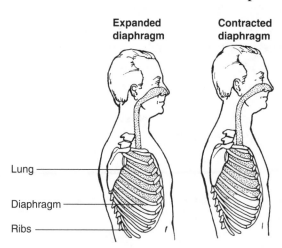

Expanded diaphragm

Contracted diaphragm

Lung

Diaphragm

Ribs

Tell him to hold in the air for 1 or 2 seconds and then let it out as slowly as he took it in. Have him use his stomach muscles to push out (exhale) every last bit of air. This contracts and lowers the diaphragm.

Splinting the ribs

Have the person either sit up straight or lie on his side with his knees bent. If necessary, he can splint his ribs by holding a pillow to his chest or by having a caregiver hold a towel around his chest and back.

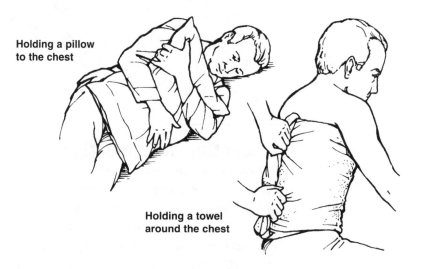

Holding a pillow to the chest

Holding a towel around the chest

Coughing

Tell the person to take a deep breath to increase pressure. Then he should tighten his abdominal muscles as he coughs vigorously. Have him spit out any secretions into a facial tissue, if he can, and discard the soiled tissue in a plastic-lined wastebasket.

Preparing to suction

The doctor or nurse will show you the correct way to suction the back of the mouth. Use the step-by-step procedure shown here as a reminder. If a problem develops, refer to the trouble-shooting tips at the end of this chapter.

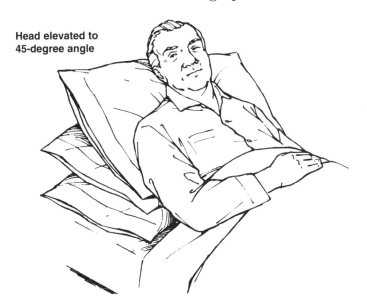

Head elevated to 45-degree angle

1 If the person you're caring for has never been suctioned, tell him that suctioning won't hurt, but it may make him feel like coughing or sneezing. To prevent this, tell him to try to relax and to breathe deeply through his nose during the procedure. Now, help him sit up. If you're using a hospital-type bed, elevate the head of the bed to a 45-degree angle. Turn the person's head toward you, and use pillows to support his back and neck.

2 If the catheter and disposable glove are packaged separately, open the catheter package before you put on the glove but don't remove the catheter yet. Now, hold the glove by its cuff, and slip it on the hand you'll be using to handle the suction catheter. Once you've put on the glove, don't touch anything but the suction catheter with your gloved hand. Now, using your gloved hand, remove the suction catheter from its wrapper or airtight container.

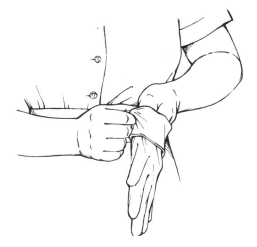

3 If the suction catheter has a control valve, attach the catheter directly to the connection tubing. Make sure you keep the catheter in your gloved hand.

Attaching the suction catheter to the tubing

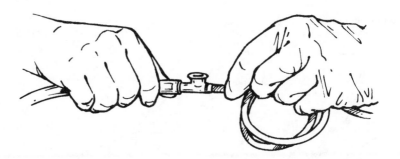

4 If the suction catheter doesn't have a control valve, attach the suction catheter to a Y-connector before you attach it to the connection tubing.

Attaching the Y-connector

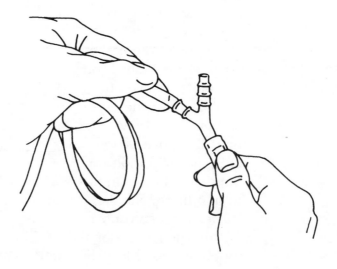

5 Turn on the machine. Then turn the regulator dial to set the suction pressure ordered by the doctor. The setting usually is – 80 and –120 mm Hg. Don't set the dial above –120 mm Hg. (If your suction machine doesn't have a regulator dial, simply turn on the machine.)

Now, with your gloved hand, dip the catheter tip in the water. This makes it easier to insert.

To test the machine, place a finger of your nongloved hand over the suction catheter's control valve or the Y-connector's opening and suction a little water through the catheter. This test allows you to tell whether or not the suction machine is working properly and will help secretions to pass through the catheter once you begin suctioning.

Testing the suction machine

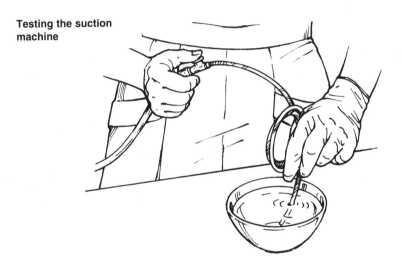

Suctioning the back of the mouth

1 Now you're ready to begin suctioning the back of the mouth. Insert the moistened suction catheter into the person's mouth, and advance it along one side until it reaches the back of the mouth.

Caution: Don't keep your finger over the control valve or Y-connector opening during insertion. This will create suction pressure while you're inserting the catheter and can damage the lining of the mouth.

Inserting the catheter

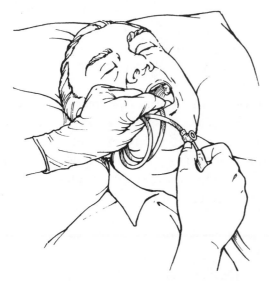

If the person begins to gag, immediately stop inserting the catheter. If he doesn't stop gagging, remove the catheter, and let him take several deep breaths before you insert it again. If you can't remove the catheter, just leave it in place. It will act as an airway until the gagging stops. Then continue insertion.

2 With the machine on and your finger over the suction catheter's control valve or Y-connector opening, slowly withdraw the catheter.

As you withdraw it, roll the catheter between your thumb and index finger. This motion prevents you from damaging the mucous lining. Don't take more than 10 to 15 seconds to withdraw the catheter.

Withdrawing the catheter

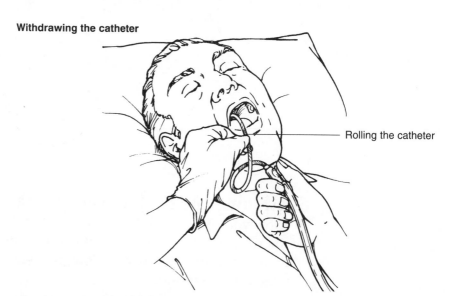

Rolling the catheter

3 If the catheter becomes clogged with secretions while you're suctioning, remove the catheter and place the tip in the water. With the machine on and your finger on the catheter's control valve or Y-connector opening, draw some water into the catheter. This should clear it. Then reinsert the catheter into the person's mouth and continue suctioning.

4 After you withdraw the catheter, place the tip in water, keep your finger over the control valve or Y-connector opening, and let the machine run a few seconds longer. This helps clear the catheter and connection tubing.

To help the person relax, have him take several slow, deep breaths. If he continues to have breathing problems, repeat the suctioning procedure. If he no longer has difficulty breathing, turn off the suction machine.

If you're using a disposable catheter, discard it and the glove in a plastic-lined wastebasket. Clean the water container in hot water so that it'll be ready for future use. Every 8 hours, or as often as necessary, remove, empty, and rinse the collection bottle and connection tubing.

If you're using a reusable catheter, see "Making a suction catheter germ-free."

Suctioning the back of the nose

If you're planning to suction the back of the nose, follow the same basic procedure as for suctioning the back of the mouth. The major differences between the two procedures are the way you position the person and the way you insert the suction catheter. If a problem develops, refer to the trouble-shooting tips at the end of this chapter.

1 If the person has never been suctioned, explain to her that suctioning won't hurt, but it may make her feel like coughing or sneezing. Help her relax, and tell her to breathe deeply through her mouth during the procedure. Now, help the person sit up. If you're using a hospital-type bed, elevate the head of the bed to a 45-degree angle. Tilt back the person's head, and use pillows to support her back and neck.

2 If the catheter and disposable glove are packaged separately, open the catheter package before you slip on the glove but don't remove the catheter. Now, put on the glove

**Head elevated to
45-degree angle**

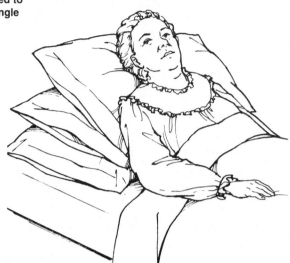

and remove the suction catheter as described in step 2 of "Preparing to suction."

3 Because you can't see when the catheter reaches the back of the nose, you need to determine how much of the catheter to insert before you begin. To do this, hold the catheter alongside the person's face, but make sure it doesn't touch her face. Align the tip of the catheter with the tip of the person's nose, and measure the distance on the catheter from the tip of the person's nose to her earlobe. Use your thumb to mark the spot. This length is the amount of tubing you should insert.

**Measuring
the tubing
needed**

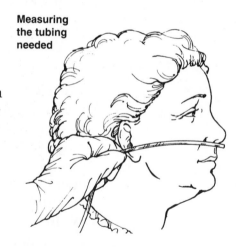

4 Attach the suction catheter to the connection tubing. If the suction catheter doesn't have a control valve, attach the catheter to the connection tubing with a Y-connector. Test the suction machine as described in step 5 of "Preparing to suction."

**Inserting the
catheter**

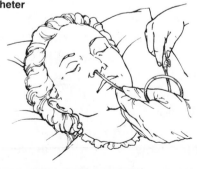

5 Gently insert the catheter through one nostril, aiming the catheter tip downward, until you've inserted as much as you measured off with your thumb.

Caution: Don't keep your finger over the control valve or Y-connector opening during insertion. This will create suction pressure while you're inserting the catheter that could damage the lining of the nose.

6 If the catheter becomes clogged with secretions while you're suctioning, remove the catheter and place the tip in the water. With the machine on and your finger on the catheter's control valve or Y-connector opening, draw some water into the catheter. This should clear it. Then reinsert it into the person's nostril.

7 With the machine on and your finger over the control valve or Y-connector opening, slowly withdraw the catheter. As you withdraw the catheter, roll it between your thumb and index finger to prevent damaging the lining of the nose. Don't take longer than 10 to 15 seconds to withdraw the catheter.

Withdrawing the catheter

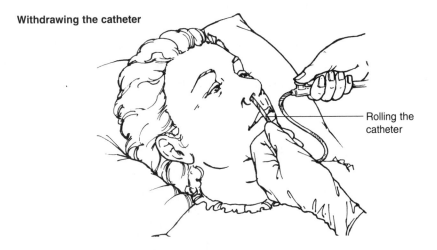

Rolling the catheter

8 After you withdraw the catheter, place the tip in water, keep your finger over the control valve or the Y-connector opening, and let the machine run a few seconds longer. This helps clear the catheter and connection tubing.

Tell the person to take several slow, deep breaths to help her relax. If she continues to have breathing problems, repeat the suctioning procedure. If she no longer has difficulty breathing, turn off the suction machine.

If you're using a disposable catheter, discard it and the glove in a plastic-lined wastebasket. Clean the water container in hot water so that it'll be ready for future use. Every 8 hours, or as often as necessary, remove, empty, and rinse the collection bottle and connection tubing.

If you're using a reusable catheter, see "Making a suction catheter germ-free."

Making a suction catheter germ-free

1 Place the suction catheter in a clean saucepan. Add water to cover the catheter. Bring the water to a boil, and let it boil, uncovered, for 5 minutes.

2 Turn off the burner, and cover the pot with a clean lid. This allows the suction catheter to cool but protects it from household germs.

3 Wash your hands, and remove the catheter from the cooled pot. Place it in a clean, airtight jar, such as a mason jar, and store it for future use.

Boiling for 5 minutes

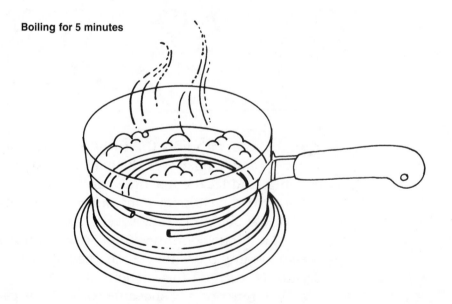

Troubleshooting tips

If you have problems while suctioning, use the following chart to help identify and solve them—or better yet, avoid them.

Diagnosing problems

PROBLEM	HOW TO SOLVE IT	HOW TO AVOID IT
You begin suctioning and discover that the machine doesn't work.	• Make sure the machine is plugged in. • Make sure the machine is turned on. • Make sure the rubber stopper or lid on the collection bottle is on tight. • Make sure the tubing and catheter connections aren't loose. • Make sure the suction catheter isn't twisted.	• Check the equipment carefully before you begin suctioning. • Draw some sterile water through the suction catheter before you insert it to make sure the machine's working.
As you're suctioning, the person begins to cough continuously, and you're unable to remove the suction catheter.	• Don't use force to remove it if gentle tugging doesn't work. • Disconnect the suction catheter from the connection tubing, and let the person breathe through it. • When the coughing does stop, quickly remove the suction catheter and reassure the person.	• Suction the person as little as possible. • Discontinue suctioning whenever difficulties appear likely, and call the doctor.
The person sounds congested, but you're unable to suction any secretions.	• Stop suctioning immediately, and call the doctor.	• Ask the doctor if he recommends using a humidifier in the person's room. • Have the person drink lots of fluids. Also, he should avoid milk or milk products, such as cheese, because they can thicken secretions.

(continued)

Diagnosing problems *(continued)*

PROBLEM	HOW TO SOLVE IT	HOW TO AVOID IT
While you're suctioning the back of the mouth of a person who's had a stroke, he becomes uncooperative.	• Try to calm the person by speaking soothingly to him. • Get someone to assist you in holding the person's mouth open.	• Turn the person from side to side at regular intervals so that secretions can drain from his mouth naturally. • Encourage him to cough up secretions by demonstrating what you want him to do.
You notice pink-tinged secretions while you're suctioning the person.	• Stop suctioning immediately, and call the doctor. Ask the doctor about using a smaller suction catheter.	• Have the person drink lots of fluids. • Review the way you're suctioning to make sure you're doing it correctly.

When to call the doctor

Sometimes, you may be unable to clear secretions from a person's airway by suctioning. Or you may notice a change in the color, odor, consistency, or amount of the secretions during suctioning. These signs could indicate a serious health problem. Immediately stop suctioning and call the doctor if any of the following situations occur:
• The secretions are bloody or tinged with blood.
• The secretions have a foul odor.
• The suction catheter needs to be cleared frequently because the secretions are excessive or thick.
• The person's breathlessness doesn't improve when you complete the suctioning procedure.
• The person sounds congested, but you're unable to suction any secretions.
• The person needs to be suctioned more often than the doctor recommends.
• The person's skin, lips, or fingernail beds look blue during suctioning.

18 Tracheostomy Care

Learning about a tracheostomy

A tracheostomy is a small opening, or stoma, that the doctor makes during surgery in the part of your throat called the trachea, or windpipe. A tube inserted into the tracheostomy makes it easier for you to breathe because it keeps your windpipe, or airway, open. You can also receive extra oxygen and remove mucus through the tracheostomy (trach) tube, if you need to. The illustration on the next page shows where the trach tube fits in your throat.

Your tracheostomy may be temporary or permanent, depending on your condition. If it's temporary, the doctor will allow the stoma to close when you're able to breathe normally again. If your tracheostomy is permanent, the doctor will suture, or sew, the edges of the stoma to your skin so that a permanent stoma will form. After the stoma heals, you may no longer need a trach tube to keep your airway open, but you'll still need to care for your tracheostomy properly.

Having a tracheostomy doesn't need to cramp your style. Whether temporary or permanent, a tracheostomy can help you lead a full, healthy life.

Learning about trach tubes

Most trach tubes are made of plastic and have three major parts: an outer tube, an inner tube, and an obturator.

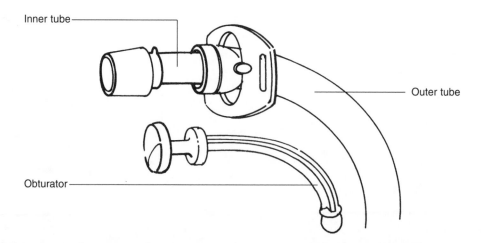

Inner tube

Outer tube

Obturator

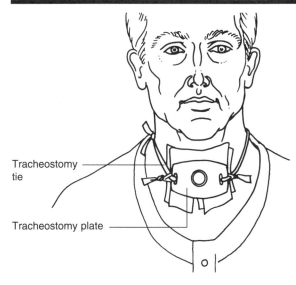

Tracheostomy tie

Tracheostomy plate

How a trach tube works

The obturator fits inside the outer tube and serves as a guide when the doctor slips the outer tube into the trachea. After the outer tube is inserted, the obturator is removed and the inner tube is inserted. The obturator can be inserted into the stoma in an emergency if the tube accidentally comes out of your throat. A tracheostomy tie threaded through loops on both sides of the tracheostomy plate holds the tube in place. A small lock secures the inner tube in place when you turn it.

What a cuff does

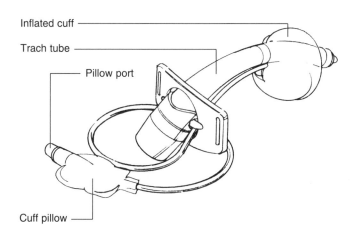

Inflated cuff

Trach tube

Pillow port

Cuff pillow

Many trach tubes have one or two balloon-like cuffs that can be inflated after the tube is inserted. A cuffed trach tube is less likely than an uncuffed tube to come out of your throat accidentally—for example, if you cough violently or if the trach tie comes loose. The cuff creates a seal that keeps air from leaking around the trach tube. The cuff will also help prevent you from accidentally aspirating, or inhaling, food, liquid, or anything else other than air into your airway.

To inflate the cuff, use a syringe to inject a small amount of air into the cuff's pillow port. (For guidelines on measuring cuff pressure, contact the home health care nurse or respiratory therapist.) The cuff pillow should inflate slightly. If the pillow is flat, the trach cuff has a leak. Notify the home health care nurse immediately.

Determining tube size

The doctor will decide which size tube is right for you based on your age, the amount of swelling (if any) around the stoma, and the size of your neck muscles. For example, if your neck is muscular, you'll need a trach tube that's larger and longer than average.

Reviewing care supplies

To care for your tracheostomy, you'll need to stock up on some or all of these supplies:
- scissors
- spare trach tube
- trach tube brush
- two basins
- trach bib
- cotton swabs
- tweezers
- 3% hydrogen peroxide solution
- sterile water or normal saline solution.

The doctor or nurse will tell you which of these supplies to use and where to get them. (A medical supply company or a drugstore carries most of these items.)

Cleaning the inner cannula

To prevent infection, remove and clean the inner cannula regularly, as the doctor orders.

1 Gather this equipment near a sink: a small basin, a small brush, mild liquid dish detergent, a gauze pad, a pair of scissors, and clean trach ties (twill tape).

Or open a prepackaged kit that contains the equipment you need. Now, wash your hands. Position a mirror so that you can see your face and throat clearly.

2 Unlock the inner cannula, and remove it by pulling steadily outward and downward.

Prepare to clean the soiled cannula immediately for rein-

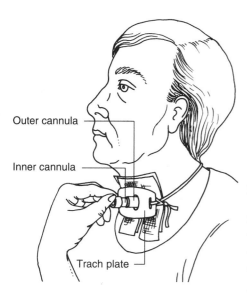

Outer cannula

Inner cannula

Trach plate

sertion. (Or put the soiled cannula aside and slip a clean inner cannula inside the outer cannula.)

If you start to cough, cover your stoma with a tissue, lean forward, and relax until the coughing stops.

3 Next, clean the soiled cannula. Here's how. Soak the cannula in mild liquid dish detergent and water. Then clean it with a small brush. If the cannula is heavily soiled, try soaking it in a basin of 3% hydrogen peroxide solution. You'll see foaming as the solution reacts with the secretions that are coating the cannula. When the foaming stops, clean the cannula with the brush.

You can obtain a special trach tube brush at a medical supply company or a pharmacy. However, the small brushes used to clean coffee pots work just as well. They're inexpensive and available at hardware stores. Just make sure to use the brush only for your trach tube.

4 Rinse the inner cannula under running water. Make sure you've removed all the cleaning solution. Shake off the excess water, and reinsert the clean, moist cannula immediately. Don't dry it; the water droplets that remain help lubricate the cannula, making reinsertion easier. Remember to lock the inner cannula in place.

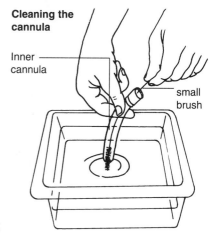

Cleaning the cannula

Inner cannula

small brush

Making trach ties and securing the trach tube

You can make your own trach tie with tracheostomy twill tape, but you may need another person to help you secure it.

Here's how.

1 Remove both twills from their wrapper, and knot one end of each to prevent fraying. Make folds about 1 inch (2.5 cm) below the knots you've made. Cut a ½-inch (1.3-cm) slit up the middle of each fold.

Knotting the twills

Cutting the twills

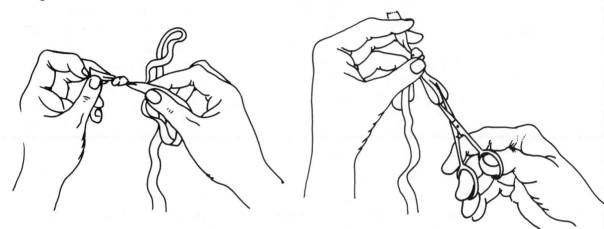

2 Hold the trach plate steady as your helper takes one twill and slips the end that isn't knotted through the trach plate slot from the bottom. Then he should feed it through the slit you've made and gently pull the twill taut. He should secure the second twill the same way. If you're threading the twills yourself, you'll need to look in a mirror so you can see what you're doing.

Threading the twills through the trach plate

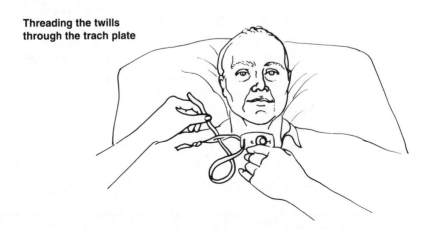

Tying the twills

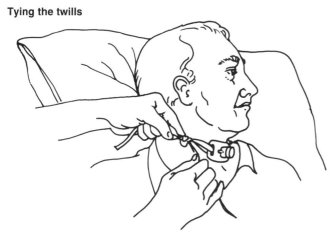

3 Have your helper tie both twills together on the side of your neck. He should put a finger underneath the tie to act as a spacer while setting the knot. To avoid a bulky knot that could irritate the skin, have him wrap one twill around the other several times before he makes the knot or use a double bow. Whichever method he uses, he should wrap a piece of tape around the knot to make it more secure. Finally, fit a trach bib in place around the trach plate.

Making a trach bib

A trach bib will help collect any discharge that drains from the stoma and prevent skin irritation around the stoma. You can use either a standard gauze pad or a nonstick, nonshredding gauze pad to make a trach bib. Just follow these steps.

1 Unwrap a 4-inch by 4-inch (10.2-centimeter by 10.2-centimeter) gauze pad and unfold it. Then fold it in half lengthwise, and turn down the corners to form a center opening about 1 inch to 2 inches (2.5 centimeters to 5 centimeters) long.

Folding the gauze pad lengthwise

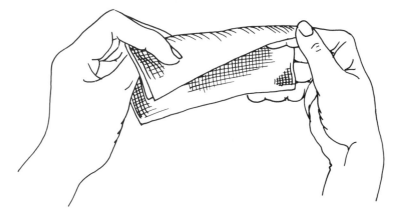

Turning down the corners

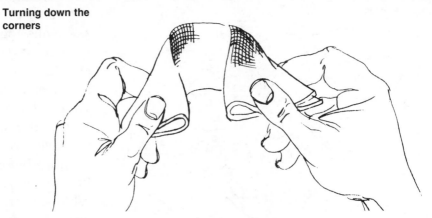

2 Cut a slit through both the pad and its wrapper as far as the pad's center. Then cut a hole in the center just big enough to go around the trach tube, and remove the wrapper.

Cutting to the center of the pad

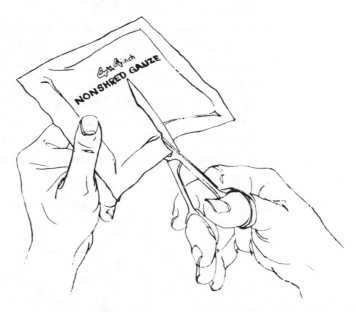

3 Carefully insert the bib under the trach plate. When it's in place, it should look like one of the examples shown below. If heavy discharge is draining from the stoma, insert the bib from below.

Standard gauze bib

Nonshredding gauze bib

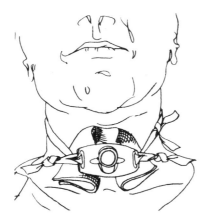

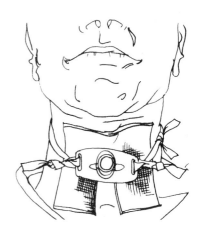

Suctioning the tracheostomy

To remove secretions that accumulate in the tracheostomy, use these directions to help you remember how to suction.

1 Gather the following equipment:
- suction machine
- connection tubing
- basin
- water
- suction catheter.

Note: If you're suctioning your own tracheostomy, you won't need disposable sterile gloves. However, if you're performing this procedure on someone else, wear gloves. You may also choose to use gloves if you have a respiratory tract infection. You should suction your trach tube whenever you can't cough up mucus or other secretions that block your airway.

You can sterilize normal tap water by boiling it for 5 minutes. As the water cools, put a lid on the pot so that the water stays germ-free. Keep a supply of sterile water in a glass jar that's been sterilized by boiling. You can also buy sterile water.

Also keep a bulb syringe nearby in case the suction machine malfunctions or the power fails.

Wash your hands thoroughly. Then fill the basin with sterile water and set it aside.

2 Turn on the suction machine, and adjust the regulator dial to the proper setting. The setting usually should be between –80 and –120 mm Hg but no higher than –120 mm Hg.

3 Remove the suction catheter from its wrapper or airtight container.

4 Now, attach the suction catheter to the control valve on the suction tubing if the control valve isn't part of the suction catheter.

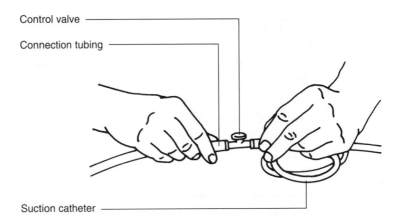

Control valve

Connection tubing

Suction catheter

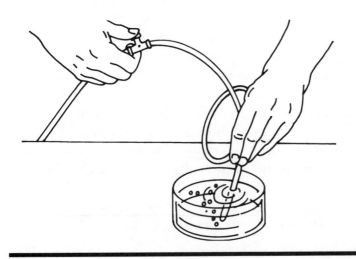

5 Dip the catheter tip into the sterile water. This will make the catheter easier to insert.

6 Take a few deep breaths, and then gently insert the moist catheter 5 inches to 8 inches (12.7 centimeters to 20.3 centimeters) into the trachea through your trach tube or stoma until you feel resistance.

Caution: Be careful not to cover the catheter's control valve during insertion. This will create suction pressure that could damage the lining of the trachea.

Inserting the catheter

Withdrawing the catheter

Rolling the catheter

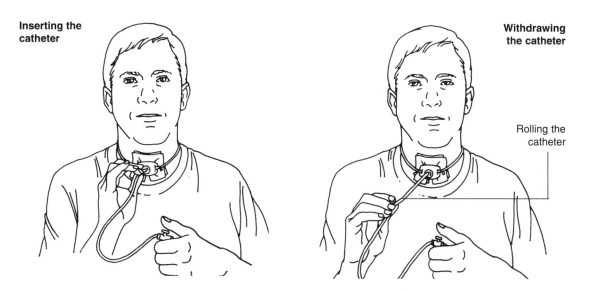

7 With your thumb, alternately cover and uncover the catheter's control valve to start and stop the suction. As you do this, slowly withdraw the catheter from the trachea, rolling it between your thumb and fingers as you go. Withdrawing the catheter should take no longer than 10 seconds. (Longer than that steals oxygen from your lungs.)

8 After you withdraw the catheter with your finger over the control valve, put the tip in the water and let the suction machine run a few seconds longer to clear the suction catheter and connection tubing. Then turn off the suction machine and disconnect the catheter from the connection tubing. If you're using a disposable catheter, discard it in a plastic-lined wastebasket.

If you're using a reusable catheter, sterilize it according to the manufacturer's instructions. Also, clean the basin and the collection receptacle.

Reinserting your trach tube

Suppose you accidentally cough out your trach tube. Don't panic. Follow these simple steps to reinsert it.

1 Remove the inner cannula from the dislodged trach tube. If you're using a cuffed tube, be sure you deflate the cuff first.

Inserting the obturator

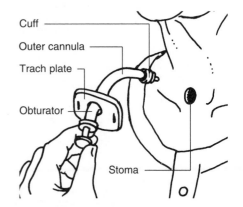

2 Insert the obturator into the outer cannula. Then use the obturator to reinsert the trach tube into your stoma.

3 Hold the trach plate in place, and immediately remove the obturator.

Then insert the inner cannula into the trach tube. Next, turn the inner cannula clockwise until it locks in place. Chances are you'll cough or gag while you're doing this, so be sure to hold onto the trach plate securely.

Removing the obturator

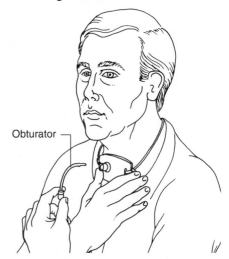

4 Now, insert the tip of a syringe without a needle into the tube's pillow port or cuff. Inflate the cuff, as the doctor orders. The inflated cuff will help prevent the tube from accidentally being dislodged again.

5 After inflating the cuff, secure the trach ties and tuck a trach bib under the trach plate.

Using a trach collar

If you have a tracheostomy, you'll use a humidifier to add moisture to the oxygen and a trach collar to breathe it. The humidifier attaches to your oxygen system the same way a humidifier bottle does when a nasal cannula or face mask is being used. Special wide oxygen tubing connects the trach collar to the humdifier.

A family member or other caregiver will help you put on the collar and set up the oxygen supply. The following instructions explain how.

Adding moisture to the oxygen

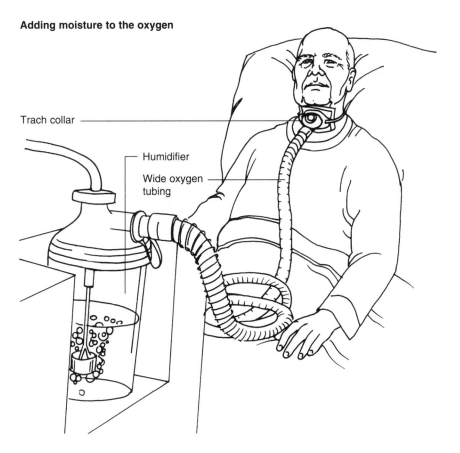

Trach collar

Humidifier

Wide oxygen tubing

Attaching the tubing

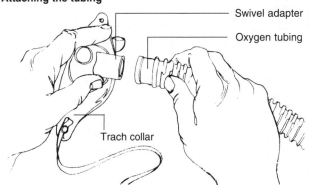

Swivel adapter

Oxygen tubing

Trach collar

1 Attach one end of the oxygen tubing to the humidifier. Attach the other end of the tubing to the swivel adapter on the trach collar.

2 Next, set the oxygen to the flow rate and concentration the doctor has prescribed. Make sure the oxygen is flowing freely through the tubing.

3 Snap the elastic strap on one side of the collar, and place the collar's center opening, or exhalation port, directly over the trach tube.

Positioning the collar

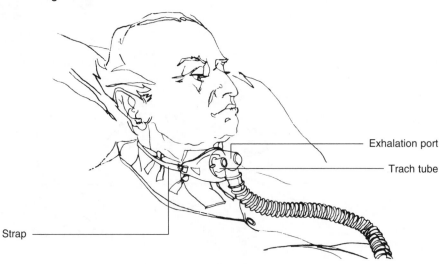

Exhalation port

Trach tube

Strap

4 Now, slip the free end of the elastic strap around the back of your neck, and insert it through the opening on the collar's other side. Gently pull the strap to adjust the fit.

Adjusting the strap

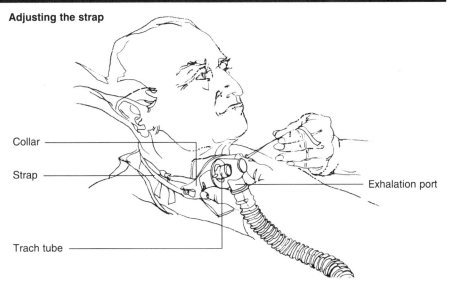

Collar

Strap

Exhalation port

Trach tube

5 Position the tubing so that moisture buildup can't flow toward the tracheostomy. Remember, you can move the swivel adapter to either side. Take care not to block the exhalation port with bed linen.

Using the trach collar safely

To use the trach collar safely, follow these guidelines:
• Empty moisture buildup at least once every 2 hours. If moisture is allowed to collect, it can drain into the tracheostomy and make you choke.
• Remove the trach collar every 4 hours and clean it with water. If mucus collects in the collar, your stoma can become infected.

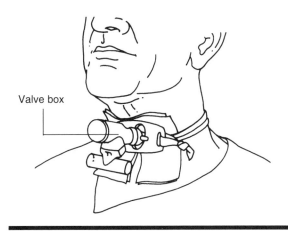

Valve box

Using tracheostomy attachments

Here are four tracheostomy attachments that may meet your special needs.

One-way trach valve box

This attachment allows you to speak with the trach tube in place. The valve box fits directly into the trach tube opening. When you inhale, the one-way valve lets air through the trach tube into your lungs. When you exhale, the force of your breath closes the valve. This diverts air through your larynx so that you can speak.

Artificial nose

This attachment fits directly into the trach tube and humidifies the air you breathe. When you exhale, aluminum foil that's rolled inside the artificial nose traps moisture. Then, as you inhale, the moisture evaporates.

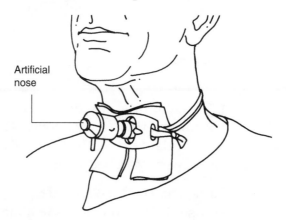

Tracheostomy button

A tracheostomy button closes off the trach tube so that you can breathe normally. The button consists of two main pieces: a short outer tube that fits into the stoma and reaches the trachea and a solid inner tube that completely closes off the tracheostomy.

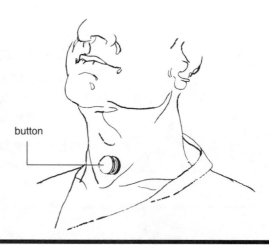

Tracheostomy plug

Like a tracheostomy button, this attachment helps wean you from the tracheostomy. The plug fits into the outer tube of most small-diameter trach tubes. By adjusting the plug, you can gradually decrease the tube's diameter until the tube is completely closed.

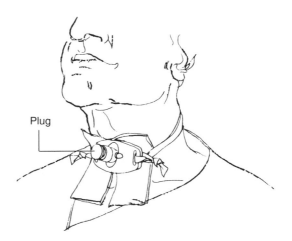

Plug

Living with a tracheostomy

You'll find that daily living with a tracheostomy involves making a few changes in your normal routine. Here's how to adjust.

Eating

If you have a cuffed trach tube, the doctor will tell you whether to keep the cuff inflated or to deflate it when you eat. What's the difference? Some doctors prefer to keep the cuff inflated so that you won't accidentally aspirate food or liquid into your airway while you eat. Other doctors disagree, contending that an inflated cuff bulges into the food tube, or esophagus, making it hard to swallow. Whichever method you use, be sure to call the doctor if you have problems eating. To make eating easier, follow these guidelines:

• Eat soft or pureed foods; liquids may be hard for you to swallow.

• Take small bites and chew thoroughly before swallowing.

• If your condition permits, sit upright in a chair while you eat.

• Be sure to keep suction equipment nearby in case you aspirate food or liquid.

Wearing a stoma shield

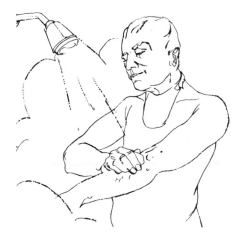

Showering

To protect your stoma while you're showering, wear a stoma shield. Or simply direct the stream of water to hit below the level of your stoma.

Coughing and sneezing

A tracheostomy may decrease your normal reflex to cough. But you'll need to remember to cough regularly so that your airway won't get blocked with secretions from your lungs. Follow these guidelines:

• Take a deep breath before you cough.

• Cover your tracheostomy when you cough so that mucus and secretions will collect in a tissue.

• Bend over when you cough to expel the secretions more easily.

• Keep tissues nearby, and remember to cover your nose and tracheostomy when you sneeze.

Communicating

Keep a small bell and writing materials nearby so that you can call for help and communicate your needs. You may want to use picture cards, a small chalkboard, or hand signals to express yourself.

If you have a cuffed trach tube, you won't be able to speak while the tube is in place. Why? Because the cuff prevents air from passing over your larynx, or voice box. When the tube is removed, you'll be able to speak normally again (unless your larynx has been removed). In the meantime, you may be able to speak when the cuff isn't fully inflated. If your condition permits, temporarily block the trach tube's opening with your finger to speak. Or use a one-way trach valve box or trach plug.

Getting out of the house

Feeling some anxiety about socializing and resuming your usual activities is normal when your tracheostomy is new. These tips will help:

• If you feel self-conscious about your appearance, conceal your stoma with a shirt and tie, a scarf, or jewelry.

• During the winter, wear a foam filter to warm the air you breathe. The filter will also help screen out air pollutants and prevent foreign objects, such as hair and food particles, from entering the stoma.

• To shield your stoma and cover the filter, wear a crocheted bib. Change the filter and the bib when they get dirty. You can also wear a scarf or a shirt with a closed collar that covers the opening, but be sure it's made of porous material, such as cotton.

Saving energy

Because you have a tracheostomy, you'll need to avoid any activity that makes you breathe harder or faster. These guidelines will help you save energy.

• If you're used to being physically active, ask the doctor to recommend less strenuous ways to exercise.

• Avoid rushing by planning your day carefully. For example, if you have an activity scheduled for the morning, get up a little earlier. That way you'll have time to get ready without hurrying.

• Spread out your activities over the day. For example, don't do all your chores in the morning. Save some for the afternoon or the next day, and rest between activities.

• Breathe deeply at least every 2 hours while you're awake. Remember to use your abdominal muscles. Breathing out should take twice as long as breathing in.

• Breathe deeply while performing any active movement, such as sweeping or mopping, or any activities that require you to raise your arms, such as lifting packages or combing your hair. Coordinate your movements with breathing.

Note: Whenever possible, avoid working with your arms raised, which can tire you more quickly. Work with objects at waist level instead.

19   Respiratory Therapy

Using an incentive spirometer

An incentive spirometer encourages you to breathe deeply and provides instant feedback to show how well you're doing.

Several types of incentive spirometers are available. The type shown below has one ball. All of them are used in the same way. Just follow these steps.

1 Sit up as straight as you can to help your lungs fully expand. Hold the spirometer's mouthpiece in one hand and the meter in your other hand. Position your hands so that the instrument is nearly level with your mouth.

Holding the spirometer correctly

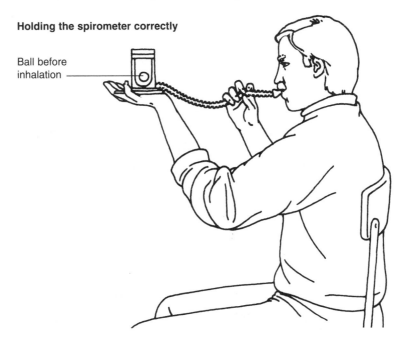

Ball before inhalation

2 Exhale normally. Now, place your lips tightly around the spirometer's mouthpiece.

3 With the spirometer at its lowest setting, slowly inhale through the mouthpiece as much as you can. Watch the ball in the spirometer to see how deeply you've inhaled. A rising ball usually marks your progress.

The more fully you expand your lungs, the higher the ball will rise. Now, hold your breath and count to 3 (even though the ball drops).

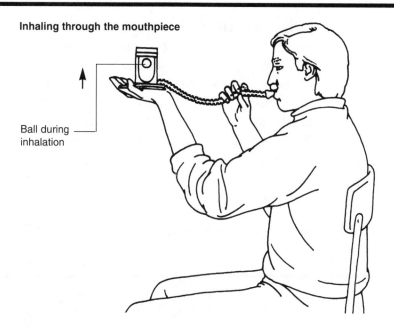

Inhaling through the mouthpiece

Ball during inhalation

4 Finally, remove the mouthpiece from your mouth and exhale normally. Rest for a moment. Repeat the exercise about 10 times, resting after each time.

As you increase your lung capacity, you'll see the ball rise higher. And as you master one level on the spirometer, aim for the next higher level.

Using a humidifier or vaporizer safely

A humidifier or vaporizer may help you breathe easier. These devices add moisture to dry air, helping to soothe an irritated airway and break up congestion.

To ensure safety, most health care professionals recommend using a cool-mist humidifier. If you use a vaporizer, you'll need to take precautions to prevent accidental steam burns. To use either unit, follow these guidelines.

1 Read the manufacturer's directions carefully. Check the unit, especially the power cord, for signs of damage.

2 Fill the unit's water tank to the correct level with cool, clean tap water or distilled water. Assemble the unit as directed in the instruction booklet.

3 If you use a humidifier, place the unit on a flat surface several feet away from the bed.

If you use a vaporizer, place the unit on the floor—not on a table or chair, where it might be knocked over and spill hot water. Also, don't have the steam vent pointing directly at you.

4 Before plugging in the unit, make sure the power cord lies safely away from such objects as radiators or heaters. And make sure no one can step on or trip over it.

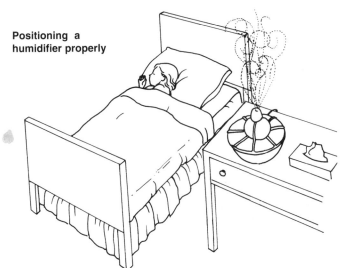

Positioning a humidifier properly

5 Check the unit periodically to make sure it's working properly. Refill the water tank as necessary. Also, at least every hour, make sure the bed linen isn't damp with excess moisture. If it is, change the sheets, and move the unit slightly farther away from the bed.

6 Unplug the power cord when you're not using the humidifier or vaporizer. And never move or tilt the unit without first turning it off and unplugging it.

7 Empty and clean the humidifier or vaporizer daily. In a humidifer, germs can breed and thrive in any remaining water. In a vaporizer, mineral deposits from hard water may build up and block steam flow. Follow the manufacturer's directions for cleaning the unit. Wipe it dry after each use.

Overcoming shortness of breath

When you're having trouble breathing, performing special exercises will help you feel better. Practice these exercises twice a day for 5 to 10 minutes until you get used to doing them.

Abdominal breathing

1 Lie comfortably on your back, and place a pillow beneath your head. Bend your knees to relax your stomach.

2 Press one hand on your stomach lightly but with enough force to create slight pressure. Rest the other hand on your chest.

Using your hands to monitor your breathing

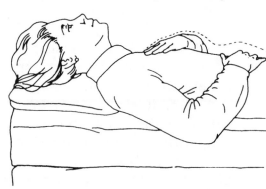

3 Now, breathe slowly through your nose, using your stomach muscles. The hand on your stomach should rise during inspiration and fall during expiration. The hand on your chest should remain almost still.

Pursed-lip breathing

1 Breathe in slowly through your nose to avoid gulping air. Hold your breath as you count to yourself: one-1,000; two-1,000; three-1,000.

2 Purse your lips as if you're going to whistle. Now, breathe out slowly through pursed lips as you count to yourself: one-1,000; two-1,000; three-1,000; four-1,000; five-1,000; six-1,000.

You should make a soft, whistling sound as you breathe out. Exhaling through pursed lips slows down your breathing and helps get rid of the stale air trapped in your lungs.

When performing pursed-lip breathing during activity, inhale before exerting yourself; exhale while performing the activity.

If the recommended counting rhythm seems awkward, find one that's more comfortable. Keep in mind that you must breathe out longer than you breathe in.

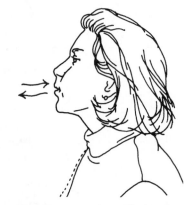

Exercising for healthier lungs and easier breathing

These exercises improve the airflow through your lungs. But keep in mind that these exercises are performed in addition to chest physiotherapy—not in place of it.

Breathing exercises

The abdominal breathing exercise described on the previous page can help you breathe more efficiently. You should do this exercise while you're resting or performing activities that don't make you breathless. Practice it until it becomes second nature.

The next exercise can help you combat breathlessness during physical activity:

Reach up and inhale, expanding the chest. Bend down and exhale, compressing the chest. Repeat several times.

For any exercise, inhale during the relaxation phase, and exhale during the exertion phase.

Try to establish a normal breathing ratio—that is, taking slightly longer to exhale than to inhale. For example, when climbing stairs, take three steps per inhalation and four steps per exhalation.

Importance of posture

Good posture promotes efficient breathing and prevents back pain. To check your posture, follow these guidelines.

Stand sideways in front of a full-length mirror. Lift your shoulders up and back, hold your head erect, and keep your lower back slightly arched. Don't flex your back, contract your abdomen, or round your shoulders.

Posture exercises

The following exercises will improve the posture, strengthen the back muscles, and stretch breathing muscles. Do them 3 times a week in twin sessions of 10 times each (10 repetitions, pause, 10 more repetitions).

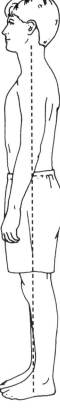

Imaginary line showing good posture

Shoulder pinch

Sit with your back straight and your elbows raised to about shoulder level. Pull your elbows back, and pinch your shoulder blades together.

Elbows raised to begin   **Elbows pulled back**

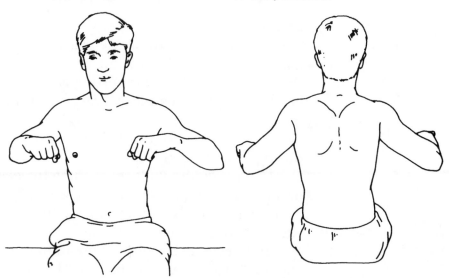

Shoulder depression

Sit with your back straight. Tilt your head to the right while pulling your left shoulder down. Then tilt your head to the left while pulling your right shoulder down.

Back arch

Lie face down in bed with your elbows pointing to the sides. Inhale, lifting your back, shoulders, and head off the bed. Hold this position for 16 seconds while breathing. Then return to a face-down position as you exhale.

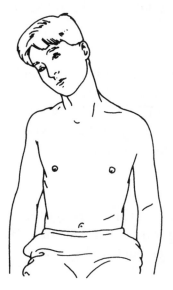

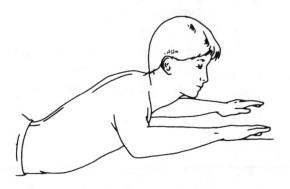

Pectoral stretch

Stand in a doorway or a corner. Place your palms or your forearms on the wall, rotating your shoulders about 90 degrees backward. Then lean into the corner or doorway, keeping your back straight and flexing only at the ankles for a count of 60.

Abdominal stretch

Lie on your back with a pillow underneath your shoulder blades and your upper and lower back. Relax your abdominal muscles, and stretch them over the pillow for about 5 minutes.

Chest mobility exercises

These exercises increase the strength and flexibility of the chest wall muscles. Do them 3 times a week in twin sessions of 10 times each.

Side bends

Stand with your feet about 12 inches (30.5 centimeters) apart and your arms extended to the sides. Bend to the right side as you exhale, and return to the center as you inhale. Now, bend to the left side as you exhale, and return to the center as you inhale.

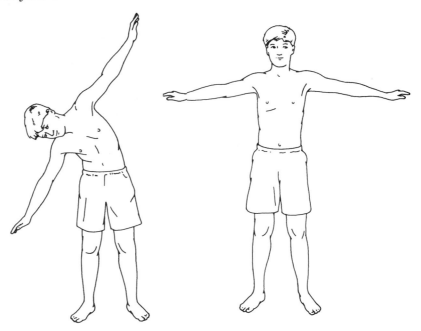

Trunk rotation

Sit with your arms raised to about shoulder level and your elbows bent. Twist to the right while exhaling, and return to the center while inhaling. Now, twist to the left while exhaling, and return to the center while inhaling. Keep your hips facing forward.

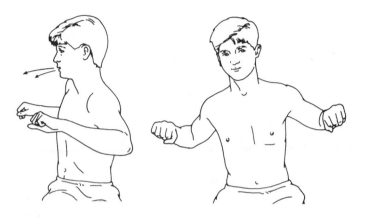

Aerobic exercises

This form of exercise helps lower the heart rate (because the heart muscles work more efficiently), helps clear mucus from the lungs, and can increase your activity level. It can also be lots of fun.

Keep in mind that any moderate exercise performed continuously for at least 20 minutes is considered aerobic—for example, walking, swimming, jogging, bicycling, dancing, playing basketball or soccer, or jumping rope.

Increase the duration of your exercise gradually. For maximum benefit, you should exercise at least three times a week at your target heart rate. (The doctor or physical therapist can give you a minimum and maximum pulse rate to guide you.)

Performing chest physiotherapy

Chest physiotherapy helps make your breathing easier. This treatment has three parts: postural drainage, percussion, and coughing.

You'll be able to perform postural drainage and coughing yourself, but you'll need the help of a family member or friend to percuss your back.

Postural drainage lets the force of gravity drain mucus from the bottom of your lungs. Then percussion helps move thick, sticky mucus from the smaller airways of your lungs into the larger airways. Coughing—the last and most important step—clears mucus from your lungs.

When to perform chest physiotherapy

Unless the doctor tells you differently, perform chest physiotherapy when you get up in the morning and before you have dinner or go to bed. When you have more mucus than usual (for example, during a respiratory tract infection), perform this therapy more often.

Before therapy

Don't eat for 1 hour before performing chest physiotherapy to avoid abdominal bloating and the risk of choking on vomited food. If the doctor tells you, use your inhaler 10 to 15 minutes before percussion to improve its effectiveness.

Avoid wearing tight or restrictive clothing around your chest, neck, or stomach. Wear a light shirt or gown to avoid friction from percussion.

Postural drainage

1 Place a box of tissues within easy reach. Also, stack pillows on the floor next to your bed.

2 Next, lie on your stomach over the side of your bed. Support your head, chest, and arms with the pillows you've placed on the floor. Stay in this position for 10 to 20 minutes, as tolerated.

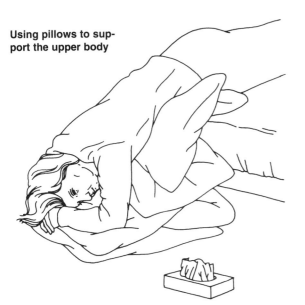

Using pillows to support the upper body

Percussion

1 Remain in the postural drainage position. Have a family member or friend position his hands in a cupped shape, with his fingers flexed and thumbs pressed tightly against the side of his index fingers.

Positioning hands for percussion

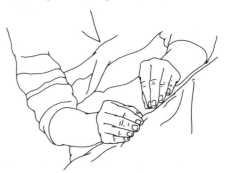

2 Next, have him rhythmically pat your back for 3 to 5 minutes, alternating his cupped hands. He can start on one side of the back, just above the waist, and percuss upward, changing sides as he continues. Percussion will feel firm but shouldn't hurt. You should hear a hollow sound like a horse galloping.

Coughing

1 While remaining in the postural drainage position, take a slow, deep breath through your nose. Hold the breath as you count to yourself: one-1,000; two-1,000; three-1,000.

2 Briefly cough three times through a slightly open mouth as you breathe out. An effective cough sounds deep, low, and hollow; an ineffective cough sounds high-pitched.

3 Take a slow, deep breath through your nose and breathe normally for several minutes. Repeat this coughing procedure, as tolerated.

4 After chest physiotherapy, return to an upright position slowly to prevent light-headedness and, possibly, fainting.

Performing forced exhalation techniques

The doctor has ordered a type of chest physiotherapy called forced expiratory technique (FET) to help you clear your lungs during exhalation (breathing out).

How FET works

FET combines deep breathing and normal breathing with long, controlled exhalations.

This treatment forces air behind the mucus in your airways to help keep them open. It also helps to move mucus into the windpipe so that you can cough it up more easily.

FET isn't hard to learn. Just remember, you must concentrate during the long exhalations. Otherwise, the mucus won't move.

When to perform FET

Perform FET after being in the postural drainage position, before or after coughing, or after an aerosol treatment (explained below) to maximize airway clearance.

You can also use it as a separate treatment, repeating each cycle five to six times or until your lungs are clear (15 to 20 minutes).

How to perform FET

1 Sit in a comfortable position, and place one hand on your abdomen.

2 Take two or three slow, moderately deep breaths, expanding your lower chest and abdomen. Try to breathe in through your nose and out through your mouth.

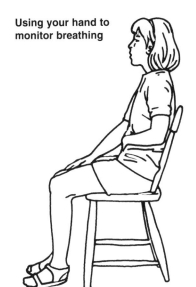

Using your hand to monitor breathing

3 Then inhale gently and slowly, expanding your lungs about halfway. Pause.

4 Keep your mouth in an O shape and the back of your throat open. Then force the air out, using your stomach muscles. But don't force it out too hard. Repeat until you cough up some mucus.

5 Repeat steps 2 through 4 until your lungs are clear.

Did I do it right?

If you've done FET correctly, you'll make a "ha" sound when coughing or you'll hear a crackling sound before mucus is coughed up.

If you do FET too hard or for too long, you'll have a hacking, dry, nonproductive cough or you'll hear a hiss, wheeze, grunt, or catch. You may also get a sore throat. If you perform FET too gently, nothing will happen.

Using aerosol equipment

Aerosol equipment consists of a compressed air machine and disposable plastic parts (mouthpiece, mask, syringes, and medicine cups). The equipment must be kept scrupulously clean. If it isn't, bacteria can enter your lungs along with the mist.

Here's how to clean the plastic parts and maintain the air compressor.

Cleaning the plastic parts

You don't need to clean the parts every time they're used, but you should rinse them in warm or cool water after each treatment.

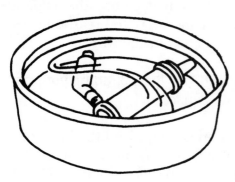

Soaking the plastic parts in vinegar and water

Clean the parts daily, following the doctor's recommendations or those of the equipment manufacturer. Or use the following procedure:

1 Wash the plastic parts daily in warm water and a mild dishwashing detergent and then rinse them. The air compressor doesn't require cleaning. Never submerge it in water.

2 After rinsing the parts, soak them for 30 minutes in a solution of 1 cup white vinegar and 3 cups warm water. Rinse well in cool water.

3 Let the parts air-dry before placing them in a clean storage container. Be sure to replace them every month.

Maintaining the air compressor

Keeping the compressor in perfect working order promotes better treatments and extends the life of the compressor. How often you have the compressor serviced depends on the type of compressor you have and the manufacturer's recommendations.

Troubleshooting equipment problems

If the machine isn't producing enough mist, the problem may be a simple one that you can solve yourself. For example, you might need to:
• change the air filter
• tighten the connections
• try a new aerosol cup.

If these measures fail, take the compressor to your medical equipment supplier for checking. It may need internal cleaning, but if the compressor is 8 to 10 years old, you'll probably need to replace it.

Performing aerosol treatment

1 Place the correct amount of medication into the plastic medicine cup and secure the cap.

2 Attach the mouthpiece or mask to the medication chamber. Then attach the tubing to the medication chamber and the air machine.

3 Turn on the machine. Breathe slowly and deeply until all the medication has evaporated. (Shake the medication chamber to make sure you've taken all the medication.)

4 Turn off the machine, and clean the equipment.

Using a hand-held inhaler

To use a hand-held inhaler, follow these steps.

1 Shake the inhaler, holding it so that the canister is above the mouthpiece.

2 Take a deep breath and exhale completely.

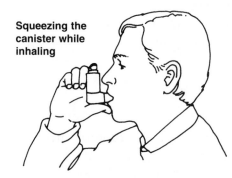

Squeezing the canister while inhaling

3 Hold your mouth on or near the mouthpiece, squeeze the canister downward, and inhale the mist that comes out of the mouthpiece.

4 Hold your breath for a few seconds when inhaling (to enhance the placement and action of the drug), and wait 1 minute before inhaling again. Be careful not to inhale too early or too late. Make sure to inhale the mist; don't swallow it.

5 Rinse your mouth with water after each use. Your nose and throat may be dry and you may have an unpleasant taste in your mouth after you inhale the medication.

6 Take the mouthpiece off the canister and rinse it daily. Clean the inhaler according to the manufacturer's directions.

Don't use the inhaler more than the prescribed number of times. Also, be careful not to get the spray in your eyes because it may temporarily blur your vision.

Using an inhaler with a holding chamber

To dilate your bronchial tubes, you need to inhale a medication called a bronchodilator through an inhaler that's placed in the mouth. Attached to the inhaler is a holding chamber that allows the medication to penetrate deep into the lungs.

The most common types of holding chamber are the InspirEase System and the aerochamber. Here are instructions for using an inhaler with either of these devices.

InspirEase System

This system consists of a holding chamber that collapses and inflates during inhaling and exhaling. To use the inhaler with this device, follow these steps.

1 Insert the inhaler into the mouthpiece, and shake the inhaler. Then place the mouthpiece into the opening of the holding device, and twist the mouthpiece to lock it in place.

2 Extend the holding device, exhale, and place the mouthpiece in your mouth.

3 Firmly press down on the inhaler once. Then inhale slowly and deeply, collapsing the bag completely. If you breathe incorrectly, the bag will whistle. Hold your breath for 5 to 10 seconds, and then exhale slowly into the bag. Repeat the inhaling and exhaling steps.

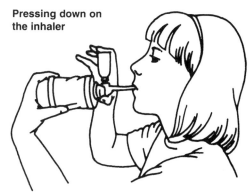

Pressing down on
the inhaler

4 Wait 5 minutes. Then shake the inhaler again and repeat the dose, following steps 2 and 3.

Aerochamber system

This system uses a small cylinder called an aerochamber to trap medication. To use the inhaler with this device, follow these steps.

1 Remove the caps from the inhaler and the mouthpiece of the aerochamber. Then insert the inhaler mouthpiece into the wider rubber-sealed end of the aerochamber. Shake the entire system.

Pressing down on
the inhaler

2 Exhale. Place the aerochamber in your mouth, and close your lips. Depress the inhaler once. Inhale slowly and deeply. Hold your breath and count to 10.

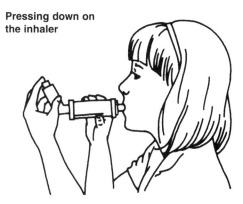

3 Wait 5 minutes. Then shake the entire system again, and repeat step 2.

Using a turbo-inhaler

Inhaling medication through this "whirlybird" device will help prevent asthma attacks.

Caution: Never use the turbo-inhaler more often than the doctor prescribes.

1 Wash and dry your hands. Unwrap one capsule so that it's ready to use. Then hold the inhaler so that the mouthpiece is on the bottom. Slide the sleeve all the way to the top.

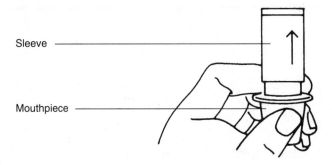

Sleeve

Mouthpiece

2 Open the mouthpiece by unscrewing its tip counterclockwise. Inside you'll see a small propeller on a stem.

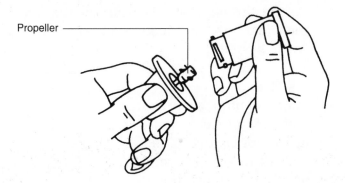

Propeller

3 Firmly press the colored end of the medication capsule into the center of the propeller. Avoid overhandling the capsule, or it may soften.

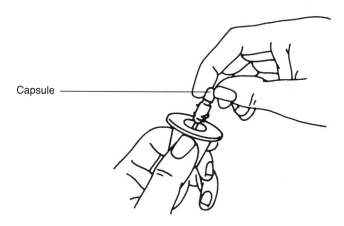

Capsule

4 Now, screw the device together securely, and hold it with the mouthpiece at the bottom.

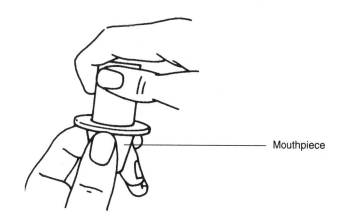

Mouthpiece

5 To puncture the capsule and release the medication, first slide the sleeve all the way down and then slide it up again. Do this step only once.

6 Make sure every-thing is secure. Then hold the device away from your mouth, and exhale as much air as you can.

7 Now, tilt your head backward. Place the mouthpiece in your mouth and close your lips around it.

Quickly inhale once to fill your lungs. Inhaling through the mouthpiece spins the propeller, releasing the medication, which will then reach your airways.

8 Hold your breath for several seconds. Then remove the device from your mouth, and exhale as much air as you can. Repeat step 7 and this step several times, until all the medication in the device has been inhaled. Never exhale through the mouthpiece.

Exhaling before using the inhaler

Holding your breath after inhaling

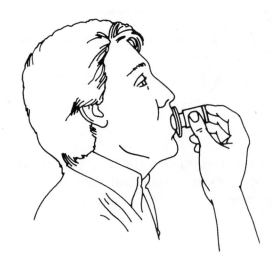

Exhaling with mouthpiece removed

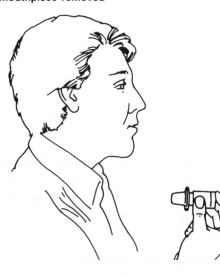

9 Discard the empty medication capsule. Then place the entire turbo-inhaler in its metal can, and screw on the lid.

At least once a week, remove the turbo-inhaler from the can, take it apart, and rinse it thoroughly with warm water. Make sure it's completely dry before you reassemble it. Leave the capsules wrapped until needed to keep them from deteriorating too rapidly.

Using continuous positive airway pressure

When you sleep, your tongue or relaxed fatty tissue in your throat can block your breathing, causing sleep apnea. To help you breathe more easily, the doctor may order continuous positive airway pressure (also called CPAP) to keep this tissue out of your airway.

How CPAP works

While you sleep, you'll wear a mask that fits snugly over your nose and supplies pressurized air. A flow generator feeds compressed air through the mask. You'll regulate the air pressure with a valve that you'll set for the level that will prevent your apnea.

Before using CPAP, you'll undergo a sleep study. This will help the doctor calculate the pressure level that's right for you. Then he'll prescribe a custom-fitted CPAP unit for your use at home.

Using CPAP

The nurse (or equipment supplier) will show you how to set the machine for the prescribed pressure. She'll also teach you how to check for leaks or kinks. Then she'll show you how to clean the mask and change the air filter.

Your symptoms should subside quickly after you start using CPAP. Remember to keep using the device every night, even after you feel better. Otherwise, sleep apnea could recur.

Using CPAP while you sleep

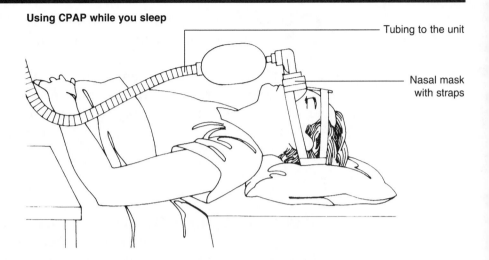

Tubing to the unit

Nasal mask
with straps

Troubleshooting equipment problems
• Keep the names and telephone numbers of the doctor and equipment supplier handy.
• If your mask doesn't fit properly, your skin may become red and chafed and escaping air may irritate your eyes. Call the equipment supplier and ask for a new mask.
• If you suspect that the CPAP device may be giving you an earache, a runny nose, or sinus pain, consult the doctor. Also let the doctor know if your symptoms don't subside or if they recur.
• If you have a mechanical or an electrical problem with the equipment, notify the equipment supplier at once.

Caring for a person on a ventilator
If the person you're caring for can't breathe on his own or if his respiratory efforts fail to expand his chest and deliver oxygen to his lungs, the doctor may order mechanical ventilation (a vent, or ventilator). Before a ventilator can be used, the person must have an endotracheal tube (ET), a tracheostomy tube, or a noninvasive form of delivery, such as a continuous positive airway pressure mask, in place.

Follow these steps if the person you're caring for is on a ventilator. Ensure that the person can reach you by using a bell or some other device.

1 Check all connections between the ventilator and the person. Make sure the ventilator alarms are turned on.

2 Verify that the ventilator settings are correct and that the ventilator is operating at those settings.

3 Check the in-line thermometer to make sure the temperature of the air being delivered is close to body temperature, between 89.6° and 98.6° F (32° to 37° C).

4 Check the water level in the humidifier, and refill it if necessary. Check the corrugated tubing for condensation. If condensation is present, drain it into another container and discard it. (Don't drain the humidifier.)

5 Check the person's breathing pattern and respiratory status. Look at chest expansion, noting symmetry (similarity of both sides) and breathing depth. Watch for signs of distress or discomfort. Also observe the person closely for changes in level of his consciousness.

6 Check the person's blood pressure, heart rate, and respiratory rate as ordered or when a change occurs in his condition. Take his temperature at least daily (more frequently if it's elevated). If vital signs change significantly, report such changes to the doctor immediately.

7 Suction the person as necessary, noting the amount, color, odor, and consistency of the secretions.

8 If possible, weigh the person, and report a weight gain of 5 pounds (2.3 kilograms) or more within a week.

9 Have emergency telephone numbers nearby. Call the doctor or respiratory therapist if you have any questions or problems.

Providing supportive care

If the person you're caring for is on a ventilator, he'll need additional supportive care. This may include maintaining his airway, meeting his medication and nutritional needs, sustaining mobility and communication, and providing mouth care.

Suctioning the airway

• Clear the person's airway as needed. Indications for suctioning include frequent coughing, secretions in the tube, and activation of the equipment's high-pressure alarm.

• Before you begin suctioning the person, explain the procedure to help reduce his anxiety. Warn him that he'll have an urge to cough. Reassure him that he'll receive extra oxygen during the procedure.

• Note the amount, color, and consistency of the secretions, and write down your findings.

Providing medications

• Give the person all the medication that the doctor has ordered.

• If aerosol treatments are ordered, place the medication into a small-volume nebulizer, and insert the nebulizer into the inspiratory line of the ventilator circuit. Connect the administration tubing to the nebulizer port of the ventilator.

• Monitor the person for adverse reactions. After treatment, suction the person, if necessary.

• Check the person's nutritional status throughout treatment. Depending on his condition, provide parenteral or enteral nutrition, as ordered.

Promoting mobility and communication

• Reposition the person every 2 hours to help mobilize respiratory secretions and to make him comfortable. Whenever possible, help him sit in a chair near the ventilator.

• If the person can turn himself, encourage him to change positions frequently. Repositioning prevents pressure ulcers and improves lung aeration.

• Perform chest physiotherapy as ordered. This therapy helps move secretions to the larger airways, where they can be removed through suctioning or coughing.

• Maintain the person's muscle tone by performing range-of-motion exercises. Explain each exercise, and encourage him to participate, if possible. Plan exercises related to his specific needs and tolerance.

• If the person is well enough, set up a writing board or other communication tool so that he can convey his questions and concerns. Place the call bell within easy reach.

• Explain that the alarms on the equipment (the ventilator, cardiac monitor, and pulse oximeter) will immediately alert you to any situation that needs attention.

Providing mouth care

• Brush the person's teeth or rinse his mouth at least every 4 hours.

• Sponge the lining of his mouth to keep it clean and moist and to make him more comfortable, as needed.

20   Feeding Tubes and Pumps

Learning about feeding tubes

The body's cells need fuel to produce energy. Food produces that fuel after the body breaks it down into forms the cells can use. This conversion of food is called digestion.

Sometimes, a person can't take in all the nutrients the body needs by chewing and swallowing. That's when the feeding tube may be needed to get food into the body. The doctor might order tube feeding if:

• a person's throat is blocked—for instance, from surgery or a tumor.

• chewing or swallowing becomes difficult—for instance, after head or neck surgery or because of a broken jaw.

• a person is too weak or confused to eat—for instance, after a stroke or serious illness.

• the body needs extra nutrients to speed healing—for instance, if the person is badly burned.

• the person is unconscious.

How food travels through the gastrointestinal tract

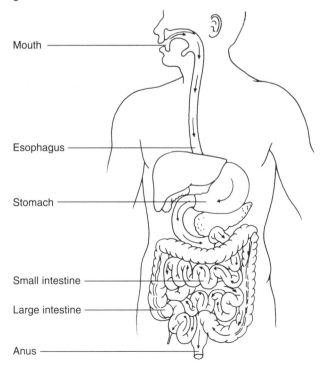

Mouth

Esophagus

Stomach

Small intestine

Large intestine

Anus

The feeding tube may be inserted through the mouth (orogastric) or nose (nasogastric) or through a surgical opening into the stomach (gastrostomy) or small intestine. The most common types are nasogastric and gastrostomy tubes.

If the person you're caring for needs tube feeding, you can provide him with this special care at home. A home tube feeding system includes formula (liquid food), a delivery set—a feeding bag, clamps, syringe, and tubing—to carry the formula to the person's feeding tube, and an intravenous (I.V.) pole or a hook from which to hang the delivery set. Tube feedings can be given intermittently or continuously. If the person you're caring for needs continuous feeding, you'll also need an enteral infusion pump to deliver a steady, constant flow of formula.

Preparing for an intermittent tube feeding

Called intermittent feedings because the procedure isn't continuous, these liquid meals supply nourishment when the person in your care can't chew or swallow, or can't ingest sufficient food to meet nutritional needs.

Gather the following equipment:
- feeding formula
- measuring, mixing, and pouring devices
- warm water
- bulb or piston syringe
- feeding bag.

1 If the formula is in the refrigerator, take it out and let it warm to room temperature. (Formulas come premixed or in a powder or liquid form to be mixed with water. The doctor will tell you which type of formula to use and how to feed it to the person.) Or warm the formula by placing the container in a basin of tepid water. *Note:* Never warm the formula over direct heat, and always follow the manufacturer's directions for storing and reusing. If the formula isn't premixed, measure and mix it as directed for one feeding only.

2 Position the person properly by raising his head to at least a 30-degree angle (higher if his condition permits). You can use pillows or a backrest if you're not using a hospital bed.

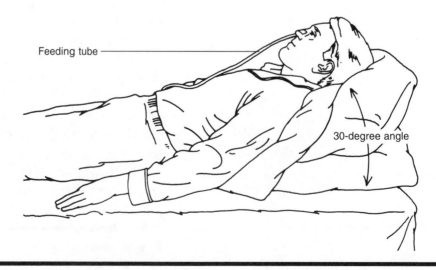

Feeding tube

30-degree angle

Drawing up gastric fluid

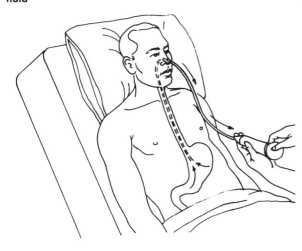

3 Verify the tube's position in the person's stomach by drawing up gastric fluid into the syringe. To do this, first remove the feeding tube's cap or plug. If you're using a bulb syringe, gently squeeze and hold the bulb. Attach the syringe to the end of the feeding tube, and release the bulb. If you're using a piston syringe, pull back on the barrel. This should draw some gastric juices—yellow-green fluid— through the tube.

If you can't draw any fluid, the tube may be pressed against the stomach wall or curled in the stomach. Help the person move or turn. Then try again to draw up some fluid. If you're still unsuccessful, call the doctor.

If you're able to draw fluid into the syringe, squeeze the bulb or push in the barrel of the piston syringe to return the fluid to the stomach.

Checking stomach sounds with a stethoscope

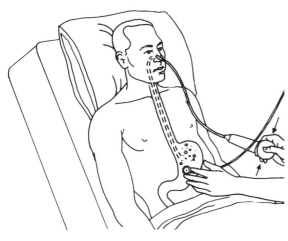

4 Perform a second verification of the tube's position by listening to the person's stomach sounds with a stethoscope. If he has a nasogastric tube, pay special attention to this test to make sure that the tube is correctly positioned in his stomach and hasn't drifted into his lungs. Now, reattach the syringe to the feeding tube, and either squeeze the bulb or push in the barrel to inject a small amount of air into the tube. If you hear a gurgling sound through the stethoscope, this means that air is entering the stomach and the tube is clear. Now, clamp the tube, and remove the syringe. If you don't hear a gurgling sound, call the doctor.

Giving an intermittent tube feeding

After you've checked tube placement, assemble the feeding bag or syringe, tubing, and roller clamp. You'll need an I.V. pole or hook to hold the feeding bag. Now, follow these steps.

1 Attach one end of the tubing to the feeding bag. Then clamp the tubing shut. Pour in the prescribed amount of formula, and hang the bag from the I.V. pole or hook. Unclamp the tubing, and slowly run the formula through it to remove all air bubbles. Then reclamp the tubing. Now attach the other end of the tubing to the person's nasogastric or gastrostomy tube. (You may need a connector.)

Hang the bag at the height that allows the feeding formula to flow freely. Set the flow rate to provide the feeding amount prescribed by the doctor. Unclamp the tubing to start the flow.

Feeding elements in place

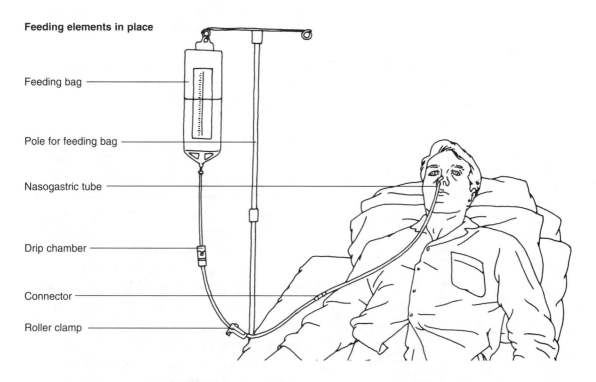

Feeding bag

Pole for feeding bag

Nasogastric tube

Drip chamber

Connector

Roller clamp

If you're using a syringe, pinch off the feeding tube with your fingers or a clamp, and attach the syringe. Remove the syringe's bulb or plunger, and pour in the prescribed amount

Unclamping the tube

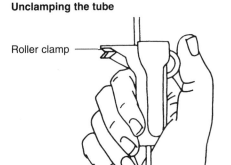

Roller clamp

of formula while holding the syringe at the level of the person's head.

Unclamp the tube to start the flow. When the syringe is three-quarters empty, pour in more formula.

2 Write down what time the flow began and when it's scheduled to end. Always give a tube feeding as slowly as possible. If you give it too quickly, the person may get diarrhea.

3 During the feeding, check the feeding bag and tubing to make sure the flow doesn't stop or change. Squeeze the feeding bag every now and then to prevent clogging or settling.

If you're using a syringe, never allow it to empty completely until the end of the feeding to prevent air from entering the tube and the person's stomach.

Ending the Feeding

After you've fed the person the prescribed amount of formula for the right length of time, you're ready to end the feeding.

1 Clamp the feeding bag, and disconnect it from the person's nasogastric or gastrostomy tube. Then pour 2 ounces (59 millileters) of water into the bulb or piston syringe after you've attached it to the feeding tube.

If you're using a syringe, pour 2 ounces (59 milliliters) of water into the syringe before it completely empties of formula.

Allow the water to flush the feeding tube. This clears away any leftover formula that could stick to and clog the tube.

Once you've flushed the feeding tube, clamp the tube shut. If the person has a nasogastric tube, replace the cap or plug, and tape or pin the tube to the person's clothing until the next feeding. If he has a gastrostomy tube, apply the plug or gauze dressing, as directed. If the person complains of nausea, leave the feeding tube unclamped and uncovered until the feeling passes.

Flushing the feeding tube

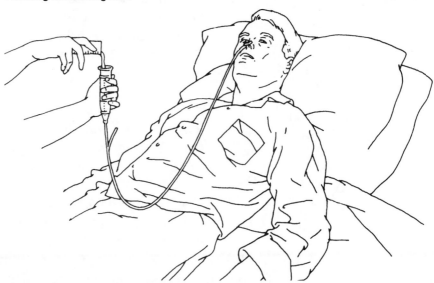

2 Keep the person in a sitting position for about 30 minutes to help prevent him from vomiting or inhaling any leftover formula. If he's uncomfortable sitting, help him lie on his side. Prop up his head with pillows, or partially elevate the head of the bed.

If the feeding bag or syringe is reusable, wash it with warm water, dry it, and store it.

Preparing for a continuous tube feeding

Giving continuous tube feeding to the patient you're caring for isn't difficult. The nurse and equipment supplier will show you how. Then use the following information to review their instructions.

Getting ready

Make sure the person's feeding tube is clear (unblocked) and in the correct position for delivering food.

Wash your hands thoroughly with soap and water. Then prepare the formula as directed by the doctor, and help the person sit up. Now, remove the cap or plug on the feeding tube, and follow these steps.

Schematic drawing of fluid withdrawal

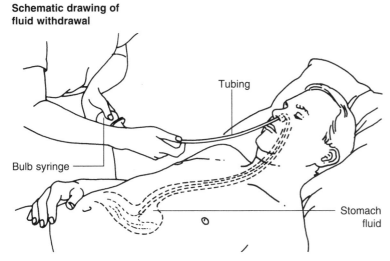

Tubing

Bulb syringe

Stomach fluid

1 If you're using a bulb syringe, gently squeeze and hold the bulb while you attach the syringe to the feeding tube. Then release the bulb.

If you're using a piston syringe, attach the syringe's barrel to the feeding tube, and then gently pull back on the plunger.

With either type of syringe, some stomach fluid should be drawn up through the tube. This shows that the tube's in the correct position. If no fluid appears, the tube may be pressed against the intestinal wall or curled in the small intestine. Try to reposition the tube by helping the patient move or turn. Then try again to draw up some fluid. *Caution:* If no fluid appears, call the home health care doctor or nurse before proceeding.

2 Make sure the tube is clear. To do this, squeeze the syringe's bulb or push in its plunger to return the fluid to the stomach. Then flush the feeding tube with 2 ounces (59 milliliters) of water at body temperature. If water flows easily through the tube, the tube is clear.

If the patient has a nasogastric tube, pay special attention to the steps above to be sure the tube is still positioned correctly in the stomach and hasn't drifted into the lungs.

3 To double-check, reattach the syringe to the feeding tube, and either squeeze the bulb or push in the plunger to inject a small amount of air into the tube. Then listen to the patient's stomach with a stethoscope.

If the tube's clear and positioned correctly, you'll hear whooshing or gurgling as air enters the stomach. (If you don't hear these sounds, call the home health care doctor or nurse before proceeding.)

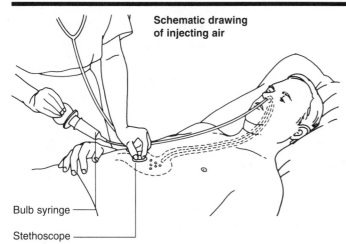

Schematic drawing of injecting air

Bulb syringe

Stethoscope

4 Now, clamp the tube, and remove the syringe. Gather the rest of the equipment:
- infusion pump and stand
- delivery set (feeding bag and tubing)
- tube connector
- I.V. pole or hook.

Giving a continuous tube feeding

Follow the pump manufacturer's directions for attaching the tubing to the feeding bag and for filling, closing, and hanging the feeding bag and working the pump.

1 Be sure to clamp the tubing after attaching it to the feeding bag.

Pump and stand

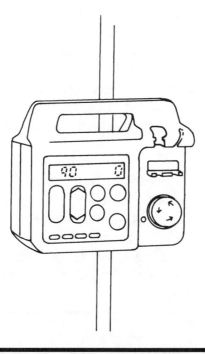

Food delivery set

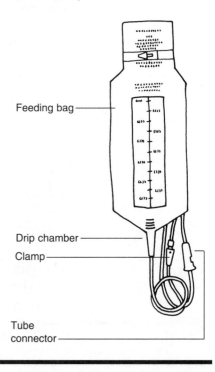

Feeding bag

Drip chamber

Clamp

Tube connector

2 If the feeding bag–tubing apparatus has a drip chamber, open the clamp and squeeze the drip chamber until it's half-filled with formula—don't fill it completely. Then run the formula through the tubing to remove all the air.

Eliminating air bubbles

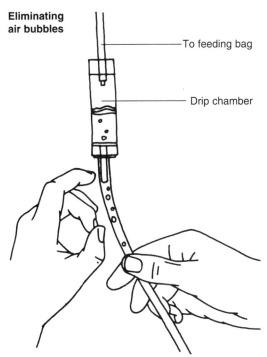

To feeding bag

Drip chamber

3 Eliminate any air bubbles by flicking the tubing with your fingers. Continue flicking the bubbles all the way up the tubing to the drip chamber so that air doesn't go into the person's stomach.

4 With the pump plugged in, set or check the flow rate on the controls according to the doctor's orders and the manufacturer's directions. Then open the flow clamp and the clamp on the feeding tube. Switch on the pump to begin the formula's flow.

5 During the feeding, check the feeding bag and tubing regularly to be sure the formula continues to flow smoothly. Remember to do the following:
• Squeeze the feeding bag every so often to help prevent clogging or settling.
• Listen for the pump to beep or stop, which it will do if the tubing becomes blocked or the feeding bag empties.
• Watch to see that the feeding bag always contains formula so that air doesn't enter the person's stomach. (Even though the feeding bag empties, most pumps continue pumping air instead of food.)
• Examine the pump setting regularly to be sure it's still correct. Adjust the flow rate, if necessary.
• Check to make sure that the tube leading to the stomach stays in place.

Changing the feeding bag

Because the person you're caring for requires continuous feedings, you'll need to replace the empty feeding bag with a full one. Here's how.

1 Cover one end of the tubing that's supplied with the new feeding bag with a sterile gauze pad. Secure the pad with a rubber band until you're ready to attach that end to the tube leading to the person's stomach.

Positioning the rubber band

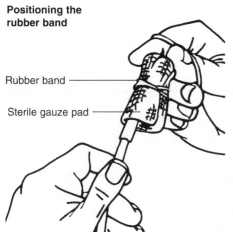

Rubber band —

Sterile gauze pad —

2 Attach the other end of the tubing to the new feeding bag, and fill the bag with formula as the manufacturer directs. Then clamp the tube.

3 Turn off the pump. Clamp the old feeding bag and its tube. Disconnect them at the connector site.

4 Remove the old feeding bag from the pump, and attach the new feeding bag as the manufacturer directs. Make sure to let the formula run through the tubing to remove any air.

5 Now, remove the gauze pad from the end of the tubing connected to the new feeding bag, and connect the tubing to the feeding tube.

6 Open the clamped tubes, and turn on the pump to start the formula's flow. Then wash, rinse, and dry the old feeding bag and tubing if they're reusable.

Giving medication through a nasogastric tube

Gather the following equipment:
• medication and medication cup
• bulb syringe
• small funnel (optional)
• clamp (or you can use your fingers)
• warm water.

1 Read the instructions on the medication container's label. Then pour the correct dose into the medication cup. Have the person sit up, and tell him to remain in a sitting position for 30 minutes after receiving the medication.

Precaution: Watch the person closely while you're giving the medication. If he shows sign of discomfort, stop at once. Call the doctor for instructions.

2 Make sure the nasogastric tube is positioned correctly in the person's stomach. (See steps 4 and 5 of "Preparing for an intermittent tube feeding.") If the tube isn't positioned correctly, don't give the medication. Instead, call the doctor for instructions.

3 Once you're sure the tube is positioned correctly, close it off using the clamp or pinch it with your fingers. Then attach the syringe or funnel to the end of the tube. (If you're using a syringe, remove the bulb.)

4 Pour the medication into the syringe or funnel, and unclamp the tube. Let the medication flow through the tube by gravity; never force it.

Before all the medication has gone down the tube, pour 1 to 2 ounces (29.6 to 59 milliliters) of water into the syringe or funnel. (Pour only ½ to 1 ounce (15 to 29.6 milliliters) of water for an infant or a child.)

5 Control the medication's flow either by raising or lowering the syringe or funnel or by pinching the tube and then releasing it.

Closing the tube

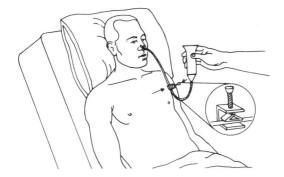

Controlling the flow by raising or lowering the syringe

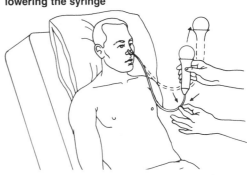

6 After you've given all the medication and the water, remove the syringe or funnel and reclamp or recap the tube. (If the person feels sick to his stomach, leave the tube open until the feeling passes.) Remind the person to remain in a sitting position for 30 minutes.

Recap the medication container. Then rinse all the equipment and store it safely.

Caring for a person with a nasogastric tube

If you're caring for a person who has a nasogastric tube, you'll need to change the tape that holds the tube in place every day. You'll also need to provide regular nasal care to keep the tube from irritating the person's nostril. Here's how to give the person the special care he needs.

Applying the tape

Take a 2-inch (5-centimeter) strip of 1-inch-wide (2.5-centimeter) tape and split it lengthwise. Leave a small tab intact at one end. Place the tab over the bridge of the nose. Then spiral the two small split ends around the tubing. Be sure the tubing isn't pulling or pressing on the nostril. Secure the two split ends with another strip of tape. Commercially prepared tape tabs are available, but they may be more expensive.

Taping over the bridge of the nose

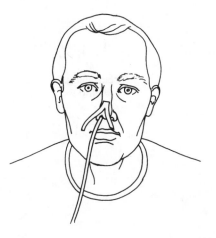

Spiralling the tape around the tubing

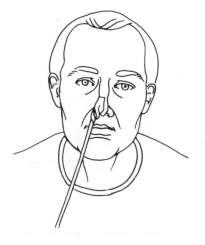

Note: Never tape the tubing to the person's forehead. This causes pulling on the tube and could create a pressure ulcer inside the person's nostril.

If the tape won't stick to the person's skin, rub his skin with tincture of benzoin. When it dries but still feels tacky, place the tape over the skin.

Checking the tape

Check the tape regularly during the day. If it's loose, apply new tape so that the tube won't slide in and out of the person's nostril.

To keep the tubing from dangling or tugging, wrap tape around its end and leave a tab free. Or loop a rubber band around the tubing. Then safety-pin the tab or rubber band to the person's clothing just below shoulder level.

Changing the tape

Change the tape daily. Remove it gently, and clean the skin under it with soap and water to wash off the adhesive. Dry the skin, and apply fresh tape. Hold the nasogastric tubing securely while it's untaped.

Providing nasal care

Clean the person's nostrils every day with cotton-tipped applicators moistened with warm water. This removes any crusted mucus and soothes the person's nose. Also, check the nostril where the tubing enters the nose for bleeding or skin irritation. Then apply a water-soluble lubricant, such as K-Y jelly, to the tube where it enters the nostril. (Don't use a petroleum jelly, such as Vaseline.) Reapply the lubricant as needed.

Providing mouth care

A person who's being tube-fed needs special mouth care. His mouth and throat can become dry and sore because he's breathing through his mouth, not drinking fluids, and not producing the saliva that normally comes from chewing food. To help the person keep his mouth and throat moist and comfortable, follow these tips.

• Encourage the person to breathe through his nose.

• Remind him to brush and floss his teeth or to clean his dentures every morning and night.

• Offer mouthwash or warm salt water for the person to gargle to soothe mouth dryness or a sore throat.

• Use petroleum jelly to prevent to relieve dry lips.

If the person can't care for his own mouth, you'll need to provide mouth care for him at least every 4 hours or as often as the doctor recommends. Here's how.

1 Gather the equipment you'll need: a soft toothbrush, toothpaste or tooth powder (with fluoride, unless your drinking water is fluoridated), a glass of cool water, a small basin, and a towel. Help the person sit up, and tuck the towel under his chin. Dip his toothbrush in the water, and apply toothpaste to it.

2 Brush the surface of each tooth with 8 to 10 strokes, moving from the gums to the tooth crowns. Use short, vibrating strokes where the gum meets the tooth.

Also brush his tongue and the roof of his mouth to help remove thickened saliva that can collect here.

3 Give the person some cool water and a basin to rinse his mouth and remove the toothpaste foam and any particles. Wipe his lips and chin with a towel.

Giving medication through a gastrostomy tube

Gather the following equipment:

Attaching the syringe to the gastrostomy tube

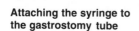

• medication and medication cup
• bulb syringe or small funnel
• warm water
• 4-inch by 4-inch (10.2 by 10.2-centimeter) sterile gauze pad
• rubber band
• 2-inch-wide (5-cm) surgical tape.

1 After you've read the instructions on the medication container's label, pour the correct amount of medication into the medication cup.

Unclamp or uncap the tube, and attach the

syringe or small funnel to the end of it. (If you're using a syringe, remove the bulb.) To make sure the tube isn't clogged, pour about 1 ounce (30 milliliters) of water into it. (For an infant or a child, pour only about ½ ounce [15 milliliters] of water into the tube.) If the water doesn't drain into the stomach by gravity, twist the tubing gently to unclog it. If this doesn't work, stop the procedure and call the doctor for instructions.

2 Pour the medication into the syringe or funnel, letting it flow into the person's stomach by gravity. Don't force it. If the medication backs up in the tube or oozes out around the tube, stop giving the medication. Then call the doctor for instructions.

After you pour all the medication down the tube, pour in about 1 ounce (29.5 milliliters) of water (about ½ ounce [15 milliliters] for an infant or child). Then remove the syringe or funnel, and reclamp or recap the tube.

Clearing the tube with water

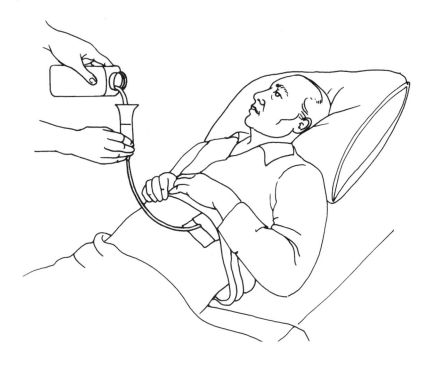

3 Wrap a gauze pad around the end of the tube, and secure the pad with a rubber band. This will keep the end of the tube clean.

Check the site where the tube enters the person's body. If medication has seeped out around the tube, call the doctor for instructions.

Store the medication container safely. Be sure to rinse all the equipment carefully.

Caring for a person with a gastrostomy tube

The area where the gastrostomy tube enters the body needs special care to avoid skin irritation or infection. Here's how to proceed.

Providing skin care

Wash the skin around the tube with mild soap and warm water at least once daily or as often as necessary. Examine the skin several times a day. If you see leakage of gastric or intestinal fluid, immediately apply a warm, moistened towel to soften any encrusted fluid. Then wash, rinse, and dry the skin. Apply ointment to the skin near the opening, if the doctor orders.

Changing the dressing

Change the tube-site dressing daily when you wash the skin and whenever it gets wet or soiled. Don't use scissors to cut off the dressing; you might cut the tube or the sutures hold-

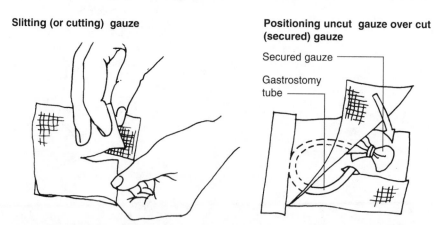

Slitting (or cutting) gauze

Positioning uncut gauze over cut (secured) gauze

Secured gauze

Gastrostomy tube

ing it in place by mistake.

Before applying a fresh dressing, make sure the end of the tubing is covered with gauze. Then position precut drainage sponges (or two 4-inch by 4-inch [10.2 centimeter by 10.2-centimeter] gauze pads cut halfway through the middle) around the tube so that the slit sides overlap. This protects the skin from gastric leakage. Then cover the slit pads and any ointment with uncut gauze pads. Secure the dressing with nonallergenic tape.

Solving common problems

Certain problems may arise when you're tube-feeding a person. For example, the feeding tube may become blocked or displaced. Or the person you're caring for may develop diarrhea, constipation, or other stomach discomfort. Sometimes you can solve these common problems yourself. Here's how.

Blocked tube

If the formula or water doesn't flow through the tube or if the person complains of nausea, vomiting, swelling, or stomach discomfort, the tube may be blocked. To try to unblock the tube, follow these tips:
• Change the person's position to shift a tube pressed against the stomach wall.
• Check each part of the feeding system, including all connections.
• Flick the tubing to remove air bubbles.
• Squeeze the feeding bag to stir up settled formula.
• Flush the tube with water.
• If you're using a pump, turn it off and check for mechanical problems as the manufacturer directs. If a pump feeding still doesn't flow, try gravity.

If the tube remains blocked, notify the home health care doctor or nurse so that the tube can be replaced.

Displaced tube

Occasionally, a tube gets out of position. Be sure to check the tube's position before and, if necessary, during continuous feeding. Stop the feeding and notify the doctor if the person vomits, gags, or chokes during feeding—these signs could signal a displaced nasogastric tube.

Diarrhea

Diarrhea is the most common side effect of tube feeding. To prevent it, try the following tips:
• Give smaller, less-concentrated feedings, slower and more frequently, as the doctor orders.
• Don't feed the person cold formula.
• Prevent bacteria from contaminating the formula by handling and storing the formula correctly.

If diarrhea is a side effect of medications the person's taking, the doctor may be able to change the prescription or prescribe a remedy.

Constipation

Many feeding solutions are low in fiber, so the person may have fewer bowel movements. But if he also has difficulty passing stools—constipation—notify the doctor. He may order a formula with more fiber or recommend that you give the person more water between or during feedings.

Nausea, cramps, and swelling

Nausea, cramps, and swelling typically occur when a person's stomach takes a long time to empty after a feeding. This can happen if the person's fed too much formula or if the formula's too highly concentrated or fed to the person too quickly.

To relieve nausea, help the person change his position. If that doesn't work, try stopping the feeding for an hour or so or slowing the flow rate. To prevent cramps, always give formula that has been warmed to room temperature. To counteract swelling and accompanying nausea, help the person walk around, if his condition permits.

When to call the doctor

Certain problems that arise during tube feeding require a doctor's help. Call the doctor if any of these situations occurs:
• the feeding tube remains blocked or dislodges.
• the person has persistent diarrhea, constipation, nausea,

cramps, or swelling.
• the person vomits, gags, or chokes during a feeding.
• the person's legs, feet, and hands become swollen.
• while checking the position of the feeding tube, you can't withdraw gastric fluid.
• you withdraw more than 1 ounce (30 milliliters) of fluid or the gastric fluid you withdraw is bloody or abnormal in color.

Also call the doctor if the person you're caring for develops any of the problems described below. Sometimes, these problems can signal a serious change in his condition.

Bleeding

Blood in the person's nostrils or around the gastrostomy tube could indicate internal bleeding. Also, be alert for less obvious signs of internal bleeding, such as bloody or dark black (tarry) stools, brown or rust-colored urine, or stomach drainage that resembles coffee grounds.

Coughing and difficult breathing

These signs could mean that fluid from formula feedings has entered the person's lungs—a condition that can lead to life-threatening pneumonia. Other, less common signs of fluid in the lungs include chest pain, coughing up rust-colored sputum, fever, chills, and a change in skin color, particularly lips and nailbeds that turn blue.

Fluid in the lungs can result when undigested formula collects in the stomach, flows back up into the throat (reflux), and is inhaled into the lungs (aspiration). To help prevent this, keep the person's head elevated at least 30 degrees during a feeding and for at least 30 minutes after a feeding. In addition, don't withdraw more than 1 ounce (30 milliliters) of gastric fluid when you check the position of the person's feeding tube.

Skin irritation

Signs of skin irritation, such as tenderness, redness, and swelling, where the feeding tube enters the person's body could mean that the tube isn't positioned properly. Unless the irritated area is treated, this condition can lead to infection, which may produce fever and leakage of pus around the feeding tube.

Changes in weight

Gradual weight loss may indicate that the person is getting too few calories to meet his energy needs. On the other hand, gradual undesirable weight gain may mean that the person's caloric intake is too high. In either case, you'll need to check with the doctor. He may need to adjust the amount or concentration of the person's feedings.

21 Cast Care

Understanding cast use

Wearing a cast for the coming weeks—although annoying and inconvenient—will keep the affected bones, muscles, and ligaments from moving so that they can heal properly.

The doctor has applied a cast for one or more of the following reasons:
- to keep the ends of a broken bone (fracture) together so that the bone can heal.
- to keep severely strained muscles and ligaments together so that they can heal.
- to keep a body part from moving after surgery or an amputation.
- to correct a deformity, such as congenital hip displacement or clubfoot.

Understanding bone healing

A broken bone starts to heal the moment the break occurs. But rigid bone tissue fragments take a long time to reestablish a firm union. That's why you should continue your rehabilitation program, even after your injured bone seems normal again. Here are the stages a broken bone goes through when it heals.

1 Blood collects around the broken bone ends, forming a sticky, jellylike-mass called a clot. Within 24 hours, a mesh-like network forms from the clot. This becomes the framework for growing new bone tissue.

Blood collects at the site

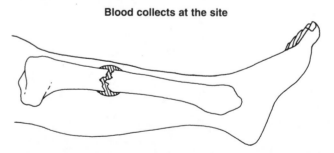

2 Osteoclasts and osteoblasts—the cells that do the bone healing—invade the clot. Osteoclasts start smoothing the jagged edges of bone. Meanwhile, osteoblasts start bridging the gap between the bone ends. Within a few days, these cells form a granular bridge, linking the bone ends.

Cells start bone healing

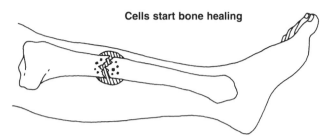

3 Six to ten days after the injury, the granular bridge of cells becomes a bony mass called a callus and, eventually, hardens into solid bone.

But for now, the callus is fragile, and abrupt motion can split it. That's why keeping a broken bone from moving while it's healing is so important.

Callus forms

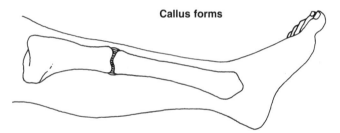

4 Three to ten weeks after the injury, new blood vessels start bringing calcium to the area to harden the new bone tissue. During this process, called ossification, the ends of the bones "knit" together.

After ossification, the bone becomes solid and is considered healed. Although the cast may be removed, up to 1 year may pass before the healed bone is as strong as it was before it broke.

Bone hardens

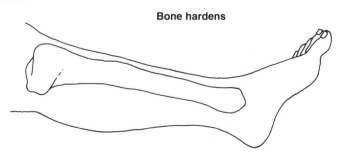

Calculating healing times

"How long will it take for my broken bone to heal?" That's a common question asked by people with fractures. The chart below lists approximate healing times. Your fracture may require more or less time to mend than average. You can speed your recovery by complying with the prescribed treatment and rehabilitation program.

AVERAGE HEALING TIME IN WEEKS

Collar bone	6
Upper arm	
Neck	6
Shaft	12
Forearm	
Both bones	12
One bone	6
Hand	6 to 10
Finger	3
Hip	12
Upper leg	16 to 24
Lower leg (tibia)	
Plateau	8
Shaft	16 to 24
Ankle	8 to 12
Lower leg (fibula)	
Shaft	8
Ankle	8
Heel	8 to 12
Foot	8
Toe	3

Caring for your cast

Think of your cast as a temporary body part—one that needs the same attentive care as the rest of you. While you wear your cast, follow these guidelines.

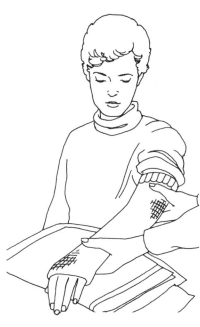

Drying

The doctor may apply a cast made of plaster, fiberglass, or a synthetic material. The wet material must dry thoroughly and evenly for the cast to support your broken bone properly. At first, the wet cast will feel heavy and warm. But don't worry—it'll get lighter as it dries.

To speed drying, keep the cast exposed to the air. Fiberglass and synthetic casts dry soon after application, but plaster casts take 24 to 48 hours to dry. Drying a plaster cast in less time will make it more comfortable sooner.

Make sure the pillows you use to raise the cast have rubber or plastic covers under the pillowcase. Place a thin towel between the cast and the pillows to absorb moisture. Never place a wet cast directly on plastic.

To make sure the cast dries evenly, change its position on the pillows every 2 hours; use your palms, not your fingertips. (You can have someone else move the cast for you, if necessary.) To avoid creating bumps inside the cast that could cause skin irritation or sores, don't poke at the cast with your fingers while it's wet. Also, be careful not to dent the cast while it's still wet.

Keeping the cast clean

After the cast dries, you can remove dirt and stains with a damp cloth and powdered kitchen cleaner. Use as little water as possible, and wipe off any moisture that remains when you've finished.

Protecting the cast

Avoid knocking the cast against a hard surface. To protect the foot of a leg cast from breakage, scrapes, and dirt, place a piece of used carpet (or a carpet square) over the bottom of the cast. Slash or cut a V-shape at the back so that the carpet fits around the heel when you bring it up toward the ankle. Hold the carpet in place with a large sock or slipper sock. Extending the carpet a little beyond the toes also helps to prevent them from being bumped or stubbed.

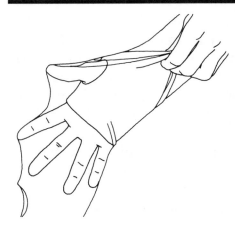

Preventing snags

To keep an arm cast from snagging clothing and furniture, make a cast cover from an old nylon stocking. Cut the stocking's toe off, and cut a hole in the heel. Then pull the stocking over the cast to cover it. Extend your fingers through the cut-off toe end, and poke your thumb through the hole you cut in the heel. Trim the other end of the stocking so that it's about 1½ inches (3.8 centimeters) longer than the cast, and tuck the ends of the stocking under the cast's edges.

Caring for your skin

Wash the skin along the cast's edges every day, using a mild soap. Before you begin, protect the cast's edges with plastic wrap. Then use a washcloth wrung out in soapy water to clean the skin at the cast's edges and as far as you can reach inside the cast. (Avoid getting the cast wet.) Dry the skin thoroughly with a towel, and then massage the skin at and beneath the cast's edges with a towel or pad saturated with rubbing alcohol. (This helps toughen the skin.) To help prevent skin irritation, remove any loose plaster particles you can reach inside the cast.

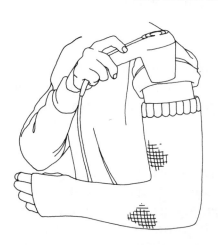

Relieving itching

No matter how much the skin under the cast may itch, never try to relieve the itching by inserting a sharp or pointed object into the cast. This could damage your skin and lead to infection. Don't put powder or lotion in your cast either or stuff cotton or toilet tissue under the cast's edges (this may cut down on your circulation).

Here's a safe technique to relieve itching: Set a hand-held blow dryer on cool and aim it at the problem area.

Staying dry

If you have a plaster cast, you'll need to cover it with a plastic bag before you shower, swim, or go out in wet weather. You can use a garbage bag or a cast shower bag, which you can

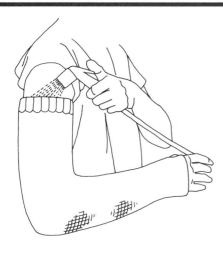

buy at a drugstore or medical supply store. Above all, don't get a plaster cast wet. Moisture will weaken or even destroy it. If the cast gets a little wet, let it dry naturally, such as by sitting in the sun. Don't cover the cast until it's completely dry.

If you have a fiberglass or synthetic cast, check with the doctor to find out if you may bathe, shower, or swim. If he does allow you to swim, he'll probably tell you to flush the cast with cool tap water after swimming in a chlorinated pool or a lake. (Make sure no foreign material remains trapped inside the cast.)

To dry a fiberglass or synthetic cast, first wrap the cast in a towel. Then prop it on a pad of towels to absorb any remaining water. The cast will air-dry in 3 to 4 hours; to speed drying, use a hand-held blow dryer.

Using a sling
The doctor may want you to wear a sling temporarily to support and rest your sore shoulder. Ask him when and how often you can remove the sling.

Signing the cast
Family members and friends may want to sign their names or draw pictures on the cast. That's OK, but don't let them paint over large cast areas. Why? Because this could make those areas nonporous and damage the skin beneath them.

Troubleshooting your casted arm or leg
After you leave the hospital, you'll need to check for possible problems with your casted arm or leg, such as wound drainage and excessive swelling. Get in the habit of checking your cast every day.

Watch for wound drainage
When a cast also covers a wound, you can expect some red or reddish brown drainage during the first 48 hours after the cast is applied. Drainage may stain the cast or, if it leaks

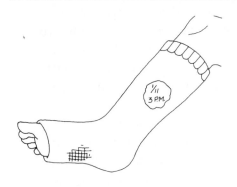

from the cast's ends, the bed linens. If drainage occurs, use a felt-tipped pen to outline it on the cast. Jot down the date and time, too.

Drainage may signal a problem that requires the doctor's attention. Notify the doctor if the drainage:
• stains the cast or bed linens bright red.
• occurs even though the cast wasn't applied over a wound (pressure from the cast may have caused a sore).
• changes in odor or color (this may indicate infection).
• spreads.

Test sensation and movement

Several times a day, check for changes in sensation by touching the area above and below the cast. Is the area numb? Do you feel tingling or pain?

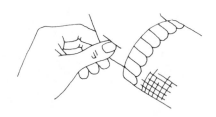

Wiggle the fingers or toes on the casted arm or leg. If you can't move your fingers or toes or you have more pain than usual when you move them, contact the doctor.

Check circulation

Press a fingernail or large toenail on the casted limb until the color fades. Then let go. If normal flesh color doesn't return quickly (within 3 seconds), contact the doctor at once. Repeat this check at least three times a day.

If your fingers or toes are cold, try covering them. If that doesn't warm them, contact the doctor.

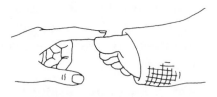

Cope with arm or leg swelling

A little swelling of a casted limb is normal, but a lot isn't. To help prevent excessive swelling, keep the cast raised above heart level as much as possible on two regular-sized pillows. Apply ice as directed by the doctor. If your leg is in a cast, sit or lie down and raise the leg on pillows. If your arm is in a cast, prop the arm so that your hand and elbow are higher than your heart. (Call the doctor if raising the cast doesn't reduce the swelling.)

Check for severe swelling above and below the cast several times daily. To do this, compare the casted arm or leg with the uncasted arm or leg.

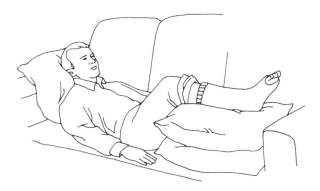

Relieve skin irritation

After the cast dries completely, rough edges may cause skin irritation. To smooth them, try these techniques.

If the cast is fiberglass, smooth rough edges by filing with a nail file. If the cast is plaster, "petal" rough edges using adhesive tape or moleskin. This prevents the material from catching on clothing or being peeled off accidentally.

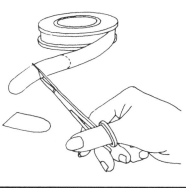

1 Cut several 4-inch by 2-inch (10-centimeter by 5-centimeter) strips of tape or moleskin. Trim the ends that will be outside the cast so that they're rounded, like toenails.

2 Place the first strip, rounded end down, on the outside of the cast.

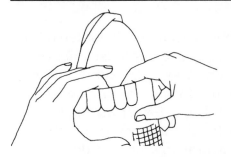

3 Tuck the straight end just inside the cast edge. Smooth the tape or moleskin with your finger to remove any creases, which can also irritate your skin.

4 Apply the remaining strips. Overlap them, as needed, until you've covered all the cast's rough edges.

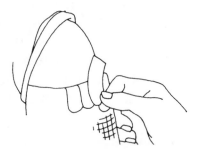

Exercises for a casted arm or leg

The doctor may recommend exercises for any joint of a casted arm or leg that is not covered by the cast. Exercising a joint will help keep the entire arm or leg strong and will help to prevent or reduce swelling.

The doctor will tell you which exercises to do. As he directs, do the exercises at least three times a day, several times each. If you feel pain when you do an exercise or have trouble moving any joint, call the doctor.

Finger exercises

Hold up the hand on your casted arm and separate (spread) the fingers; then bring them back together.

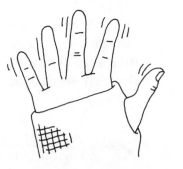
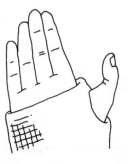

Next, hold up your hand, and touch the little finger and thumb together. Repeat with the other three fingers. Finally, bend all the fingers on your hand up and down, as though waving goodbye.

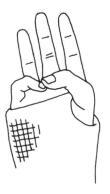

Shoulder exercise

Hold your casted arm down at your side with your palm facing your body. Now, swing the arm out and up until it's even with your shoulder; then bring it back to your side. Next, swing the arm across your chest toward your other arm. If necessary, use your unaffected arm to help lift up the injured arm to shoulder level. Then bring the casted arm back to your side.

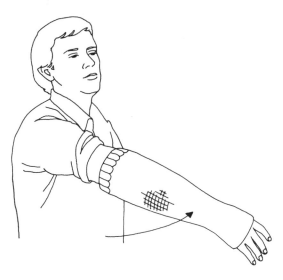

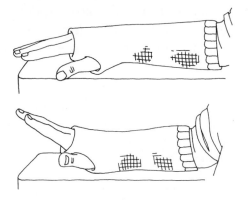

Wrist exercise

Rest the forearm of your casted arm on the arm of a chair. Extend your hand straight out with your palm down. Slowly bend your wrist up and down to raise and lower your hand.

Ankle exercises

Make a circle with the foot on your casted leg, moving it first clockwise and then counterclockwise. Next, stretch your foot so that your toes are pointing toward you. Then reverse this position so that your toes are pointing away from you.

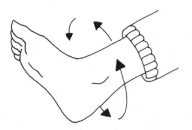

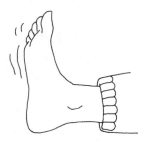

Toe exercise

Flex and wiggle your toes.

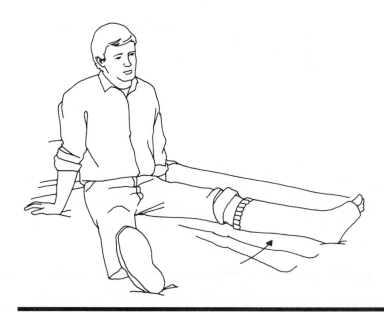

Hip exercises

Sit in the middle of the bed with both legs extended in front of you. Slowly move the casted leg as far to the side as it'll comfortably go. Then slowly move it back to its original position. Next, lie flat on your back, and bend the casted leg at the knee. Move it to your chest and then back to the bed.

When your cast is removed

Cast removal is fast and painless. The doctor will probably remove the cast only when the broken bone has healed. But he may have to remove it earlier if the broken bone requires additional movement, if the cast becomes damaged or tight, or if abnormal drainage signals a problem. Never try to trim or remove the cast yourself.

1 Using a specially designed handsaw, the doctor will first cut one side of the cast and then the other. (The handsaw swiftly cuts through stiff plaster, but it won't cut skin.)

Cutting the cast

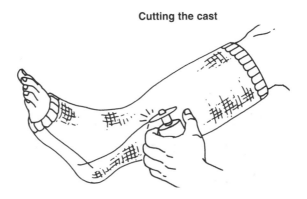

2 After cutting the cast, the doctor will open the cast pieces with a spreader. Then he'll cut through the cast padding with special scissors, revealing skin that's covered with yellow or gray scales—an accumulation of dead skin as well as oil from glands near the skin surface. The arm or leg will probably also appear thinner and flabbier than the arm or leg that wasn't casted, and it may ache and feel weak. But don't worry! With a little exercise and good skin care, the arm or leg will soon return to normal.

3 After removing all the padding, the doctor will wipe the arm or leg with an alcohol-saturated pad to remove debris. When you return home, continue this practice, which will gradually loosen all the accumulated dead skin. Wash the arm or leg every day with mild soap and water, dry it thoroughly, and then wipe it with an alcohol-saturated pad.

22 Urinary Catheters and Nephrostomy Tubes

Learning about urinary catheters

A urinary catheter or nephrostomy tube may be inserted to drain urine. A urinary catheter drains urine from the bladder; a nephrostomy tube allows urine to drain from the kidney.

An indwelling (or Foley) urinary catheter is held in place in the bladder by a small balloon. This type of catheter empties the bladder continuously. Only a health care professional can insert or remove an indwelling catheter.

An intermittent (or straight) urinary catheter is used to periodically empty the bladder. If the doctor has ordered this type of catheter for you, you'll probably be instructed how and when to insert it. If you become ill or can't insert the catheter yourself, someone else will need to do this for you.

Catheters come in a variety of sizes. The doctor or home health care nurse will tell you which size is right for you.

Urinary system

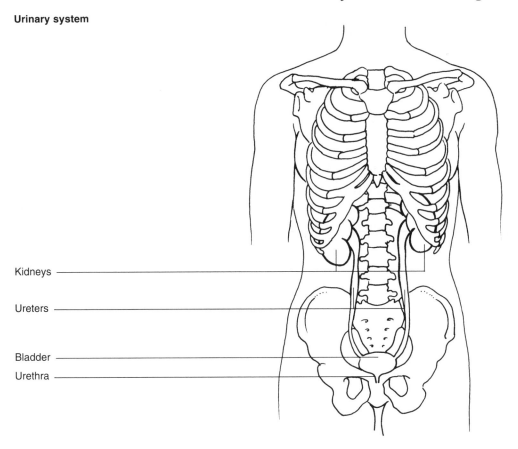

Kidneys

Ureters

Bladder

Urethra

Caring for your urinary catheter

Your catheter is a tube that will continually drain urine from your bladder so that you won't need to urinate. To care for your catheter, follow these guidelines.

Removing the tube from its sleeve

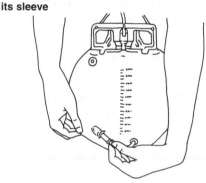

Emptying the drainage bag

The drainage bag usually should be emptied every 8 hours.

1 Unclamp the drainage tube, and remove it from its sleeve without touching the tip.

2 Then let the urine drain into the toilet or a measuring container, if required. When the bag is empty, swab the end of the drainage tube with povidone-iodine solution.

Swabbing the tube

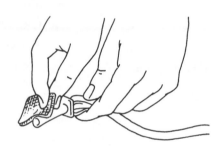

3 Reclamp the tube, and reinsert it into the sleeve of the drainage bag.

Don't let anyone else empty your drainage bag unless you have a designated caregiver who performs your catheter care. If the doctor has requested it, record the amount of urine drained.

Washing and drying around the catheter insertion

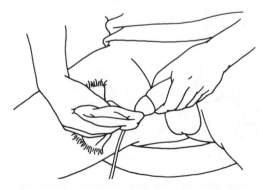

Caring for your skin

Use soap and water to wash the area around the catheter twice daily. Also wash your rectal area twice daily and after each bowel movement.

Periodically check the skin around the catheter for signs of irritation, such as redness, tenderness, and swelling.

Maintaining good drainage

To maintain good drainage from the catheter, frequently check the drainage tube for kinks and loops. Never disconnect the catheter from the drainage tube for any reason. Also, keep the drainage bag below bladder level, whether you're lying down, sitting, or standing.

Reporting problems early

Contact the doctor immediately if you have any problems, such as urine leakage around the catheter, pain and fullness in your abdomen, scanty urine flow, or blood in your urine.

Above all, never pull on the catheter or try to remove it yourself.

Leg bag

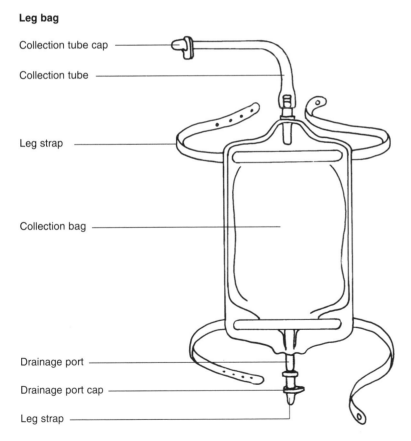

Collection tube cap

Collection tube

Leg strap

Collection bag

Drainage port

Drainage port cap

Leg strap

Attaching a leg bag

If you have an indwelling catheter and drainage bag, you may increase your ability to move around by replacing the drainage bag with a leg bag.

1 You'll need a leg bag device (which consists of a collection bag, a short collection tube, a drainage port, and two straps), several povidone-iodine swabs, and adhesive tape.

Begin by emptying the drainage bag in use, following the procedure on the previous page.

2 Remove the cap from the end of the leg bag collection tube, which is to be attached to the catheter.

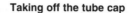

Taking off the tube cap

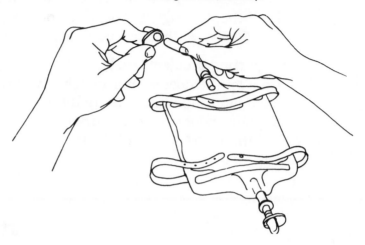

3 Clean the end of the leg bag collection tube with a povidone-iodine swab. Start at the opening of the tube, and wipe away from it to prevent germs from getting into the tube.

Cleaning the tube

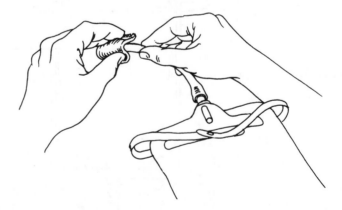

4 Using your fingers or a surgical clamp, pinch the end of the indwelling catheter closed. Disconnect the catheter and drainage tube by carefully twisting them apart. Make sure you do this without pulling on the catheter.

Separating the catheter and drainage tube

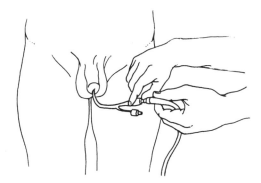

5 Quickly attach the indwelling catheter to the collection tube you've just cleaned. Keep the catheter pinched closed until it's securely attached to the collection tube.

Attaching the catheter to the collection tube

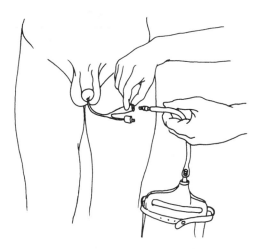

6 Place the leg bag on the outside or front of your upper leg. This placement won't interfere with walking. Secure the upper strap around your upper thigh. Secure the lower strap just above your knee. Don't fasten the straps too tightly. Doing so may cut off some of the blood flow below the straps, and you may notice the lower leg becoming discolored.

Attaching the leg bag

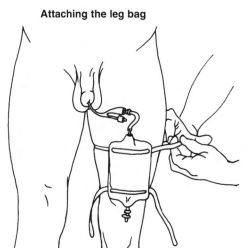

7 Tape the catheter tubing to your thigh so that it has some slack in it. This will reduce tension on the urethra.

Never lie down or raise your leg above your hips while wearing a leg bag. This can cause urine to flow back into your bladder and result in an infection.

Taping the catheter tubing

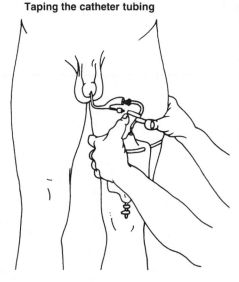

8 Clean your leg bag every night by soaking it in a solution of one part white vinegar to seven parts water. This cleans and deodorizes the bag. You can use a leg bag for up to 1 month before replacing it.

Emptying a leg bag

1 Wash your hands. Then remove the stopper on the leg bag, and drain all the urine either into the toilet or, if the doctor orders it, into a measuring container so that you can record the amount. Don't touch the drain tip with your fingers or with the container.

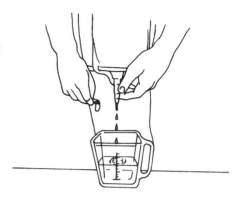

2 After all the urine has drained, swab the drain tip and the stopper with a povidone-iodine swab. Replace the stopper.

Attaching a bedside drainage bag

Before going to bed, replace the leg bag with a bedside drainage bag. This bag holds more urine so that you can sleep for 8 hours without emptying it.

To replace the leg bag, first empty it. Now, clamp the catheter, and swab the connection between the catheter and the leg bag with povidone-iodine. Then disconnect the leg bag, and connect the catheter to the bedside drainage tube and bag. Finally, unclamp the catheter.

Using nonallergenic tape, tape the drainage tubing to your thigh on the side of the bed where you want to hang the drainage bag. (Shave your skin in that area before-

Swabbing the connection

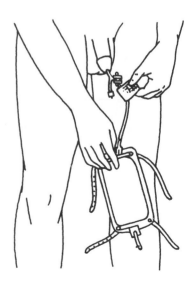

hand, if necessary.) Leave some slack in the line so that you won't pull on the catheter when you move your leg. A man should tape the drainage tubing to the inner thigh, opposite the base of the penis. A woman should tape the drainage tubing to the inner thigh below the vaginal area.

When you get into bed, arrange the drainage tubing so that it doesn't kink or loop. Then hang the drainage bag by its hook on the side of the bed. To ensure proper drainage and to reduce the risk of infection, keep the bag below your bladder level at all times, whether you're lying, sitting, or standing.

Positioning the tubing and bedside drainage bag

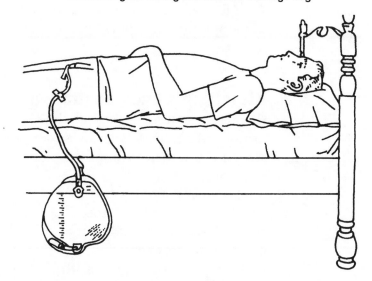

Cleaning the drainage bag

When you've finished emptying the drainage bag, wash it with soap and water, and rinse it with a solution of one part white vinegar and seven parts water to clean and deodorize it. You can use a drainage bag for up to 1 month before replacing it.

Preventing bladder infection

Your indwelling catheter increases your risk of developing a bladder infection. You can prevent or at least control infection by taking the following precautions.

Report warning signs

Contact the doctor immediately if you have any of the following warning signs:
- fever above 100° F (37.7° C)
- cloudy urine
- discharge around the catheter
- pain in the bladder area.

Don't give infection a chance

You may not always be able to prevent a bladder infection, but you can reduce your chances for infection by following these guidelines.
- Drink at least eight 8-ounce glasses (about 1.9 liters) of fluid a day. Include cranberry juice, which keeps urine acidic.
- Take the medication prescribed by your doctor.
- Wash the catheter area with soap and water twice daily to keep it from becoming irritated or infected. Also wash your rectal area whenever you have a bowel movement. Dry your skin gently but thoroughly.
- A woman should always wipe from front to back after bowel movements. Do the same when washing and drying the genital area. This prevents contamination of the catheter and urinary tract with germs from the rectum.
- Once a day, wash the drainage tubing and bag with soap and water. Rinse it with a solution of one part white vinegar to seven parts water.
- Empty your leg drainage bag every 3 to 4 hours. Empty your bedside drainage bag at least every 8 hours.
- Always keep the drainage bag below bladder level.
- Never pull on the catheter. Disconnect it from the drainage tubing only to clean the bag.
- Contact the doctor immediately if you have urine leakage around the catheter, abdominal pain and fullness, scanty urine flow, or blood or particles in your urine.
- Never try to remove the catheter yourself unless the doctor

or home health care nurse has given you instructions.
• Keep your follow-up appointments with the doctor.

Dealing with a blocked indwelling catheter

Learning to care for an indwelling catheter at home takes time and practice. Even if you're careful, the catheter can still become blocked.

How do you know if the catheter's blocked?

Suspect blockage if urine hasn't drained for 2 hours even though you've been drinking plenty of fluids. Other signs are damp underwear that smells of urine, lower abdominal pressure, and the urge to urinate.

How do you unblock the catheter?

• First, straighten any kinked tubing.
• Next, try changing position. (Drainage can stop if the catheter lies against the bladder wall. Changing your position can restart the drainage.)
• Or try lowering the drainage bag—it won't drain if it's above bladder level.
• Last, try irrigating the catheter.

Irrigating a blocked indwelling catheter

1 Assemble the equipment: irrigation solution (as ordered by the doctor), irrigation solution container (not the one you use to collect urine), drainage container, bulb syringe, two alcohol swabs, gloves, a plastic bag (to protect linens), and a 4-inch by 4-inch (10.2-centimeter by 10.2-centimeter) gauze pad. Make sure these items are clean.

Note: You can buy prepackaged kits that contain this equipment. If you're ill or have an infection, you'll want to wear gloves and a face mask.

Preparing the irrigant

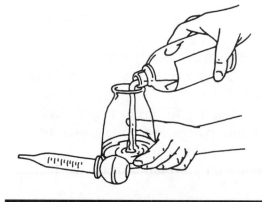

2 Place the plastic bag, covered by a towel, under your buttocks. Expose the indwelling catheter. Open the gauze pad

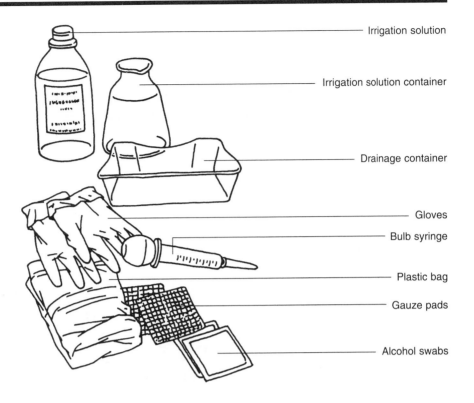

Irrigation solution

Irrigation solution container

Drainage container

Gloves

Bulb syringe

Plastic bag

Gauze pads

Alcohol swabs

package and place it on the towel without touching the gauze.

Then pour the amount of irrigation solution prescribed by the doctor into the collection container. Draw 30 to 50 milliliters of the solution into the bulb syringe.

3 Open the alcohol swab wrapper. Then put on the gloves. To avoid spreading germs, don't let the gloves touch anything other than the clean equipment.

Cleaning the connection

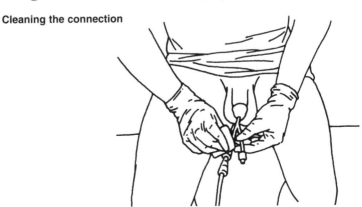

Remove the alcohol swab from its wrapper, and use it to clean the area where the catheter connects with the drainage tube.

4 Disconnect the catheter and drainage tube by carefully twisting them apart. Make sure you do this without pulling on the indwelling catheter. Use one hand to place the end of the drainage tube on the gauze pad to keep it clean as you hold the indwelling catheter in the other hand.

Disconnecting catheter and drainage tube

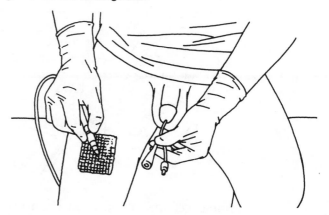

5 Insert the tip of the bulb syringe into the indwelling catheter. Then gently and slowly squeeze the solution into the catheter. *Note:* Don't apply forceful pressure to squeeze the bulb syringe.

Instilling irrigation solution

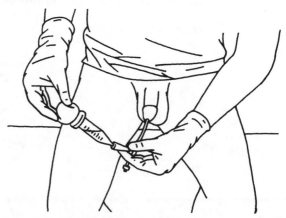

6 Remove the syringe, and let the solution flow into the drainage container. Don't let the catheter tip touch the drainage container. Also, don't draw up any of the solution after it's drained into the container.

Draining the solution

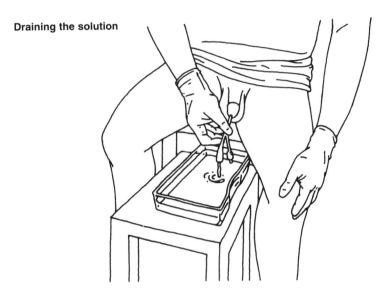

7 After all the solution has drained, wipe the end of the catheter with the unused alcohol swab. Wait a few seconds to let the alcohol evaporate, and then reconnect the catheter and the drainage tube.

Thoroughly clean the container and bulb syringe in hot water to prepare them for reuse. Remember, use the irrigation solution container only to collect solution. Never use it to collect urine.

Reconnecting the catheter and drainage tube

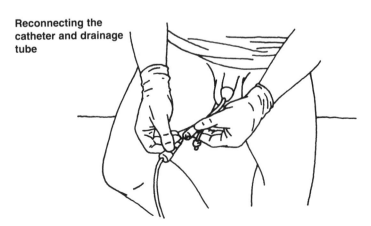

Removing an indwelling catheter

If the home health care nurse or doctor tells you to remove the catheter, follow these instructions.

Syringe attached to inflation port

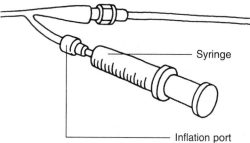

— Syringe

— Inflation port

1 Deflate the balloon on the end of the catheter. (Not doing so can injure your bladder and urethra.) To do this, attach a syringe without a needle to the unattached end of the tubing's Y-shaped portion (inflation port).

If the inflation port doesn't have a special tip that the syringe fits into, put a needle on the syringe and puncture the port.

Cutting the catheter, a last-resort action

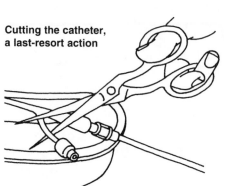

2 Gently pull back on the plunger. The water in the balloon will flow into the syringe, deflating the balloon.

If that doesn't work, try this method only as a last resort: Place a small basin under the inflation port to catch the fluid from the balloon. Then cut the catheter in two just above the inflation port. Now the water in the balloon will escape into the basin.

3 When the balloon is deflated, pull gently on the catheter to remove it. *Important:* If the catheter doesn't come out easily, don't force it. Instead, call the doctor or visiting nurse for help.

Catheterizing yourself (male)

1 Gather the equipment: catheter, water-soluble lubricant, basin for collecting urine, clean washcloth, soap and water, paper towels, and plastic bag. Then wash your hands thoroughly. During the procedure, touch only the catheter equipment to avoid spreading germs.

2 Wash your penis and the surrounding area with soap and water. Then pat dry.

Lubricating the catheter

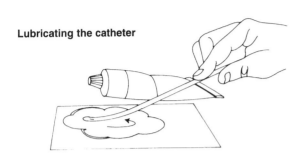

3 Open the tube of lubricant, and squeeze a generous amount onto a paper towel. Then roll the first 7 to 10 inches (18 to 25 centimeters) of the catheter in the lubricant.

4 Put one end of the catheter in the basin or toilet. Hold your penis at a right angle to your body, grasp the catheter as you would a pencil, and slowly insert it into the urethra. If you meet resistance, breathe deeply. As you inhale, continue advancing the catheter 7 to 10 inches (18 to 25 centimeters) until urine begins to flow. Allow all urine to drain into the basin or toilet.

Inserting the catheter

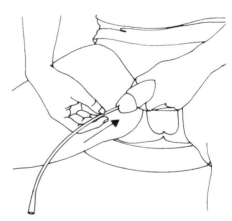

5 When the catheter stops draining, pinch it closed and slowly remove it. Empty the basin, if used; then rinse and dry it. Wash the catheter in warm soapy water, rinse it inside and out, and dry it with a clean towel. Place it in a plastic bag until the next use. (After you've used the catheter a few times, the doctor may tell you to boil it in water for 20 minutes to keep it germ-free.)

Catheterizing yourself (female)

1 Gather the equipment: catheter, water-soluble lubricant, basin for collecting urine, clean washcloth, soap and water, paper towels, and plastic bag. Then wash your hands thoroughly. During the procedure, touch only the catheter equipment to avoid spreading germs.

2 Separate the folds of your vulva with one hand, and using the washcloth, thoroughly clean the area between your legs with warm water and mild soap. Use downward strokes (front to back) to avoid contaminating the area with fecal matter. Now, pat the area dry with a towel.

Washing to avoid contamination

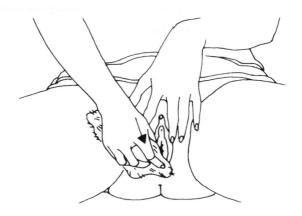

3 Open the lubricant, and squeeze a generous amount onto a paper towel. Then roll the first 3 inches (7.6 centimeters) of the catheter in the lubricant.

4 Put one end of the catheter in the basin or toilet. Spread the lips of the vulva with one hand, and using the other hand, insert the catheter in an upward and backward direction about 3 inches (7.6 centimeters) into the urethra (located above the vagina). If you meet resistance, breathe deeply. As you inhale, advance the catheter, angling it slightly upward until urine begins to flow. Allow all urine to drain into the basin or toilet.

Inserting the catheter

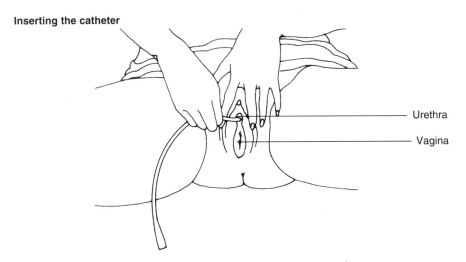

Urethra

Vagina

5 When the catheter stops draining, pinch it closed and slowly remove it. Wash it in warm soapy water, rinse it inside and out, and dry it with a clean towel. Place it in a plastic bag until the next use. (After you've used the catheter a few times, boil it in water for 20 minutes to keep it germ-free.)

Caring for a nephrostomy tube

A nephrostomy tube allows urine to drain from the kidney into a drainage bag. This bag is attached to the tube's free end with a length of tubing.

Because the nephrostomy tube goes directly into the kidney, you'll need to take proper care of the tubing and bag each day to prevent infection.

Changing the tubing and drainage bag

1 Gather the equipment: a clean drainage bag and connecting tube, disposable gloves, and alcohol swabs. Wash your hands, and put on the gloves.

Important: Always keep the drainage bag lower than the nephrostomy tube.

2 Disconnect the nephrostomy tube from the used tubing and drainage bag. Don't use your fingernails to disconnect the tubing. Clean the end of the nephrostomy tube with an alcohol swab. Also clean the end of the tubing that connects the new drainage bag to the nephrostomy tube.

3 Attach the ends of the nephrostomy tube and the connecting tube securely. Don't touch the end of either tube. Check the tubing periodically for kinks.

Cleaning the bag and tubing

1 Wash the used bag and tubing with a weak detergent solution daily. Avoid a biodegradable or chlorine product because it may erode the bag.

2 Twice weekly wash the bag and tubing with a solution of one part vinegar to three parts water to prevent crystalline buildup. Rinse them with plain water, and hang them on a clothes hanger to air-dry.

Changing the dressing

Change the dressing daily, as the doctor orders.

1 Gather the necessary equipment: Desitin powder, sterile gauze pads, and adhesive tape. Then wash your hands, and remove the old dressing.

2 Gently wash around the tube with soap and water. Inspect the skin around the tube. If any redness is present, apply Desitin powder.

If you notice white, yellow, or green drainage, with or without odor, suspect infection, and report it to the doctor. If you see drainage that looks or smells like urine, the tube may be displaced. Report this to the doctor.

3 Fold several sterile gauze pads in half, and place them around the base of the tube. Cover them with an unfolded gauze pad. Apply adhesive tape to secure the gauze pads to your skin. Remove the gloves, and wash your hands.

Placing gauze around the tube

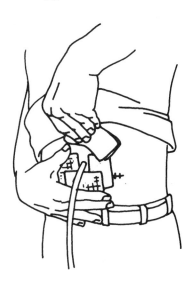

23 Dialysis Care

Native A-V Fistula

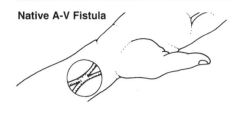

Graft A-V Fistula

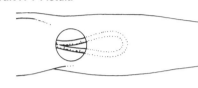

Caring for an arteriovenous fistula site

The surgeon may create a permanent vascular access site in the forearm to allow hemodialysis. This involves the creation of an arteriovenous (A-V) fistula—making a connection between an artery and a vein. The connection can either be made directly between an artery and a vein in the forearm (native A-V fistula) or involve grafting a vein from the forearm or leg or the use of a synthetic blood vessel to bridge the artery and vein (graft A-V fistula). Blood then flows through the artery into the vein.

Postoperative care

If you have a native A-V fistula, after your incision heals well, do exercises for a few months to help enlarge the vein that will be used for hemodialysis. Squeeze a tennis ball, soft putty, or a sponge to increase blood flow through the fistula vein, which enlarges it. Perform the squeezing exercise for 20 minutes three times daily.

Squeezing ball to increase blood flow

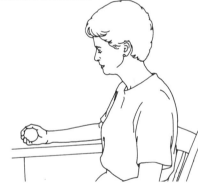
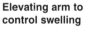

If you have a graft A-V fistula, expect swelling around the graft area. Elevate your arm on pillows to help the swelling subside.

With either type, protect your arm from bumping into hard or sharp objects. Avoid heavy lifting until the incision has healed and the stitches have been removed (10 to 14 days after surgery).

Check the fistula at least three times daily—in the morning, at noon, and at bedtime—for blood flow. Interrupted flow indicates clotting. Place your fingers directly over the vein above the incision (or directly over the graft). Expect a tingling sensation or wavelike pulsation, called a thrill. Caused by blood rushing through the fistula, the thrill should feel the same every time.

Elevating arm to control swelling

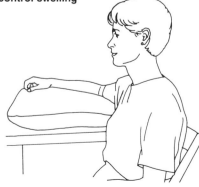
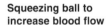

Another way to check the fistula for blood flow is to listen with an ear or a stethoscope directly over the vein or graft segment for the sound of blood flowing. Called a bruit, this sounds like the ocean's roar.

If the thrill or bruit sounds different or you can't hear it, contact the doctor. If the doctor discovers a clot, he may remove it so that hemodialysis can continue.

Avoid wearing constrictive clothing over or above the fistula. Never allow anyone to place a tourniquet on or take a blood pressure reading in the arm with the fistula. Avoid sleeping on that arm.

Check the incision daily for signs of infection, and notify the doctor right away if you notice redness, swelling, tenderness, or drainage. Keep your arm clean and dry until the wound is healed. Don't let anyone except the dialysis nurse take blood samples from the arm with the fistula.

After hemodialysis

If you have a native A-V fistula, the vein requires several months to enlarge before the fistula will be usable. If you have a graft A-V fistula, hemodialysis can begin as soon as swelling subsides, the incision heals, and your body tissues accept the graft. This takes about 2 weeks.

When the fistula is ready for hemodialysis, the dialysis nurse will use a special cleaning procedure to reduce the risk of infection at the access site. After each treatment, when the needles are removed, apply pressure to the site for 5 to 10 minutes to ensure that the bleeding has stopped. The nurse will apply an adhesive bandage, which you should remove after 6 hours. If the bandage remains in place too long, the site may become infected.

Notify the dialysis nurse of any signs of infection (redness, swelling, pus, or drainage). Check for infection every day until the needle sites heal.

If bleeding from a needle site occurs after you leave the dialysis unit or while you're at home, apply pressure until it stops. Then apply a clean bandage, and keep it in place for 6 hours. Report the bleeding at the next dialysis session. If the bleeding won't stop easily, return to the dialysis unit or go to the hospital emergency department.

Learning about peritoneal dialysis

Peritoneal dialysis removes impurities from your blood when your kidneys aren't working properly.

Before dialysis

The nurse will take your blood pressure twice—once while you're standing and once while you're lying down. She'll also weigh you. Then she'll tell you to urinate, which will help you feel more comfortable and will protect your bladder.

Next, the doctor will create an opening in your peritoneal cavity, which is near your stomach. (First, he'll numb the area with an anesthetic.) He'll insert a slender tube called a catheter into the opening.

The catheter is used to transfer a special warmed solution into your peritoneal cavity. The solution collects impurities that cross through your peritoneum (a membrane that acts like a filter). After a specified time, the solution is drained from your body.

Both you and the nurse (or the dialysis technician) will wear masks during dialysis to prevent possible infection. After the nurse connects the inflow and the drainage tubings, she'll hang the solution bag above you on an intravenous (I.V.) pole and the drainage bag below your bed.

Transferring dialysis solution into the peritoneal cavity

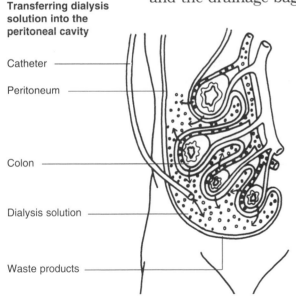

Catheter

Peritoneum

Colon

Dialysis solution

Waste products

During dialysis

To start dialysis, the nurse will open a clamp to allow the solution to flow into your peritoneal cavity, where it will remain for a prescribed time. Then it will drain into the collection bag. The procedure will be repeated until the right amount of solution has been instilled for the prescribed number of cycles.

To ensure your progress, the nurse will take your blood pressure, check your breathing, examine the tubing, and change your catheter dressing whenever it's soiled or wet.

After dialysis

The nurse will disconnect the tubing and cover the catheter with a sterile protective cap. She'll apply ointment to the catheter site and bandage it.

Call the doctor if you notice any signs of infection (such as redness and swelling) or fluid imbalance (such as a sudden weight gain and swollen arms or legs). Take your vital signs regularly, and change the catheter dressing. And be sure to keep all your follow-up appointments.

Performing a solution exchange

You and the doctor have chosen continuous ambulatory peritoneal dialysis (CAPD) for your dialysis program. CAPD is easier to do at home than other forms of dialysis. But when you perform a CAPD solution exchange at home, you must guard against bacteria entering the dialysis system. The following instructions tell how to drain the used solution and replace it with fresh solution so that you don't contaminate the system.

Gathering the equipment

Gather the prescribed bag of peritoneal dialysate solution of the correct volume and dextrose concentration, two outlet port clamps, and a sterile CAPD prep kit. This kit contains povidone-iodine sponges, 4-inch by 4-inch (10.2-centimeter by 10.2-centimeter) sterile gauze pads (you can also use a shell clamp on the connection between the solution spike and the dialysate outflow port), nonallergenic tape, and a mask. If you must inject medication into the solution, you'll also need the necessary number of 25-gauge needles, 10-milliliter syringes, and the medication itself.

Exchanging the solution

If you want to warm the dialysate solution, wrap it in a heating pad for several hours. Warming the solution isn't essential, but you should do it if you feel cramps during infusion. Keep the protective wrap on the bag until you're ready to use it. Remember to wash your hands thoroughly before removing the outer wrap and handling the bag.

1 Remove the empty solution bag from inside your clothing. Check to be sure the shell clamp or iodine-saturated dressing is still in place. If it has become dislodged, apply an iodine sponge to the connection and cover it with a dry sterile gauze pad.

Checking the shell clamp or gauze

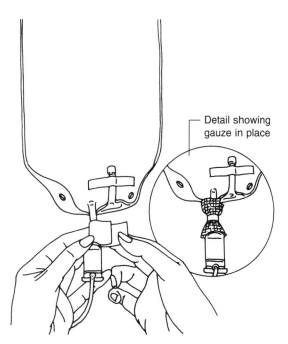

Detail showing gauze in place

2 Now, put on the mask and place the bag in the drainage position below your stomach. Open the clamp on the drainage tubing. Allow about 15 to 20 minutes for the solution to drain from your abdomen into the bag.

Draining the solution

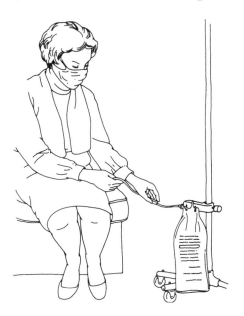

3 Meanwhile, remove the dialysate bag wrapping. Is the solution clear? If it isn't, don't use it. Read the concentration information on the label to make sure you have the right solution, and check the expiration date. Squeeze the bag firmly to test for leaks.

Checking the new solution bag

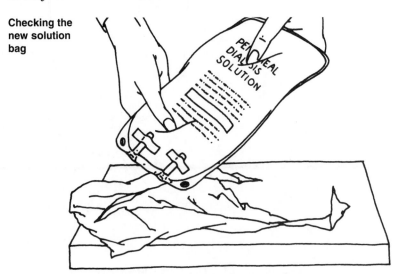

4 If the doctor has told you to add medication to the new bag, wipe the injection port with an iodine sponge and allow it to dry for a few minutes. Draw up the prescribed amount of medication. Then insert the needle through the rubber stopper of the injection port, and inject the medication. To mix the medication in the solution, turn and squeeze the bag several times. Tape the injection port so that it's out of the way.

Inserting the needle into the injection port

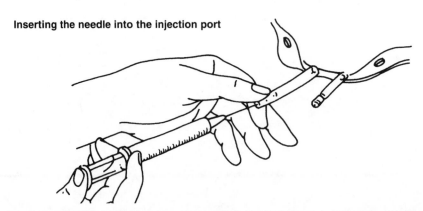

5 When the solution has finished draining, close the clamp on the tubing and place the drainage bag on a flat surface, next to the new bag. Position the used solution bag with its clear side up so that you can check the fluid for cloudiness and particles.

Position the new bag with its label side up so that you can double-check the concentration and the expiration date. Arrange the bags so that their ends extend over the edge of the work surface. Place a clamp on the outlet port of the new bag.

Double-checking the bags

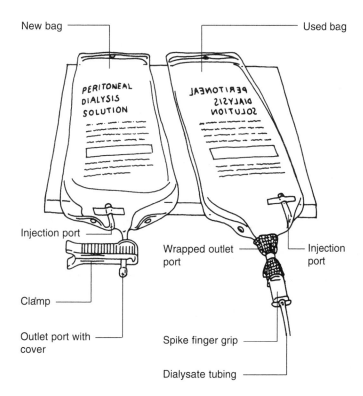

Setting up the new bag

6 Remove the iodine sponge or shell clamp from the outlet port tubing junction of the used bag. Clamp the outlet port of the used bag, being sure that it remains a safe distance from the spike junction.

• Remove the cover from the outlet port of the new bag without touching the port. Now you're ready to transfer the tubing spike.

Removing the cover

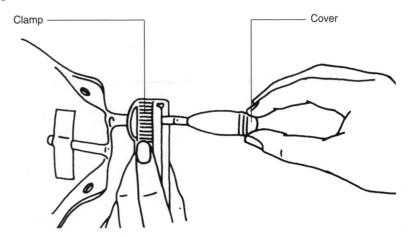

• Grasp the finger grip on the tubing spike in the drainage bag outlet port. With your free hand, hold the clamp on the outlet port of the used bag. Twist and pull the spike in the used bag to remove it from the port. Take care not to touch anything with the spike tip.

Removing the spike

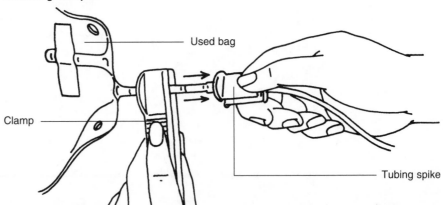

• Immediately insert the spike into the outlet port of the new bag. Apply a shell clamp or iodine sponge to the junction of the outlet port and tubing. Then remove the outlet port clamp.

Applying the clamp

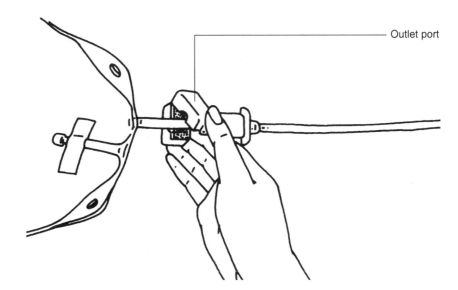

Outlet port

7 Hang the new bag on an I.V. pole. Then open the roller clamp on the tubing to allow the solution to drain into your abdomen. After about 5 minutes, when almost all the solution has drained from the bag, close the clamp. Leaving a little fluid in the bag will make it easier to fold.

Opening the clamp

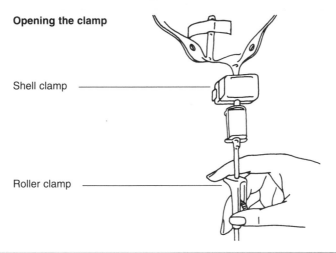

Shell clamp

Roller clamp

8 Remove the bag from the pole and place it in front of you. Fold over the connection between the spike and outlet port so that it's centered on the bag. Then coil the tubing over this connection. Next, fold the other end of the bag over the connection and tubing and place the bag inside a pouch, if you use one. Put the pouch inside your clothing.

If the doctor has ordered a drainage sample, take the used bag to the hospital laboratory for analysis. Otherwise, carefully empty the used solution into the toilet, and discard the empty bag in a trash can.

Folding the bag

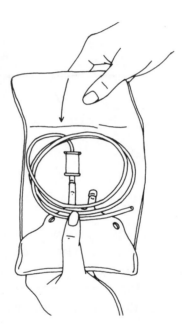

Preventing peritoneal dialysis complications
Because you'll be using peritoneal dialysis at home, you must guard against peritonitis—an infection that occurs when harmful bacteria enter the dialysis system. Follow these tips to help prevent peritonitis.

Avoid contamination
• Wash your hands before opening the dialysis system, handling the dialysis solution, or changing the dressing over the catheter.

• Change the dressing over the catheter every day and whenever it becomes wet or soiled.

• Cover your mouth or nose with a surgical mask whenever you open the dialysis system—for example, to perform a solution exchange.

• Perform solution exchanges in a clean, dry room with the doors and windows closed. Don't exchange the solution in the bathroom.

• Check dialysate drainage for cloudiness or particles—possible signs of infection.

• Make sure you have all the equipment you'll need to do the exchange before you get started.

• Ask your family to take care of the telephone and other interruptions while you're exchanging the solution, or ignore the interruptions until you're through.

• Don't use fresh dialysate solution that has excessive moisture on the outside of the bag. This could indicate a leak in the bag and possible contamination.

• Take showers instead of tub baths to prevent bacteria from entering the dialysis system. Tape a plastic cover over the site to prevent the connections from becoming contaminated.

• Follow any other instructions or restrictions recommended by the nurses and doctors.

When to seek help

• Call the CAPD unit or the doctor if the skin around the peritoneal catheter becomes red, warm, or painful or you note drainage. Also report leakage around the catheter insertion site.

• Follow the instructions you were given for care of the dialysate tubing spike if it should become contaminated by touching your hand or some other surface. This will necessitate a tubing change, which usually is done in the CAPD unit.

• Notify the CAPD unit or the doctor if you detect signs of peritonitis, such as abdominal pain, cloudy dialysate, fever, chills, nausea, vomiting, and diarrhea.

24 Stoma Care

Learning about a stoma

An ostomy, or stoma, is an opening in the bowel that's created surgically. It serves as a bypass so that you can get rid of solid body wastes or fluids without the diseased colon, rectum, or bladder.

Your stoma is part of your body—it's a small portion of your intestine that the doctor brings out through the abdominal wall and sews to the skin. The stoma's normal color is the same as the inside of your cheek. At first, the stoma will be swollen, but it will shrink as it heals. Because the stoma has no muscles, you won't be able to open and close it at will. But you can learn to control your bowel movements by irrigating the colostomy. In the meantime, you'll need to wear a colostomy pouch to collect body wastes that drain from the stoma. After you gain bowel control, you may no longer need to use a colostomy pouch, but you'll still need to give your colostomy proper care.

Types of ostomies

A colostomy is a small opening between the large intestine (colon) and the surface of the abdomen. An ileostomy is an opening in the last portion of the small bowel.

Temporary ostomies are used to rest part of the bowel and allow inflammation to decrease. Permanent ostomies may be necessary after extensive abdominal surgery. The type of ostomy you have—temporary or permanent—depends on the type, location, and extent of your disease.

A similar opening can be surgically created in your urinary tract to allow you to get rid of liquid waste. In this procedure, called urinary diversion, the ureters are either brought to the surface of the abdomen or connected to a portion of intestine that is made into an artificial bladder. The piece of intestine makes the stoma on the abdominal wall.

Common ostomy types and locations

Permanent colostomy

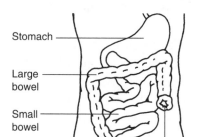

Stomach

Large bowel

Small bowel

Colostomy

Double-barrel colostomy

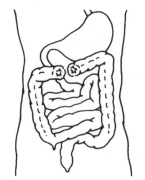

Loop colostomy

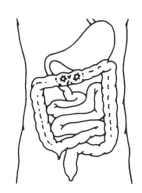

Hartman's procedure

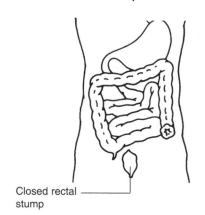

Closed rectal stump

Ileostomy

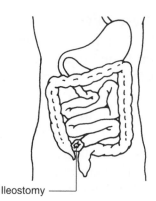

Ileostomy

Ileal conduit

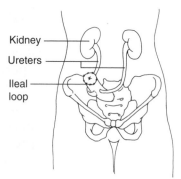

Kidney

Ureters

Ileal loop

Using ostomy equipment

Ostomy pouches are lightweight, odor-proof, and not likely to attract attention. They can be drained and don't need daily changing.

The adhesive on the pouch probably won't irritate your skin. But if your skin is extra sensitive, make sure to protect it by using a skin barrier.

Skin barriers

You can use a protective film wipe that provides a thin, clear barrier between the adhesive and your skin. Or you can choose a thicker, more protective barrier made from karaya or a pectin-based product. This barrier will fit under any pouch system to help heal irritated skin.

Contact the enterostomal therapy nurse for further information.

Applying an ostomy pouch

You can use these instructions to help you remember the steps. Choose a one-piece disposable pouch, a two-piece disposable pouch, or a two-piece reusable pouch.

Measuring the stoma

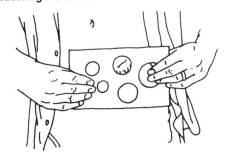

Applying a one-piece disposable pouch

1 Measure your stoma to determine the correct size of the pouch opening.

2 If the pouch opening is precut, remove the release papers from the pouch, press the pouch to your abdomen, and seal well. Attach the tail closure (a small clip that secures the pouch bottom for later drainage).

If you custom-cut your pouch, cut the opening to the correct size, remove the release papers, and then apply as above.

Applying a two-piece disposable pouch

1 Measure your stoma to determine the correct size of the faceplate opening.

2 Cut the faceplate to the correct size, remove the release papers, press the faceplate to your abdomen, and seal well. Secure the pouch to the faceplate, and attach the tail closure.

Applying a two-piece reusable pouch

1 Measure your stoma to determine the correct size of the faceplate opening.

2 Follow the manufacturer's directions to apply new adhesive to the faceplate or to your skin with each change. First, peel off one side of the adhesive disk's paper backing. Then center the disk over the faceplate, and press firmly to expel any bubbles from between the faceplate and the adhesive.

3 Peel the remaining paper backing off the adhesive disk. Center the faceplate over the stoma. Gently press around the stoma so that the adhesive sticks to your abdomen.

Secure the pouch to the faceplate, attach the supporting O-ring around the faceplate collar, and attach the tail closure.

Securing the pouch to the faceplate

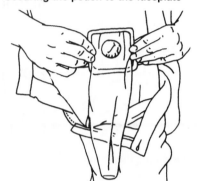

Emptying an ostomy pouch

Depending on your type of ostomy, you may need to empty your pouch from one to eight times daily. Empty it when the pouch is about one-third to one-half full.

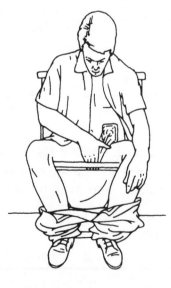

1 To begin, sit on the toilet, and direct the pouch opening into the bowl. To prevent splashing, you may want to place some toilet paper on the surface of the water or flush the toilet as you empty the pouch.

Removing the tail closure

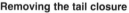

2 Turn up the bottom of the pouch and remove the tail closure. Then empty the pouch into the toilet.

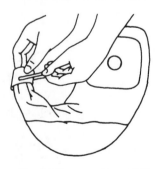

3 Slide your thumb and index finger

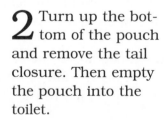
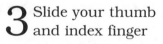

Squeezing the contents into the toilet

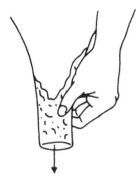

down the outside of the pouch, squeezing the contents into the toilet.

4 Use toilet paper to clean any stool from around and inside the pouch opening.

5 If desired, rinse the pouch with cool water. Remember, your pouch is odor-proof, so this step isn't necessary.

6 Now, reattach the pouch's tail closure to complete the procedure.

Cleaning the pouch's lower opening

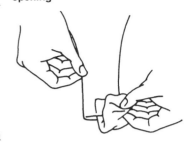

Rinsing the pouch

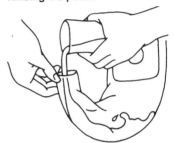

Removing an ostomy pouch

Be sure to change your pouch on a regular schedule. This will help prevent skin irritation and leakage.

How often you change the pouch depends on your type of ostomy, your activities, and the type of pouch you wear. Keep in mind that you may need to change the pouch more often in hot, humid weather. But avoid changing it daily because this can cause skin stripping and irritation. If you think that the pouch may need changing daily, contact the enterostomal therapy nurse or the doctor for guidelines.

1 Gather a wash cloth, towel or paper towels, adhesive solvent and an eyedropper (if needed), karaya powder or stoma adhesive powder, protective film wipes, and karaya or pectin-based skin barriers.

2 Remove the old pouch by gently pulling up on the adhesive with one hand while carefully pushing down on the skin with the other hand. Most disposable pouches come off easily without a solvent. If the pouch you're using requires a solvent, follow the product directions. Make sure the solvent is completely removed from your skin before applying the new pouch. If you're using a reusable pouch, set it aside to clean after you apply your new pouch.

3 Wash your skin well with warm water and pat dry. Soap usually is not needed, but if you choose to use it, rinse your skin thoroughly. Soap residue will interfere with pouch adhesion and may irritate your skin.

4 Check your skin for redness and irritation. The most common causes of irritation are stool leakage under the seal and an overly large pouch opening, which allows stool to come in contact with the skin and cause irritation. Measure the stoma routinely to ensure that the stomal opening on the pouch is correct.

If your skin is red but intact, use a protective film wipe to provide a clear, thin film between the adhesive and your skin.

If your skin is weeping, lightly dust the affected area with karaya powder or stoma adhesive powder. Wipe off any excess powder, and then cover the skin with a protective skin barrier. This may be either a karaya or pectin-based wafer cut to fit the stoma. Apply the pouch over the wafer. Many disposable pouches have a protective wafer as part of the system itself.

Skin irritation usually clears in a few days. If it doesn't, notify the enterostomal therapist or the doctor.

Cleaning a reusable pouch

To help prevent odor, clean a reusable pouch thoroughly every time you change it. You may want to have at least two pouches. That way you can clean one while wearing the other.

Here's how to clean your pouch.

1 Remove the adhesive disk from the faceplate. If some adhesive remains, try rolling the rest of it off with your fingertips. Or try loosening the adhesive with a gauze pad moistened with adhesive solvent. But always use solvent sparingly. Too much solvent may erode the faceplate.

2 After all the adhesive is off, rinse the pouch with cool tap water. Then, using a long-handled brush, scrub the inside with water and a mild soap or detergent (as recommended by the pouch manufacturer).

Using adhesive solvent

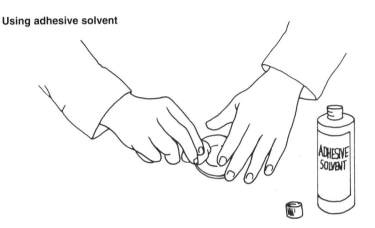

3 Rinse the pouch thoroughly with cool water. Then fill the pouch with wadded paper towels, and place it on a flat surface to dry. Or use a pouch hook to hang it over the sink. *Important:* Never dry a pouch in direct sunlight or heat.

When the pouch is completely dry, remove the paper towels, if you've used any. Store the pouch in a cool, dry place.

Rinsing the pouch

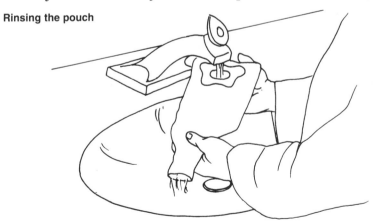

Drying the pouch

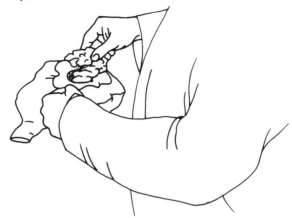

Irrigating a colostomy

Irrigating a colostomy at about the same time each day can help establish a regular bowel pattern and avoid the inconvenience of unexpected bowel movements.

Choose a time (about 1 hour) when you won't be rushed or interrupted, preferably after a meal. Follow the instructions given by the nurse or doctor. Also read the instructions that come with the irrigation kit, and review the illustrated procedure below.

Lay out your supplies in one handy place. You'll need:
• gauze pads
• water-soluble lubricant
• drainage bag
• irrigator bag with tubing and clamp
• stoma care
• gasket
• belt (if the drainage bag isn't self-adhering).

Also make sure you have an irrigation solution and a clean colostomy pouch to replace the used one.

1 Sit on the toilet or on a chair next to the toilet. Remove your colostomy pouch. Now connect the drainage bag and the gasket. Then attach one end of the belt to the gasket on the drainage bag. Hold the gasket with one hand while you

wrap the belt around your waist with your other hand. Then attach the other end of the belt to the gasket.

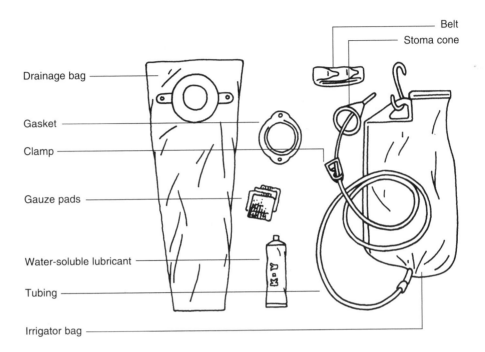

Drainage bag

Gasket

Clamp

Gauze pads

Water-soluble lubricant

Tubing

Irrigator bag

Belt

Stoma cone

2 Carefully encircle the stoma with the gasket, adjust the belt to fit, and dangle the bottom end of the drainage bag into the toilet.

Connecting drainage bag and gasket to the stoma

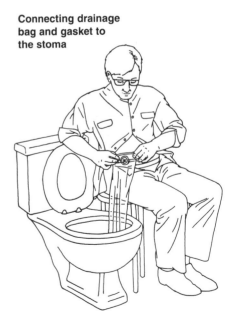

3 If you're using a stoma cone, gently twist together the end of the cone's tube and the end of the tube leading to the irrigator bag until you hear a snap.

Connecting the cone's tube and the irrigator bag's tube

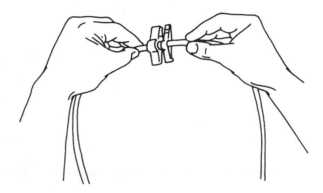

4 Fill the irrigator bag with about 1 quart (1 liter) of lukewarm water or irrigation solution, as the doctor orders. Hang the filled bag on a towel rack or a hook placed next to the toilet. During irrigation, the bag should be above your stoma at shoulder level.

Opening the control clamp

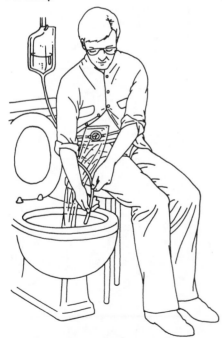

5 Hold the end of the irrigator tube over the toilet. Open the control clamp, and allow a small amount of water or irrigation solution to flow through the tubing. This will force any trapped air out of the tubing. Then close the control clamp.

6 Squeeze a small amount of water-soluble lubricant onto a gauze pad, and roll the first 3 inches (7.6 centimeters) of the tube in the lubricant.

Now, slowly slide the tube through the open top of the drainage bag and into your stoma. If you meet resistance, don't force the tube.

Instead, try to relax, and pull the tube out slightly. Unclamp the flow control, and

Inserting the tube into the stoma

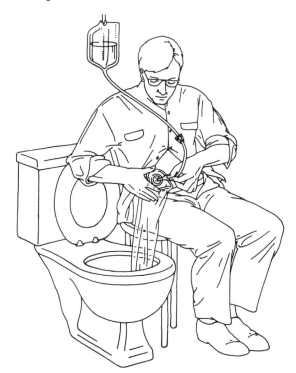

allow a small amount of water or irrigation solution to flow into the colon. Wait about 5 minutes, and then try again to insert the tube. If you have repeated trouble inserting the tube, notify the doctor.

If the doctor wants you to irrigate your colostomy with a stoma cone instead of a tube, first lubricate the tip of the cone. Then insert the lubricated tip through the open end of the drainage bag and into your stoma.

To prevent backflow, always hold the cone in place against the stoma during irrigation.

7 Open the flow clamp of the irrigator bag, and let the water or irrigation solution run slowly into your colon. This should take about 10 to 15 minutes. If you get stomach cramps, reduce the flow or stop the procedure until the cramps go away. After the fluid has entered your colon, slowly remove the tube or cone from your stoma.

8 After the initial surge of water or irrigation solution returns, you can fold the drainage bag back, clamp it shut, and do whatever you want to until all the fluid and stool have returned. It will take about 30 minutes for the colon to empty completely.

9 After the colon empties, return to the toilet. Unhook the belt and remove the drainage bag. Then clean the area around your stoma with warm water, dry the area gently, and apply a clean colostomy pouch. Finally, wash, rinse, and store the irrigation equipment for reuse.

Irrigation troubleshooting tips

You may need time and patience to learn how to irrigate your colostomy. But after you've mastered the technique, you'll find that irrigation makes living with a colostomy much easier and more comfortable. In the meantime, here's how to solve three common problems you may have when you irrigate your colostomy.

Sluggish or incomplete return

The most common reasons for this problem are not using enough water or irrigating solution and not allowing enough time for the colon to empty. Make sure you follow the doctor's orders about how much fluid to use and how much time to allow for its return. A gentle abdominal massage or walking around might help speed up the return.

Too much backflow

If fluid comes out of your colon as fast as you try to put it in, the fluid pressure may be too high. Fluid pressure is determined by the height of the irrigator bag in relation to your colon, so make sure the bag isn't higher than shoulder level.

Cramps

This problem results when the irrigator fluid is too cold or enters the colon too quickly or when the tube contains air. Make sure the fluid is lukewarm (close to body temperature), and let it flow slowly. Also make sure you remove trapped air from the tubing before irrigation.

Living with a colostomy

You'll probably wonder how a colostomy will affect your lifestyle. Here are answers to some common questions.

Will odor be a problem?

If you clean a reusable pouch or change a disposable pouch regularly, you probably won't have problems with odor. For extra security, you may want to use a pouch deodorant. Be sure to notify the doctor if your stool smells extremely foul; this could be a sign of infection or it could be related to diet.

Will I have to change the way I dress?

You'll be able to wear your regular clothes, as long as belts don't lie directly over your stoma. Colostomy pouches aren't noticeable, even under bathing suits, because they're made to lie flat against the body.

If you normally wear a girdle, choose one that stretches and is lightweight. A heavy, tight girdle may injure your stoma or cause drainage to pool around it, which may loosen the adhesive seal.

Can I participate in sports?

Check with the doctor before engaging in sports. He may want you to avoid rough contact sports, such as wrestling, ice hockey, and football. He may also advise against certain individual sports, such as weight lifting and shot putting, which put extra strain on abdominal muscles.

If you plan to swim, remember to empty your pouch and seal it securely before entering the water. You may want to wear a pouch support—for example, a wide-belted athletic supporter—under your swimsuit.

Should I wear my pouch when bathing?

In most cases, doing so is a matter of choice. Soap and water won't hurt your stoma, as long as the shower stream isn't hitting it full force. If you feel uncomfortable about stoma drainage leaking into the bath or shower, you may want to wear your pouch. If you do, make sure the adhesive seal is watertight by applying extra tape around the edge of the pouch opening.

Must I eat a special diet?

The doctor may put you on a low-residue diet for the first few weeks after surgery to give your bowel a rest. Ask him when you can return to your regular diet. If you were on a special diet before your surgery (such as one for diabetes), you'll return to it after surgery.

Foods that you had trouble digesting before surgery will probably continue to be a problem after surgery. To avoid indigestion, be sure to chew your food thoroughly and limit your intake of hard-to-digest foods, such as whole corn, nuts, and sunflower seeds.

Certain foods may cause foul-smelling gas—for example, onions, eggs, cabbage, beer, and certain cheeses. To prevent gas, consume smaller portions of these foods or avoid them entirely.

Can I travel?

With some advance preparation, you'll be able to travel whenever and wherever you want. If you travel by plane, always keep your colostomy equipment with you, in case luggage checked through to your destination gets lost en route. Also, take along enough colostomy supplies for the entire trip, if possible. If you wear a reusable pouch, you may want to pack some disposable pouches as a precaution. Find out in advance where you can buy supplies you may need as you travel. Use only potable water (water suitable for drinking) when you irrigate your colostomy.

Before a long trip, be sure to check with the doctor. He may want to prescribe medication for diarrhea or constipation, in case either develops.

If you plan a trip to a foreign country, buy or borrow an up-to-date directory of English-speaking doctors. Contact your local ostomy association for travel tips.

Can I have a baby?

A woman with a colostomy can become pregnant and have a normal pregnancy. But be sure to discuss the subject with the doctor before you become pregnant. He may recommend that you wait a year or so after surgery before becoming pregnant to give your body a chance to recover completely.

Will my colostomy affect my sex life?

If you had a satisfying sex life before surgery, it'll probably remain so after surgery. Close physical contact won't injure your stoma. And, if applied correctly, the colostomy pouch won't cause any problems. Be sure to empty the pouch before sexual intercourse. You may also want to use a pouch cover.

Women with colostomies who've had surgery in the perineal area may experience some discomfort until the wound heals. Some men with colostomies may experience temporary impotence. Men who have a colostomy because of bladder or rectal cancer, however, may have permanent nerve damage and impotence. But these conditions don't rule out a satisfying sex life. Talk with your doctor.

Occasionally, sexual dysfunction may be psychological. First, see the doctor to rule out any physical complications. Then, if you and your partner are still having trouble adjusting sexually, see a professional counselor.

What can I do about gas filling up my pouch?

For starters, avoid foods that cause gas. You might also want to try using a colostomy pouch with a gas filter. By gently pressing the pouch, you can force gas out through the filter. If you're using a pouch without a gas filter, open the closure clamp at the bottom of the pouch and drain the contents. This allows the gas to escape.

Caring for a urinary stoma

The surgeon has constructed a new passageway for urine. This passageway leads directly to the outside of the body through an opening on the abdomen called a stoma. A bag-like appliance called an ostomy bag collects the urine that drains from the stoma.

Learning about your ostomy bag

Most ostomy bags can be worn from 3 to 5 days—sometimes as long as 7 days. To prevent infection, you'll need to change the bag at least weekly. If the bag begins to leak, change it immediately to prevent infection.

To keep the weight of the bag from loosening the bag's seal against the stoma, empty the bag whenever it becomes one-third to one-half full.

At bedtime, consider connecting the bag to a larger urine collection container. This will keep the urine from stagnating in the bag and minimize the chance of infection.

Besides, when the urine drains into another container, the weight of the urine won't loosen the bag's seal.

The best time to change the bag usually is in the morning, when urine output is less. To control leakage while your bag is off, you may want to insert a thin gauze roll or a tampon into the stoma.

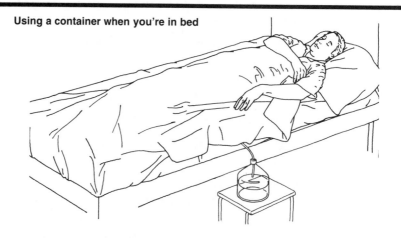

Using a container when you're in bed

Gathering the equipment

To make changing your ostomy bag easier, gather all the equipment you'll need. Whether your ostomy bag is permanent or temporary, disposable or reusable, you'll need the following supplies:
• adhesive tape and scissors
• skin barrier—either a paste or a solid seal—to protect the skin around your stoma

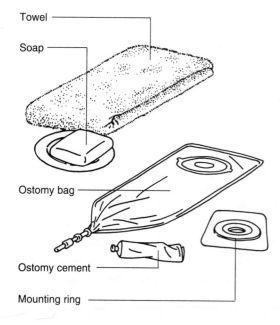

Towel

Soap

Ostomy bag

Ostomy cement

Mounting ring

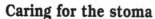

• ostomy cement or spray adhesive
• odor-proof ostomy bag with an opening at the bottom for draining urine
• mounting ring (called a faceplate) for attaching the bag
• cleaning supplies, such as soap, vinegar, and water
• gauze pads and a soft, clean towel
• electric razor (optional).

Caring for the stoma

After you remove the ostomy bag, use a vinegar and water solution (one-half vinegar and one-half water) or soap and water to wash off any crystal deposits on or around the stoma.

If you use soap, choose a nondrying, nonalkaline soap, such as superfatted or castile.

Next, rinse the area thoroughly, and pat

Patting dry the stoma area

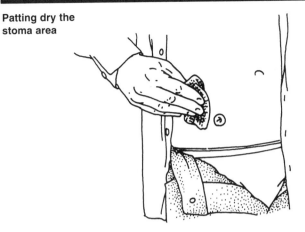

your skin dry with a towel. Any soap or moisture that remains on your skin may keep the ostomy bag from adhering.

If you notice any hairs growing around the stoma, carefully trim them with scissors or an electric razor. Don't risk cutting your skin with a razor blade.

Take meticulous care of the stoma to prevent irritation. Poor skin care may lead to a urinary tract or yeast infection. Avoid changing the ostomy bag too frequently because this can also irritate the skin.

Applying the adhesive

If you use ostomy cement, apply a thin layer around the stoma and allow it to dry.

If you use a spray adhesive, cover the stoma, and spray

Spraying adhesive onto a gauze pad

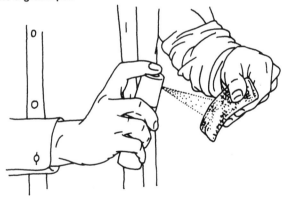

the adhesive onto the surrounding skin. Or you may decide to spray the adhesive onto a gauze pad and then dab the adhesive around the stoma.

If you use a skin barrier, measure the stoma with the cutting guide found inside the package. Select the flange size that is ¼ inch (0.6 centimeter) larger than the stoma.

Measuring the stoma

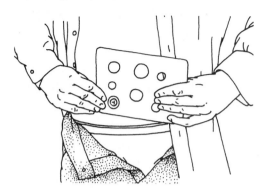

Applying the skin barrier wafer

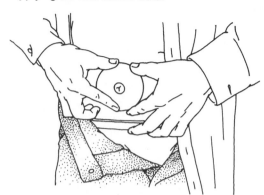

Next, trace the correct size onto the adhesive paper backing. Now, cut out a skin barrier wafer. Peel off the backing, and place the wafer over the stoma. Press the skin barrier wafer against your skin for 30 seconds to form a seal.

For more security, you may also want to apply adhesive tape around the barrier.

Attaching the ostomy bag

Remove the gauze roll or the tampon that you placed in the stoma to control leakage.

If you use adhesive, attach the ostomy bag when the adhesive becomes tacky. Center the bag over the stoma, and leave a small amount of skin exposed around the stoma.

If you use a skin barrier, attach the ostomy bag by placing the flange on the wafer and pressing firmly. You should feel the flanges snap together.

Finally, if you use an adhesive bag system, trace a circle that's ⅛ inch (0.3 centimeter) larger than the stoma onto the

Pressing firmly around the stoma

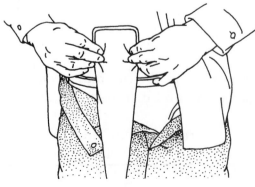

adhesive backing. Cut around the tracing and remove the backing. Next, check to be sure that the bottom drainage valve is closed.

Now, starting at the bottom, press the adhesive firmly but gently around the stoma. Be careful not to wrinkle the material. You may also want to apply adhesive tape around the faceplate.

If you want to wear an ostomy belt to

further secure the bag, be sure to wear the belt at the level of the stoma. Wear the belt loose enough so that it doesn't irritate the skin and leave red marks. (If it's loose enough, you should be able to slip two fingers between your skin and the belt.)

Controlling odor

Besides using vinegar to clean your stoma, try drinking cranberry or apple juice. Or take vitamin C tablets. All of these measures acidify urine and decrease odor.

Also, add a few drops of vinegar or commercially available ostomy deodorizer directly to the ostomy bag to eliminate odors.

Bathing with an ostomy bag

You may take a bath or shower with your ostomy bag on or off, whichever makes you feel most comfortable. With the bag off, of course, urine will flow into the bath water.

When to call the doctor

If you're bothered by occasional bouts of constipation or diarrhea, never take medicine for either without first checking with the doctor. You may be able to correct the problem by adjusting your diet. Here's how.

For mild constipation, try drinking lots of fruit juices. Also, eat more cooked fruits and vegetables.

For mild diarrhea, try returning to the low-residue diet you were on after surgery. You may find that diarrhea improves if you eat such foods as strained bananas, applesauce, steamed rice, tapioca, boiled milk, and peanut butter.

Call the doctor if constipation or diarrhea doesn't go away. Also call him if you have repeated trouble inserting the irrigation tube or if you notice any of these signs:
• bloody stools
• unusually foul-smelling stools
• stools with an unusual color
• bloody or abnormal drainage
• rash or irritation around the stoma.

Some of these problems—unusually foul-smelling or discolored stools, for example—may be related to diet or medication but may also indicate infection. The doctor will determine what's causing your problem and help you solve it by prescribing special medication, advising some diet changes, or suggesting new ways to care for and irrigate your colostomy.

Understanding special tests and interventions

The following information will tell you about special tests and interventions that may be used in the home setting. A test or an intervention may be used alone or be part of the overall treatment of an illness, such as heart problems, gallbladder surgery, diabetes, speech loss, Alzheimer's disease, concussion, AIDS, and the side effects of chemotherapy and radiation therapy.

Using a Holter monitor

A Holter monitor works like a continuous electrocardiogram by recording any irregular heartbeats you may have during the 24 hours you're wearing it. The information from this recording will help the doctor diagnose your heart's condition.

The monitor has various leads that the nurse will attach to your skin. She'll also show you how to wear the monitor on a belt or over your shoulder. If one of the leads becomes loose, secure it with a piece of tape.

While wearing the monitor, you can perform most of your usual activities. You'll even wear it to bed.

Practice these safety measures:
• Don't get the monitor wet—don't shower, bathe, or swim with it on.
• Avoid high-voltage areas and strong magnetic fields.

While you're wearing the monitor, the doctor wants you to write down your activities and feelings. (You can see sample diary entries on the next page.) Your diary will help the doctor establish a connection between the monitor tracing and your activities and feelings. Jot down the time of day when you perform an activity, such as taking medication, eating, drinking, moving your bowels, urinating, engaging in sexual activity, experiencing strong emotions, exercising, and sleeping.

If your monitor has an event button, the nurse will show you how to press it if you experience anything unusual, such as a sudden, rapid heartbeat.

Sample personal diary

DAY	TIME	ACTIVITY	FEELINGS
Tuesday	10:30 am	Rode from hospital in car	Legs tired, some shortness of breath
	11:30 am	Watched TV in living room	comfortable
	12:15 am	Ate lunch, took Inderal	Indigestion
	1:30 pm	Walked next door to see neighbor	shortness of breath
	2:45 pm	Walked home	Very tired, legs hurt
	3:00-4:00 pm	urinated, took nap	comfortable
	5:30 pm	Ate dinner, slowly	comfortable
	7:20 pm	Had bowel movement	shortness of breath
	9:00 pm	Watched TV - drank 1 beer	Heart beating fast for about 1 minute, no pain
	11:00 pm	Took Inderal, urinated, went to bed	Tired
Wednesday	8:15 am	Awoke, urinated, washed face & arms	Very tired, rapid heart beat for about 30 secs.
	10:30 am	Returned to hospital	Felt better

Helping your pacemaker help you

A pacemaker has been inserted in your chest to produce the electrical impulses that help your heart beat as it should. Follow these guidelines to make sure your new pacemaker works correctly.

Check your pacemaker daily

To do so, count your pulse beats for 1 minute after you've been resting for at least 15 minutes—a good time to count is the first thing in the morning. Call the doctor if you detect an unusually fast or slow rate or if you have chest pain, dizziness, shortness of breath, prolonged hiccups, or muscle twitching.

Check the implantation site each day. Normally, the site bulges slightly. If it reddens, swells, drains, or becomes warm or painful, call the doctor. Remember to wear loose-fitting clothing to avoid putting pressure on the site.

Follow the doctor's orders

Take your heart medication as prescribed to ensure a regular heart rhythm. Also follow the doctor's orders about diet and physical activity. Exercise every day, but don't overdo it, even if you think you have more energy than you did before getting your pacemaker. Avoid rough horseplay and lifting heavy objects. Be especially careful not to stress the muscles near the pacemaker.

Keep all scheduled doctor's appointments. Your pacemaker will need to be checked regularly at the doctor's office or over the telephone to make sure it's in good working order. Pacemaker batteries usually last about 10 years, and a brief hospitalization is necessary for replacement.

Take precautions

Always carry your pacemaker emergency card. The card lists your doctor, hospital, type of pacemaker, and date of implantation.

Don't get too close to gasoline engines, electric motors, or strong magnetic forces, such as those from a magnetic resonance imaging (MRI) machine used by hospitals for diagnostic testing. The MRI test uses a strong magnet that can damage your pacemaker. Also, don't get too close to high-voltage fields created by overhead electric lines. (*Note:* Your microwave oven won't affect your pacemaker.)

If you need dental work or surgery, mention beforehand that you have a pacemaker. You may need an antibiotic to prevent infection.

Avoid driving for 1 month after implantation, and avoid long trips for at least 3 months. If you're traveling by plane, you must pass through an airport metal detector. Before doing so, let the airport security personnel know that you have a pacemaker.

If you have a nuclear pacemaker and plan to travel abroad, the Nuclear Regulatory Commission requires that you tell the pacemaker manufacturer of your travel itinerary, means of travel, and the name of your doctor.

Checking your pacemaker by telephone

The doctor can check your pacemaker by telephone by using a special device called a pacemaker transmitter. After the nurse explains how to operate the transmitter, use these directions as a guide when you go home.

Insert the battery

Before using your transmitter for the first time, remove the battery cover and insert the battery supplied by the manufacturer. You'll need to replace the battery every 2 to 3 months.

Position the transmitter

When you're ready to use the transmitter, put its chain around your neck. Then adjust the chain so that the transmitter hangs comfortably at the middle of your chest. Open or take off your shirt (and undershirt, too) so that the transmitter's chest electrodes rest against your bare skin.

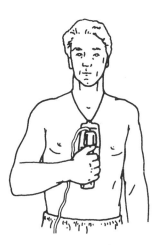

Transmit the signal

Call the doctor. When his office is ready to receive your pacemaker's signal, set the transmitter's ON-OFF switch to the ON position. Listen for a squealing sound. If you don't hear it, change the transmitter's battery before continuing.

Now, place the telephone's mouthpiece against the transmitter's speaker. Hold the telephone steady, and try to remain still for about 30 seconds.

Follow instructions

After 30 seconds, hold the telephone to your ear, and listen for further instructions. For instance, the doctor may want you to repeat the procedure while you hold a special magnet over the pacemaker. If so, take care to hold the magnet flat and steady against the pacemaker. (Or ask someone to hold it for you.) Don't use the magnet unless the doctor asks you to do so.

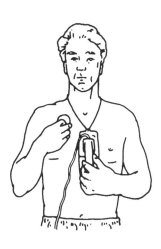

If you receive no further directions, hang up the phone. Remove the transmitter from around your neck and turn off the switch. Keep the transmitter switched off whenever you're not using it.

Caring for a T tube

Here are some instructions for taking care of a T tube at home. You'll have this tube in place for 10 to 14 days. During that time, it'll drain excess bile so that your incision will heal faster. The tube will also allow passage of any retained gallstones.

Caring for your T tube isn't difficult, but it does take time and planning. Set aside about 20 uninterrupted minutes a day to empty your drainage bag and care for your incision. To help prevent infection and promote healing, carefully follow these directions.

Gathering your supplies

Assemble the following supplies on a table or countertop:
• large measuring container
• toilet paper
• soap
• clean towel
• paper bag
• sterile paper cloth
• five sterile 4-inch by 4-inch (10.2-centimeter by 10.2-centimeter) gauze pads
• alcohol swabs
• normal saline solution
• hydrogen peroxide
• povidone-iodine solution
• sterile gloves
• povidone-iodine ointment
• scissors
• adhesive tape.

Emptying the drainage bag

Empty the drainage bag at about the same time each day or when it's two-thirds full. First, place the large measuring container within easy reach.

1 Sit on a chair, and unfasten and remove the belt that secures the drainage bag and connecting tubing to your abdomen. Uncoil the tubing, and position the spout at the bottom of the drainage bag over the measuring container. Don't pull on the connecting tubing or place too much ten-

Releasing the clamp

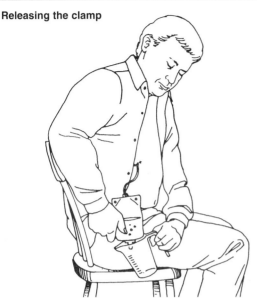

sion on it because you may dislodge the T tube.

2 To empty the drainage bag, release the clamp on the drainage spout so that the bile flows freely into the measuring container. When the bag is empty, clean the drainage spout with toilet paper. To reseal the drainage bag, close the clamp.

3 Gently coil the connecting tubing. Then position the drainage bag and tubing below the incision site. Secure the bag and tubing with the self-fastening belt. Never position the drainage bag and connecting tubing higher than your incision. This could cause the draining bile to back up into the common bile duct.

4 Note the amount, color, and odor of the drainage. Contact the doctor if you notice a significant increase or decrease in the amount of drainage or a change in the color or odor. These signs may mean complications, such as infection or T-tube obstruction.

Caring for your incision

After you've emptied and resecured the drainage bag, you're ready to clean and redress the incision site. Follow these steps.

1 Wash your hands with soap and water, and dry them with a clean towel. Carefully remove the soiled dressing, and discard it in the paper bag. Then wash and dry your hands again.

2 Open the package that contains the sterile paper cloth. Unfold the cloth, and spread it on a table or countertop. Don't touch the top surface of the cloth.

3 Open the five sterile gauze pads, and drop them onto the sterile cloth.

4 Open the packets of alcohol, normal saline solution, hydrogen peroxide, and povidone-iodine solution, and place them on the table.

5 Put on the sterile gloves. Then pick up a sterile gauze pad with your dominant hand (your "sterile" hand). Pick up the saline solution with your other hand, and thoroughly soak the gauze pad.

6 Clean the incision area with the soaked pad. Wipe outward, away from the tube, in a 3-inch (7.6-centimeter) circular pattern.

Repeat this with the hydrogen peroxide and the povidone-iodine solution, again wiping outward. Use a clean pad each time.

7 Soak a clean gauze pad with alcohol, and use it to wipe the first 6 inches (15.2 centimeters) of the tube. Start at the incision and wipe toward the drainage bag.

8 Apply a nickel-sized drop of povidone-iodine ointment over the wound site. Cover the ointment with the remaining sterile gauze pad. Be sure to apply the pad so that the slit end faces up and slides under the tube. Then tape the pad securely to your abdomen.

9 Tape a small segment of the T tube to your abdomen so that you won't accidentally dislodge the tube. Discard used supplies in a paper bag.

Watching for complications

Call the doctor if you notice any of the following signs of infection when you're caring for your tubing and incision:
• redness, swelling, or pain
• pus-like drainage.

Also contact him if you have:
• fever
• nausea or vomiting
• clay-colored stools.

Testing urine for ketones

Urine may contain waste chemicals called ketones. If so, your blood glucose levels may be too high.

You should test your urine for ketones when your blood glucose level rises above 240 milligrams per deciliter or when you're ill. Even a minor illness can dramatically affect your blood glucose levels.

The doctor will probably recommend testing every 4 hours until your blood glucose levels have stabilized or your illness is over. To test your urine for ketones, follow these steps.

1 Gather a clean container (a small plastic cup will do), a bottle of reagent strips, and a wristwatch or a clock with a second hand.

2 Collect a urine specimen in the container.

Removing reagent strip

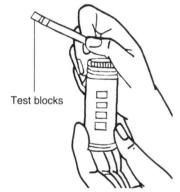

Test blocks

3 Remove one reagent strip from the bottle and replace the cap. Hold the strip so that the test blocks face up, but don't touch the blocks.

4 Dip the end of the strip with the test blocks into the urine for about 2 seconds. Then remove the strip and shake off any excess urine. (Or you can perform the test while you urinate by simply holding the strip under the urine stream for about 2 seconds.)

Dipping the strip for 2 seconds

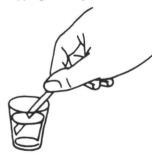

Timing the reaction

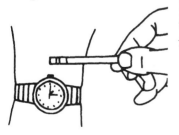

5 Now hold the reagent strip horizontally and immediately begin timing, following the manufacturer's directions.

Matching the test block with the color chart

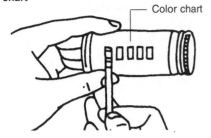

Color chart

6 After waiting the recommended time, compare the ketone test block with the ketone color chart on the bottle label.

7 Keep a record of your tests, listing the date, time, results, and other pertinent information. Call the doctor if your urine is positive for ketones.

Testing blood glucose levels

You'll be able to tell whether your diabetes is under control by testing your blood glucose level daily.

First, assemble the necessary equipment: a lancet, a mechanical device to draw blood (optional), a container of reagent strips, cotton balls, a watch or a clock with a second hand, and a pen.

Remove a reagent strip from the container. Then replace the cap, making sure it's on tight. Two types of reagent strips commonly are used to test blood glucose levels visually: Chemstrip bG and Visidex II. (You can also use a glucose meter to measure levels. If you do, be sure to follow the manufacturer's directions precisely.)

Obtaining blood

1 Choose a site on the end or side of any fingertip. Wash your hands thoroughly and dry them. To enhance blood flow, hold your finger under warm water for 1 or 2 minutes.

2 Hold your hand below your heart, and milk the blood toward the fingertip you plan to pierce. Squeeze that fingertip with the thumb of the same hand. Place your fingertip (with your thumb still pressed against it) on a firm surface, such as a table.

Piercing a fingertip

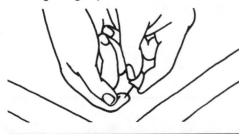

3 If you're using a lancet manually, twist off the protective cap. Then grasp the lancet and quickly pierce your fingertip just to the side of the finger pad, where you have more blood vessels and fewer nerve endings.

Milking your finger

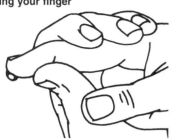

4 Remove your thumb from your fingertip to permit blood flow. Then milk your finger gently until you get a hanging drop of blood that looks large enough to cover the reagent area of the test strip. Be patient. If blood doesn't flow immediately from the puncture site, keep milking your finger before trying another site.

5 If you're using a mechanical device, follow the manufacturer's instructions precisely. To prevent a deep puncture, don't press the device too deeply into the skin surface.

Applying blood to the reagent strip

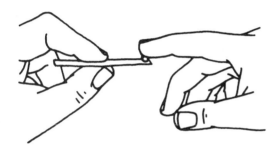

Testing blood

1 Carefully lift the reagent strip to the drop of blood. (The strip has a shiny, slippery undersurface; the blood will roll off if you don't place it on the strip correctly.) Let the blood completely cover the reagent area without rubbing or smearing it. If the blood smears, start over with a new strip.

Timing the reaction

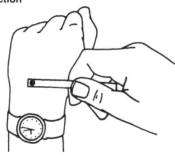

2 As you put the drop of blood on the reagent area, look at your watch or a clock. Begin timing according to the manufacturer's directions. Make sure you keep the strip level.

3 When the recommended time has elapsed, gently wipe all the blood off the strip with a clean, dry cotton ball. Wipe the strip three times, using a clean side of the cotton ball each time. Then wait the recommended time.

Wiping three times

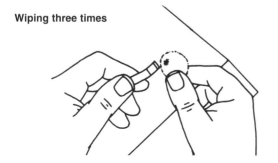

Matching the color

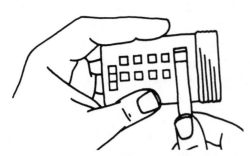

4 Now, determine your blood glucose level by holding the reagent strip next to the area of color blocks on the reagent strip container. Then match the colors on the strip with the color blocks on the container. For example, if both colors match the block labeled 180, your blood glucose level is about 180 milligrams per deciliter.

If the colors fall between two blocks, take the average of the two numbers. For example, if the colors fall between the two blocks labeled 120 and 180, your blood glucose level is about 150 milligrams per deciliter.

5 Write the date, time, and your initials on the reagent strip and store it in an empty container. Make sure you replace the cap securely. The colors on the reagent area will last for up to 1 week.

Preventing hypoglycemic episodes
Although hypoglycemia is a chronic disorder, you can keep it under control and prevent most hypoglycemic episodes. Follow these guidelines.

Stick to your diet
Eat all your meals and snacks at the prescribed time and in the prescribed amounts. Also, avoid alcohol and caffeine— they can cause your blood glucose level to drop.

Take your medicine
If the doctor prescribes medicine to control your hypoglycemia, strictly follow your schedule. Take the right amount of medicine at the right time.

Always check with the doctor who is treating your hypoglycemia before you take any over-the-counter medicine or any other prescribed medicine.

Also, inform him about any new treatments you're having for another condition.

Control stress

Reduce stress by practicing relaxation techniques, such as deep breathing and guided imagery. Change your lifestyle, if possible by working less and taking more time for hobbies, traveling, and other leisure activities.

Exercise

Take some precautions when you exercise. For example, eat extra calories to make up for those burned, don't exercise alone and don't exercise when your blood glucose level is likely to drop.
• If you have fasting hypoglycemia, your blood glucose level is likely to drop 5 or more hours after a meal.
• If you have reactive hypoglycemia, your blood glucose level will fall 2 to 4 hours after a meal.
• If you have pharmacologic hypoglycemia, ask the doctor for guidelines.
• If you're diabetic, don't inject insulin into a part of your body that you'll be exercising during the next few hours.

Carry carbohydrates

Carry a source of fast-acting carbohydrate, such as hard candy or sugar packets, with you at all times.

Know the warning signs

Note what symptoms you typically have before an episode of hypoglycemia. Make certain that your family, friends, and co-workers know that you have hypoglycemia, and be sure that they can also recognize the warning signs. Early recognition can prevent an acute episode.

Alert others

Wear a medical identification bracelet or carry a medical identification card that describes your condition and what emergency actions to take.

Preventing other diabetic complications

Controlling your diabetes means checking your blood glucose levels daily and making the following good health habits a way of life.

Heart care

Because diabetes raises your risk of heart disease, take care of your heart by following these American Heart Association guidelines:
• Maintain your normal weight.
• Exercise regularly, following the doctor's recommendations.
• Help control your blood pressure and cholesterol levels by eating a low-fat, high-fiber diet, as the doctor prescribes.

Eye care

Have your eyes examined by an ophthalmologist at least once a year. Before symptoms appear, he may detect damage that can cause blindness. Early treatment may prevent further damage.

Tooth care

Schedule regular dental checkups, and follow good home care to minimize dental problems that may occur with diabetes, such as gum disease and abscesses. If you experience bleeding, pain, or soreness in your gums or teeth, report this to the dentist immediately. Brush your teeth after every meal and floss daily. If you wear dentures, clean them thoroughly every day, and be sure they fit properly.

Skin care

Breaks in your skin can increase your risk of infection. Check your skin daily for cuts and irritated areas, and see the doctor, if necessary. Bathe daily with warm water and a mild soap, and apply a lanolin-based lotion afterward to prevent dryness. Pat your skin dry thoroughly, taking extra care between your toes and in any other areas where skin surfaces touch. Always wear cotton underwear to allow moisture to evaporate and help prevent skin breakdown.

Foot care

Diabetes can reduce blood flow to your feet and dull their

ability to feel heat, cold, or pain. Follow your nurse's instructions on daily foot care and necessary precautions to prevent foot problems.

Other care measures

Because symptoms of kidney disease usually don't appear until the problem is advanced, the doctor will check your urine routinely for protein, which can signal kidney disease. And don't delay telling the doctor if you have symptoms of a urinary tract infection (burning, painful, or difficult urination or blood or pus in the urine).

See the doctor regularly so that he can detect early signs of complications and start treatment promptly.

Using talking boards

If the person you're caring for can't speak or is having trouble speaking, use board devices that allow you to communicate with each other without speech.

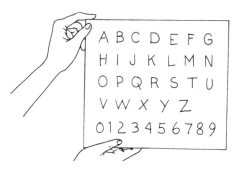

Letter-number board

The letter-number board is arranged with four rows of letters placed in alphabetical order and one row of numbers placed in numerical order 0 through 9. Tell the person to stare at the board when she wants to use it. Then ask her if she wants the first, second, third, fourth, or fifth row. By blinking once for yes and twice for no, she can answer which rows and then which letters she wants to use to spell out a message.

Phrase board

The phrase board lists common phrases that we all use, such as *Rub my back* and *Turn on the TV.* You'll want to include whatever requests you've heard the person make.

First, number each column, and then

number each phrase. List 10 phrases in each column. Then, by blinking yes or no, the person can identify the column and then the message that she wants to convey.

Powered communicator board

If the person has enough strength, she can use a straw or stick to press letters and numbers to spell out a message on a display panel or computer screen. Or she can press preprogrammed buttons on the keyboard to convey frequent requests, such as *Turn me,* without having to write the message letter by letter.

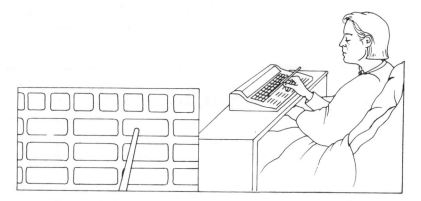

Caring for a person with Alzheimer's disease

Taking care of a person with Alzheimer's disease requires a great deal of patience and understanding. It also requires you to look at the person's environment with new eyes. Then you have to learn how to change this environment to help him function at the highest possible level.

Keeping these points in mind, use the following tips to help plan your daily care.

Reduce stress

Too much stress can worsen the person's symptoms. Try to protect him from the following potential sources of stress:
• change in routine, caregiver, or environment
• fatigue
• excessive demands
• overwhelming, misleading, or competing stimuli
• illness and pain
• over-the-counter medications.

Establish a routine

Keep the person's daily routine stable so that he can respond automatically. Adapting to change may require more thought than the person can handle. Even eating a different food or going to an unfamiliar grocery store may overwhelm him.

Ask yourself: What are the person's daily activities? Then make a schedule.
• List the activities that are necessary for his daily care, and include those that he especially enjoys, such as weeding the garden. Specify a time for each activity.
• Establish bedtime rituals. This is especially important because such rituals promote relaxation and a restful night's sleep for both of you.
• Stick as close to the schedule as possible (for example, breakfast first and then dressing) so that the person won't be surprised or need to make decisions.
• Keep a copy of the person's schedule to give to other caregivers. To help them give better care, include notes and suggestions about techniques that work for you; for instance, "Speak in a quiet voice" or "When helping Mitchell dress or take a bath, take things one step at a time, and wait for him to respond."

Practice reality orientation

In your conversation with the person, orient him to the day and the activity he'll perform. For instance, say, "Today is Tuesday, and we're going to have breakfast now." Do this every day. This keeps the person aware of his immediate environment and tells him what to expect without challenging him to remember events.

Simplify the surroundings

The person eventually will lose the ability to correctly interpret what he sees and hears. Protect him by trying to decrease the noise level in his environment and by avoiding busy areas, such as shopping malls and restaurants.

If the person mistakes photographs and images in the mirror for real people, remove the photographs and mirrors. Also, avoid rooms with busy patterns in the wallpaper or carpets because they can overtax his senses.

To avoid confusion and encourage the person's independence, provide cues. For example, hang a picture of a toilet on the bathroom door.

Avoid fatigue

Because the person tires easily, plan important activities for the morning, when he's functioning best. Save less demanding activities for later in the day. Remember to schedule a break in the morning and one in the afternoon.

About 15 to 30 minutes of listening to music or just relaxing is sufficient in the early stages of the disease. As the disease progresses, schedule longer, more frequent breaks (perhaps 40 to 90 minutes). If the person naps during the day, have him sleep in a reclining chair rather than in a bed to prevent him from confusing day and night.

Don't expect too much

Accept the person's limitations. Don't demand too much from him—this forces him to think about a task and causes frustration. Instead, offer help when needed, and distract him if he's trying too hard. You'll feel less stressed, too.

Prepare for illness

If the person becomes ill, expect his behavior to deteriorate and plan accordingly. He'll have a low tolerance for pain and discomfort.

Never rely on the person to take his own medicine. He may forget to take it or miscount what he has taken. Always supervise him.

Providing hand-to-hand contact

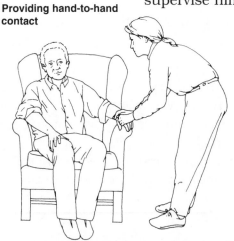

Use touch

Because the person's visual and auditory perceptions are distorted, he has an increased need for closeness and touching. Remember to approach the person from the front. You don't want to frighten him or provoke him into becoming belligerent or aggressive.

Respect the person's need for personal space. Limit physical contact to his hands and arms at first and then move to more central parts of his body, such as his shoulders and head.

Using long or circular motions, lightly stroke the person to help relieve muscle tension and give him a sense of his physical self. Physical contact also expresses your feelings of intimacy and caring.

Allowing the person to touch objects in the environment can help relieve stress by providing information. Let him handle, poke, pull, or shake objects—for example, a handbag, brush, or comb. Make sure they're unbreakable and can't harm him.

Handle problem behavior

If the person becomes restless or agitated, divert his attention with an appropriate activity. Good choices include walking, rocking in a rocking chair, sanding wood, folding laundry, and hoeing the garden. These repetitive activities don't require a particular sequence or planning. A warm bath, drink of warm milk, or back massage can also be calming.

Although problem behavior can be taxing for you, try to remember that the person can't help himself. Your understanding and compassion can increase his sense of security.

Ensure safety

• Serve food in unbreakable dishes.
• Taste the food before serving it to prevent the person from burning his tongue or mouth or himself if it is accidentally spilled.
• Remove knobs from the stove, if possible. If this isn't possible, place wide tape over the knobs to discourage their use.
• Store small kitchen appliances that can be hazardous (for example, an iron or a blender) out of reach.
• Keep knives, forks, scissors, and other sharp objects where the person can't reach them.
• Be sure the temperature on the hot water heater is set no higher than 120° F (48.8° C) to prevent burning.
• Keep your keys where the person won't find them.
• Keep medications out of the person's reach.
• Don't use throw rugs.
• Cover slippery floors with large area rugs. Tape edges down, if necessary.
• Remove mirrors unless they're make of safety glass.

• Keep walkways, floors, and stairways clear of objects.
• Don't rearrange furniture.
• Cover electrical outlets that aren't in use with masking tape or outlet safety caps.
• Cover doors with large posters or murals so that they don't look like exits. You can increase safety by installing locks at the base of the doors and using child-proof devices that go over the knobs.
• If stairs are a hazard, install a high gate in front of them.
• Remove all breakable wall hangings and pictures.
• Provide a low bed.
• Keep the house well lighted during the day, and provide night lights in the bedroom, bathroom, and connecting hallways.
• Cover sharp furniture corners with masking tape.
• Encourage use of the bathroom by marking a path on the floor in that direction with brightly colored tape.
• Mark stair edges with yellow or orange tape (yellow, orange, and red are good contrasting colors) to compensate for altered depth perception.
• Attach safety rails in the bathtub, on stairways, and beside toilets.
• Apply nonskid strips on the bottom of the bathtub and by the toilet.
• Provide the person with an identification bracelet that includes his name, address, phone number, and health problem.

Caring for a person after a concussion

Although a concussion isn't a serious brain injury, it can temporarily disrupt normal activities.

The person you're caring for can continue his recovery at home—as long as you watch him for the next 24 hours and call for medical help if necessary. Here are some guidelines.

Observe the person

Set an alarm clock to wake the person every 2 hours during his first night home. Ask him his name, where he is, and whether he can identify you. If he won't wake up or can't answer your questions, take him to the hospital emergency department right away.

Review medical instructions
Help the person follow the instructions given by the nurse for the first 48 hours after discharge. Tell him to:
• go slow and return gradually to his usual activities.
• avoid medicine stronger than acetaminophen for a headache. Also avoid aspirin; it can intensify any bleeding caused by the accident.
• try relieving a headache by lying down but keeping his head raised slightly with pillows.
• eat lightly, especially if nausea or vomiting occurs. (Occasional vomiting isn't unusual, but it should subside in a few days.)

Call for medical help
Call the doctor or return to the hospital at once if the person experiences:
• increasing irritability or personality changes
• increasing sluggishness
• confusion
• seizures
• persistent or severe headache that's unrelieved by acetaminophen
• forceful or constant vomiting
• blurred vision
• abnormal eye movements
• staggering gait.

Recognize delayed symptoms
Although the person may feel fine in a few days, new symptoms may emerge later. Called postconcussion syndrome, these symptoms may occur up to 1 year after the injury. Tell him to to watch for:
• headaches that worsen with emotional stress or physical activity
• lack of usual energy
• occasional double vision
• dizziness, giddiness, or light-headedness

- memory loss
- emotional changes (feeling irritable or easily upset, especially in crowds)
- tenseness and nervousness
- difficulty concentrating
- reduced sex drive
- easy intoxication by alcohol
- loss of inhibitions
- difficulty relating to others
- noise intolerance.

If these symptoms worsen or last longer than 3 months, urge the person to seek medical advice.

Caring for a person with AIDS

You can care for a person with AIDS (acquired immunodeficiency syndrome) at home without exposing yourself or other family members to the virus and without giving the person a new infection. How? By ensuring that no one comes into contact with the person's blood, semen, or vaginal secretions. Although the virus that causes AIDS may be detected in saliva, urine, feces, mucus, perspiration, tears, and other body secretions, no one has contracted AIDS as a result of coming into contact with these body fluids.

The precautions recommended below take time and planning, but they'll soon become second nature. Remember, though, they shouldn't be so exaggerated that the person feels isolated.

To prevent AIDS transmission at home, follow these guidelines.

Handwashing

Use soap and water to wash your hands, arms, and any other body surfaces that touch the person you're caring for before and after all personal contact and before preparing food or eating. Also remind the person to wash his hands frequently, especially before eating and after using the bathroom.

Don't touch your own body or your mouth when you're giving care to the person.

Gloves, gowns, and masks

Protective clothing isn't needed for general care or during casual contact, such as when bathing intact skin or feeding the person. It should be worn, however, in the following instances.

Use gloves when touching body secretions or excretions—for example, in blood contact during mouth, wound, or nose care or when caring for a woman who is menstruating or has just given birth.

Also wear gloves when handling soiled diapers, sheets, and clothing, when the person has vomited or been incontinent, or when caring for a person with rectal or genital lesions (sores or blisters). Remember to wash your hands after removing the gloves.

Wear a gown if you may be splattered with body fluids. Wear a mask if the person has tuberculosis and is coughing. Wear a mask and protective eyewear to prevent vomit or saliva from splashing into your eyes, nose, or mouth.

Eating utensils

Wash dishes used by a person with AIDS in hot soapy water, and dry them after washing. You needn't keep the person's dishes isolated from other dishes.

Kitchen and bathroom facilities

A person with AIDS doesn't need separate kitchen and bathroom facilities. He may use the same toilet as other family members without special precautions unless he has diarrhea or herpes lesions or is incontinent. If these conditions are present, disinfect the toilet with a solution of 1 part bleach to 10 parts water (1:10) after each use. Wait 10 minutes, and then rinse with clear water.

Cleanups

If blood, urine, or other body fluids spill, clean them up promptly with hot soapy water. Then disinfect the washed surface with the 1:10 bleach-water solution, and rinse with clear water after 10 minutes.

Soak sponges or mops used to clean up body fluids in the 1:10 bleach-water solution for 5 minutes. Don't rinse them in sinks where food is prepared, and don't use them to clean

Mopping with bleach-water solution

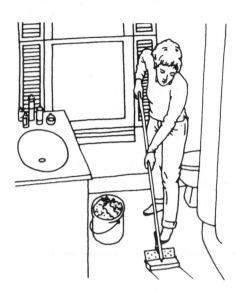

food preparation areas.

Pour mop water down the toilet. If the person uses a bedpan or an emesis basin, pour the body fluids and excretions down the toilet.

Clean the kitchen and bathroom as you normally do. To prevent growth of fungi and bacteria, wash surfaces regularly with soap and water and scouring powder. Clean the refrigerator regularly, and mop the floors at least once a week.

Disinfect the bathroom and shower floor with a commercial disinfectant or a 1:10 solution of bleach and water. Pour a small amount of full-strength bleach down the toilet. Clean up spills as soon as they occur, and don't use the same sponge to clean the bathroom and the food preparation areas.

Laundry

Wear gloves when handling soiled items. Always launder towels and washcloths after the person uses them. Seal laundry soiled with body fluids in heavy-duty, double plastic bags until you can wash them. Soak items soiled with body fluids in cold water and an enzymatic detergent. Then wash them in hot water, detergent, and 1 cup of bleach. Machine dry on hot. Wash all the person's laundry separate from the rest of your laundry.

Disposable items

Place soiled gloves, diapers, underpads, tissues, and other disposable items in heavy-duty, double plastic bags, and seal the bags securely before discarding them. Regular trash pickup usually is adequate, but follow your community's regulations for disposal.

Injection needles

Dispose of a used needle immediately in a sealed, rigid, puncture-proof plastic or metal can. Never recap or break a needle because you may stick or cut yourself. Follow your community's regulations for disposal.

Personal items

Never share the person's toothbrush, razor, or other personal items that might be contaminated with blood.

Glass thermometers can be shared as long as they're cleaned thoroughly first. Wash them with soap and cold water, soak them in ethyl alcohol (70% to 90%) for 30 minutes, and then rinse them under running water.

Controlling side effects from chemotherapy and radiation therapy

Used for treating cancer, chemotherapy and radiation therapy typically cause unpleasant side effects. You'll be able to prevent some of them. Even with unpleasant side effects, you can do things to make yourself more comfortable. Just follow the advice below.

Mouth sores

• If you're going to have radiation therapy, see the dentist beforehand.
• Keep your mouth and teeth clean by brushing after every meal with a soft toothbrush.
• Don't use commercial mouthwashes that contain alcohol, which can irritate your mouth during radiation therapy. Instead, rinse with water, water mixed with baking soda, or a mouthwash that contains equal parts of Kaolin and pectin suspension and diphenhydramine elixir. Floss daily, and

Cleaning teeth with a soft toothbrush

apply fluoride if the dentist recommends it. If you have dentures, clean them regularly.
• Until your mouth sores heal, avoid foods that are difficult to chew (such as apples) or irritating to your mouth (such as citrus juices). Also avoid drinking alcohol, smoking, and eating extremely hot or spicy foods.
• Eat soft, bland foods, such as eggs and oatmeal, and soothing foods, such as ice pops. The doctor might also prescribe medication for mouth sores.

Dry mouth

• Frequently sip cool liquids and suck on ice chips or sugarless candy.

• Ask the doctor about artificial saliva.

• Moisten your food with water, juices, sauces, and dressings to soften the food and make it easier to swallow.

• Don't smoke or drink alcohol, because they can further dry your mouth.

Nausea and vomiting

• Before a radiation treatment, try eating a light, bland snack, such as toast or crackers. Or don't eat anything—some people find that fasting controls nausea better.

• Keep unpleasant odors out of your dining area. Avoid strong-smelling foods. Also, brush your teeth before eating to refresh your mouth.

• Eat small, frequent meals, and try not to lie down for 2 hours after you eat. Sip small amounts of clear, unsweetened liquids, such as apple juice, and then progress to crackers or dry toast. Stay away from sweets and fried or other high-fat foods. Try eating bland foods.

• Take an antiemetic medication, as the doctor prescribes. Be sure to notify him if your vomiting is severe or lasts longer than 24 hours, if you're urinating less, if you feel weak, or if you have a dry mouth.

Diarrhea

• Stick with low-fiber foods, such as bananas, rice, applesauce, toast, and mashed potatoes. Stay away from high-fiber foods, such as raw vegetables and fruits and whole-grain breads. Also avoid milk products and fruit juices. Cabbage, coffee, beans, and sweets can increase stomach cramps.

• Because potassium may be lost when you have diarrhea, eat high-potassium foods, such as bananas and potatoes. Check with the doctor to see if you need a potassium supplement.

• After a bowel movement, clean your anal area gently and apply petroleum jelly to prevent soreness.

• Ask the doctor about antidiarrheal medications.

• Notify the doctor if your diarrhea doesn't stop or if you urinate less, have a dry mouth, or feel weak.

Constipation

• Eat high-fiber foods unless the doctor tells you otherwise. They include raw fruits and vegetables (with skins on), whole-

grain breads and cereals, and beans. If you're not used to eating high-fiber foods, start gradually to let your body get accustomed to the change or else you could develop diarrhea.
• Drink plenty of liquids unless the doctor tells you not to.
• If changing your diet doesn't help, ask the doctor about stool softeners or laxatives. Check with the doctor before using enemas.

Heartburn
• Avoid spicy foods, alcohol, and smoking. Eat small, frequent meals.
• After eating, don't lie down right away. Avoid bending or stooping.
• Take oral medications with a glass of milk or a snack.
• Use antacids, as the doctor prescribes.

Muscle aches or pain, weakness, numbness or tingling
• Take acetaminophen. Or ask the doctor for acetaminophen with codeine.
• Apply heat where it hurts or feels numb.
• Be sure to rest. Also, avoid activities that aggravate your symptoms.
• If symptoms don't go away and pain focuses on one area, notify the doctor.

Hair loss
• Wash your hair gently. Use a mild shampoo, and avoid frequent brushing and combing.
• Get your hair cut short to make thinning less noticeable.

Applying heat to a sore lower back

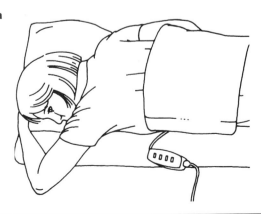

• Consider wearing a wig or toupee during therapy. Buy one before radiation begins. Or use a hat, scarf, or turban to cover your head during therapy.

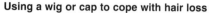
Using a wig or cap to cope with hair loss

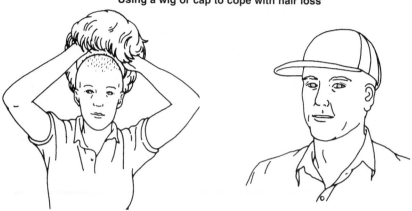

Skin problems

• For sensitive or dry skin, ask the doctor or nurse to recommend a lotion. Don't use petroleum jelly or nonprescription creams and powders. They could leave a coating that will interfere with your radiation treatments.
• Use cornstarch to absorb moisture, and avoid wearing tight-fitting clothing over the treatment area. Be sure to report any blisters or cracked skin to the doctor.
• Stay out of the sun during the course of therapy. You may even have to avoid the sun for several months afterward, so check with the doctor, especially if you're planning a vacation to a sunny area. When you can go out in the sun again, wear light clothes over the treated area, and wear a hat, too. Cover all exposed skin with an effective sunblock lotion (SPF 15 or higher).

Tiredness

• Limit activities, especially sports.
• Get more sleep.
• Try to reduce your work hours until the end of treatments. Discuss your therapy schedule with your employer.
• If possible, schedule radiation treatments at your convenience.
• Ask for help from family and friends, whether it's pitching in

with daily chores or driving you to the hospital. Most people are glad to help out—they just need to be asked.

• If you lose interest in sex during treatments, either because you're too tired or because of hormonal changes, bear in mind that sexual desire usually returns after treatments end. One special note: Avoid sex if you're receiving radiation treatments to your abdomen—intercourse may be painful. This should also improve when treatment ends.

Risk of infection

You're more likely to get an infection during therapy, so follow these tips.

• Avoid crowds and people with colds and infections.

• Use an electric shaver instead of a razor.

• Use a soft toothbrush. It will help you avoid injuring your gums—a frequent site of infection.

• Tell the doctor if you have a fever, chills, a tendency to bruise easily, or unusual bleeding.

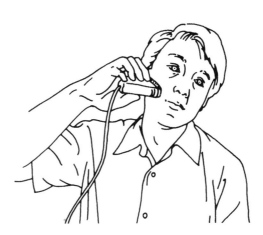

Checking fluid balance

A child's condition, particularly that of a young child, can change rapidly and insidiously when a fluid imbalance occurs. Suspect a fluid imbalance if your child has vomiting or diarrhea, if he can't swallow liquids because of a sore throat, or if he's breathing through his mouth. If he has a fever, he'll need more fluids than usual. Use this checklist to help you decide if your child is well hydrated.

• Inspect the insides of your child's mouth and lower eyelids. Do the tissues look pink and moist?

☐ Yes   ☐ No

• Watch your child closely the next time he has a crying spell. Are his eyes producing plenty of tears?

☐ Yes   ☐ No

• Watch for changes in the amount of your child's urine and bowel movements. Does the amount increase when your child drinks more fluids?

☐ Yes   ☐ No

• Pinch your child's skin gently. Does his skin quickly spring back to normal?

☐ Yes   ☐ No

• Weigh your child daily. Is he maintaining his normal weight?

☐ Yes   ☐ No

• If he's a baby, observe his fontanelles (the soft spots on top of his head). Do they appear flat, not sunken or bulging?

☐ Yes   ☐ No

If you answered yes to all these questions, your child probably is well hydrated. If you answered no to any questions, don't be alarmed, but do call the doctor immediately and discuss the symptoms with him. Remember, dehydration can cause serious problems because it upsets the body's balance of essential salts and fluids. If your child is dehydrated, follow the doctor's advice for treating the condition.

Coping with seizures

You probably have many questions about seizures and how to help your child lead a normal life.

What causes seizures? Seizures may follow a birth injury, a head injury, a high fever, or a disease that affects your child's nervous system, such as meningitis and encephalitis.

However, the cause of many seizures is never known. Rest assured, though, that they aren't contagious. No one gave them to your child, and no one can catch them from him.

Medication

Follow the doctor's instructions exactly for the dose of medication to give your child and when to give it. Taking medication exactly as the doctor prescribes will help control your child's seizures. Remember: Missed doses of medication could lead to a seizure.

When your child begins taking medication for seizures, he may seem less alert or his behavior may change. If these side effects interfere with his activities and school work, tell the doctor. He may adjust the dose or change the medication.

Activities

Has the doctor placed any restrictions on your child's activities? If so, follow his instructions. If not, take the same precautions as you would with any other child. For example, caution him to wear a helmet when he's skateboarding or bicycling. And don't let him swim alone.

Emotional support

Help your child deal with people who have misguided ideas about seizures. If you have other children, help them understand their brother's or sister's condition. Explain what they should do if their brother or sister has a seizure.

Enlist the support of your child's teacher. Tell her about

your child's seizures, and explain what to do if he has one in school. She can help your child's classmates accept him as being just like them—except that he has seizures. She can also help his classmates deal emotionally with a seizure if he has one in school.

Ask the school nurse to help if your child must take medication during school hours. Also, inform camp counselors, baby-sitters, and any other people who care for your child about his seizures and how to handle them.

Additional information

Contact the Epilepsy Foundation of America for free information for you, your child, other family members, and your child's friends. (See this book's appendix for helpful details.) You can also call the doctor if you have any questions.

Managing diarrhea

Diarrhea can disrupt essential fluid balance in anyone, especially a child. It may make a sick child's recovery take longer.

Observe your sick child carefully. You know he has diarrhea when his bowel movements increase in amount and frequency and look watery. For example, several loose, runny bowel movements over a few hours signal diarrhea.

Beware of dehydration, which can result from diarrhea. This is a dangerous condition that should be treated right away by the doctor. Here's how to recognize the signs of dehydration, how to know when to call the doctor, and how to restore lost fluids.

Pinching the skin on top of the hand

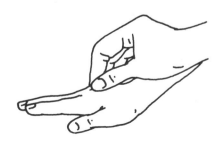

Signs of dehydration

Your child may be dehydrated if:
• he stops urinating or produces much less urine than usual
• he appears to be losing weight
• his eyes look sunken.

Try this test: Pinch the skin on top of your child's hand and let it go. If the skin remains in the pinched position instead of returning to its normal position, your child may be dehydrated.

When to call the doctor

Don't delay getting medical care for your child if:
• you notice any dehydration signs
• he's younger than 18 months and has watery bowel movements
• he's an older child whose diarrhea lasts longer than 12 hours
• his bowel movement contains blood or mucus or both.

How to restore fluids

• Encourage clear fluids for the first 24 hours after diarrhea starts. Flat soda (stir a carbonated beverage until it stops fizzing), chicken broth, and tea are good choices.
• Offer soft, bland foods, such as bananas, rice, and applesauce, as your child begins to feel better.
• Avoid giving your child milk and other dairy products, such as cheese and ice cream, when he's sick and for 1 week after he recovers. These foods may trigger another bout of diarrhea.
• Give an oral rehydrating solution if the doctor advises. This solution is available in powder form from the drugstore. (Or ask the nurse how to mix a homemade solution.) Made with pure water, the solution will bring your child's fluid balance back to normal more effectively than an ordinary liquid, such as cola.

Follow the doctor's instructions on how much to give. Don't offer any other fluid but water if you're using this solution.

Caring for a child with hemophilia

Your child has hemophilia, a lifelong bleeding disorder. With proper care, he can lead a nearly normal life, attending school regularly and taking part in most activities. Follow these guidelines to promote his health and well-being.

Prevent injury

Protect your child from injury, but avoid unnecessary restrictions that impair his normal development. For example, if your son's a preschooler, add padded patches to the knees

Preventing an injury

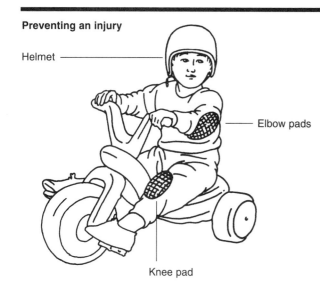

Helmet

Elbow pads

Knee pad

and elbows of his clothing to protect these joints when he falls and have him wear a helmet.

You must forbid an older child to participate in contact sports, such as football, but you can encourage him to swim or play golf.

Administer first aid

If your child is injured, administer first aid as you would for anyone else. Remember, he won't bleed any faster than normal. He'll just bleed longer. If he's not treated promptly, he may have prolonged or delayed oozing that can cause pain and disability. Injuries to the head, neck, or eyes are serious.

If your child says he has pain, starts limping, or stops using an arm or a leg, suspect that he's bleeding into a joint or muscle. Arrange for prompt treatment.

Watch for bleeding

Be alert for signs of bleeding, especially in the head area and particularly if your child has suffered a blow to his head within the past 4 to 5 days. Called intracranial bleeding, this problem causes nausea, vomiting, headache, irritability, and drowsiness.

If your child vomits blood or material that looks like coffee grounds or passes stools that are black and sticky (tarry), suspect bleeding in the stomach or intestinal area.

Blood in the urine points to kidney bleeding and should be treated by giving fluids and clotting factor.

Whenever your child is injured or appears to be bleeding abnormally, call the doctor or hemophilia treatment center immediately.

Learn to infuse clotting factors

When your child reaches age 6 or 7, you may want to learn how to give him clotting factor infusions at home. This will enable him to receive treatment as quickly as possible after you (or he) notice signs and symptoms of abnormal bleeding.

It also may eliminate the need for hospitalization.

Your son's nurse or doctor or the specialists at the hemophilia center can teach you. Once you know how to give an infusion, remember to keep the blood factor concentrate and infusion equipment handy at all times—even (or especially) during family vacations.

Receiving immunization shots

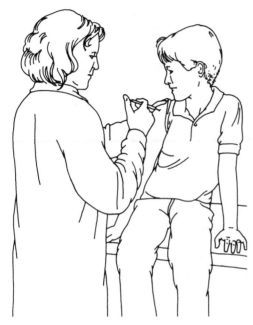

Be alert for illness

You may fear that your child may contract AIDS from blood products, but heat-treated blood products, improved quality assurance programs, and more stringent laboratory controls have resulted in AIDS-free factor concentrates. However, heat-treated factor concentrate can still infect the child with hepatitis. Watch for early signs of hepatitis, which may appear from 3 weeks to 6 months after treatment with blood components. These include headache, fever, decreased appetite, nausea, vomiting, and abdominal tenderness and pain.

Be sure your child receives the hepatitis B vaccine along with his regularly scheduled immunizations.

Take important precautions

• Make sure your child wears a medical identification bracelet or necklace at all times.

• Never give him aspirin. It may increase the frequency or severity of his bleeding episodes. Examine all medicine labels for these words: "aspirin," "acetylsalicylic acid," or "ASA." They are all names for the same medicine: aspirin.

• Teach your child to care for his teeth regularly with careful toothbrushing. This may prevent the need for future dental procedures, such as scaling, restoration, and surgery. Have him use a soft toothbrush to avoid gum injury.

Brushing carefully

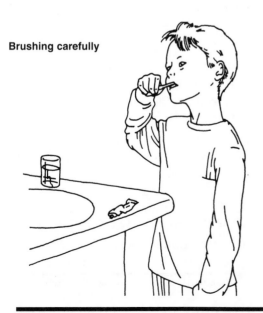

• Keep routine follow-up appointments with the doctor or at the local hemophilia center.
• To answer questions about the vulnerability of future offspring, consult a genetic counselor or contact the National Hemophilia Foundation.
• Your daughters may want to consider genetic screening, too. Such screening can detect whether they carry the hemophilia gene.

Caring for an HIV-infected child

Diagnosis of AIDS in infants is difficult because, in most instances, infants born to human immunodeficiency virus (HIV)-infected mothers will test positive for up to 15 months whether or not they are infected, because they carry maternal antibodies.

Within 12 and 15 months, however, the infant's HIV antibody levels will fall to undetectable levels. In contrast, infected infants will have persistent or rising HIV antibody levels.

You should use the same precautions for an HIV-infected child as for an HIV-infected adult. In addition, follow these special precautions:

Vaccines

Immunizations for an HIV-infected child should be given according to the usual guidelines. This includes immunizations against measles, mumps, and rubella. Vaccines against pneumonia should be given at age 2; influenza vaccinations are recommended at age 6 months and yearly thereafter. Because an immunocompromised child may lose his ability to produce antibodies, many doctors recommend periodic antibody tests and reimmunization as necessary, based on the test results.

An inactivated polio vaccine rather than the activated oral form should be given to an HIV-infected child. Polio vaccines should be administered along with pertussis vaccine and diphtheria and tetanus toxoids at ages 2, 4, 6, and 18 months and 4 and 6 years.

If active chicken pox appears, the immunocompromised

child should be seen by a doctor for evaluation and possible treatment with oral or injected acyclovir.

Fevers

An HIV-injected child can run fevers of 101° F (38.3° C) for weeks. If tests don't reveal a bacterial infection, HIV is assumed to be the cause.

To treat fevers, keep the child warm and comfortable, change the bed linens often, and use extra blankets. Give sponge baths and fluids to control the fever.

Clean the thermometer after every temperature reading. Wash it with soap and water, soak it in ethyl alcohol (70% to 90%) for 30 minutes, and then rinse it under running water. If the child has chronic diarrhea, take his temperature under his arm rather than rectally.

Nutrition

Feed an HIV-infected child a high-protein, high-calorie diet that supplies 100% to 150% of the recommended daily allowance for his weight. Try to make the food as appealing as possible.

Blood products

Before blood or blood products are given to a child with HIV infection or AIDS, they need to be irradiated to prevent the child from developing graft-versus-host disease.

Umbilical stumps

To prevent infection, clean the umbilical stump daily until it falls off or is removed.

Circumcision

An infant of a mother at high risk for HIV infection shouldn't be circumcised because of the risk of infection.

Protective clothing

Wear gloves when changing diapers, a mask and glasses if you might be splashed with body secretions or excretions, and a gown when handling an infant of a mother at high risk.

Use an artificial airway when performing cardiopulmonary resuscitation—don't use mouth-to-mouth resuscitation.

Wear gloves when handling newborns until after their first

baths and when handling the placenta.

Other considerations

The child's home environment and relationship with family members will greatly influence how he copes with his illness. Allow the child to lead as normal a life as possible. He should attend school unless he presents an infection risk to classmates or they pose a risk to him. Seek occupational therapy for older children who fall behind in motor development because of illness or work with them at home.

27   Emergency Situations

Managing an emergency

When an emergency occurs, you'll need to think quickly and act with certainty. An emergency is extremely stressful at any time, but especially if it occurs with the person you're caring for. Use the guidelines that follow to help manage specific emergency situations. (Also see Chapter 1, Preparing for an Emergency.)

Managing a hypoglycemic episode

A sudden hypoglycemic episode may affect the person's ability to recognize his symptoms and take appropriate action.

   You will have to manage the crisis for him. In such an emergency, you must raise his blood glucose level immediately to prevent permanent brain damage and even death. So be sure you have sources of glucose (sugar) available.

If the person is conscious

Give him any of the following:

FOODS AND FLUIDS	AMOUNT
Apple juice, orange juice, or ginger ale	4 to 6 ounces (118 to 177 milliliters)
Regular cola or other soft drink	4 to 6 ounces (118 to 177 milliliters)
Corn syrup, honey, or grape jelly	1 tablespoon
Hard candy	5 to 6 pieces
Jelly beans	6
Gumdrops	10

If the person is unconscious or has trouble swallowing

Give him a subcutaneous injection of glucagon. (See "Giving a subcutaneous injection" in Chapter 8, Giving Medications.) Be sure to check the expiration date on the glucagon kit frequently and replenish your supply as needed.

How to inject glucagon

1 Prepare the glucagon following the manufacturer's instructions included in the kit.

2 Select an appropriate injection site.

3 Pull the skin taut, and then clean it with an alcohol swab.

4 Using your thumb and forefinger, pinch the skin at the injection site, and then quickly plunge the needle into the skin fold at a 90-degree angle up to the needle hub.
   Push the plunger down to quickly inject the glucagon.

5 Withdraw the needle, and rub the site with an alcohol swab.

6 Turn the person onto his side. Because glucagon may cause vomiting, this position reduces the possibility of choking.

7 If the person doesn't wake up in 5 to 20 minutes, give a second dose of glucagon and seek emergency help. If he wakes up and can swallow, give him some sugar immediately. (See the chart on the previous page for a selection of foods and fluids that contain high amounts of sugar.) Do this because glucagon isn't effective for longer than about 90 minutes. Then call the doctor.

Managing a person in sickle cell crisis

Because the person you're caring for has sickle cell anemia, he's at risk for a serious complication called sickle cell crisis. If this crisis occurs, the tips below can help you treat it and maybe prevent it from recurring.

What goes wrong?

In sickle cell anemia, some red blood cells change from round shape to a sickle shape. When this happens, the sickled cells clog small blood vessels and keep blood from reaching vital organs. This condition, called vaso-occlusive crisis, causes pain and, possibly, cell damage.

Some things that cause a crisis are:
• infection, such as a cold or the flu
• dehydration—from not drinking enough fluid or from sweating, vomiting, or diarrhea
• low oxygen levels—for example, from a visit to the mountains
• temperature extremes.

Recognizing a crisis

Suspect a crisis if the person has:
• pain, especially in the stomach area, chest, muscles, or bones
• paleness, usually around the lips, tongue, and fingernails
• unusual sleepiness or irritability
• a low-grade fever that lasts for 2 days
• dark urine.

Responding to a crisis

Call the doctor and describe the person's symptoms. For a mild crisis, the doctor may suggest home care. Here's how to help the person at home.
• Apply warm, moist compresses to painful areas. Cover the person with a blanket so that he doesn't become chilled. Never use ice packs or cold compresses. These could be harmful.
• Ease pain with acetaminophen.
• Tell the person to stay in bed. Let him sit up if that's more comfortable.
• Make sure the person drinks lots of fluids so that he doesn't become dehydrated.
• Call the doctor if symptoms persist or worsen.

Preventing a crisis

Although these precautions aren't foolproof, they may help to prevent another crisis. Discuss these do's and don'ts with the person in your care.

Do's

• Stay up to date with immunizations.
• Prevent infections: Take meticulous care of wounds, eat well-balanced meals, have regular dental checkups, and learn proper tooth and gum care.
• Seek treatment for an infection.
• Drink fluids at the first sign of a cold or other infection.

Don'ts

• Avoid wearing tight clothing that could block circulation.
• Never exercise strenuously or excessively.
• Avoid drinking lots of ice water or being exposed to extremely hot or cold temperatures.
• Avoid mountain climbing, unpressurized aircraft, and high altitudes.

Using an anaphylaxis kit

Because you could have a severe reaction from insect stings or other substances, the doctor has prescribed an anaphylaxis kit for you to use in an emergency. The kit contains everything you need to treat an allergic reaction:

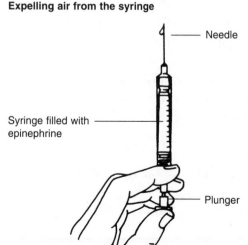

Expelling air from the syringe

Needle

Syringe filled with epinephrine

Plunger

• a prefilled syringe containing two doses of epinephrine
• alcohol swabs
• a tourniquet
• antihistamine tablets.

If an insect stings you, use the kit as follows. Also, notify the doctor immediately or ask someone else to call him.

1 Take the prefilled syringe from the kit and remove the needle cap. Hold the syringe with the needle pointing up. Then push in the plunger until it stops. This will expel any air from the syringe.

2 Clean about 4 inches (10 centimeters) of skin on your arm or thigh with an alcohol swab. (If you're right-handed, clean your left arm or thigh. If you're left-handed, clean your right arm or thigh.)

Inserting the needle

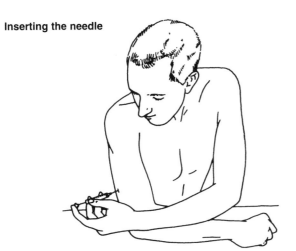

3 Rotate the plunger one-quarter turn to the right so that it's aligned with the slot. Insert the entire needle—like a dart—into the skin.

Push down on the plunger until it stops. It will inject 0.3 milliliter of the drug for an adult or a person over age 12. Withdraw the needle.

Note: The dose and administration for babies and for children under age 12 must be directed by the doctor.

4 Quickly remove the insect's stinger, if you can see it. Use a dull object, such as a fingernail or tweezers, to pull it straight out. Don't pinch, scrape, or squeeze the stinger. This may push it further into the skin and release more poison. If you can't remove the stinger quickly, stop trying. Go on to the next step.

Removing the stinger

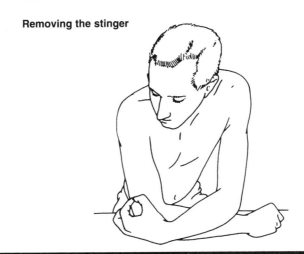

5 If you were stung on your neck, face, or body, skip this step and go on to the next one.

If you were stung on an arm or a leg, apply the tourniquet between the sting site and your heart. Tighten the tourniquet by pulling the string.

After 10 minutes, release the tourniquet by pulling on the metal ring.

Applying the tourniquet

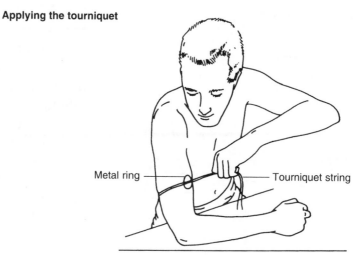

Metal ring — — Tourniquet string

6 Chew and swallow the antihistamine tablets. (For children age 12 and under, follow the dose and administration directions supplied by the doctor or provided in the kit.)

7 Apply ice packs—if available—to the affected area. Avoid exertion, keep warm, and see a doctor or go to a hospital emergency department immediately.

Important: If you don't notice an improvement within 10 minutes, give a second injection by following the directions in the anaphylaxis kit. If the syringe in your kit has a preset second dose, don't depress the plunger until you're ready to give the second injection. Proceed as before, following the instructions to inject the epinephrine.

Special instructions

• Keep your kit handy to ensure emergency treatment at all times.

• Ask the pharmacist for storage guidelines. Find out whether

the kit can be stored in a car's glove compartment or whether you need to keep it in a cooler place.
• Periodically check the epinephrine in the preloaded syringe. Pinkish brown solution needs to be replaced.
• Make a note of the kit's expiration date. Then renew the kit just before that date.
• Dispose of the used needle and syringe safely and properly.

Clearing an obstructed airway

You'll need to come quickly to the aid of a choking victim. That's because an airway obstruction, if uninterrupted, leads to brain damage and death in 4 to 6 minutes.

If the person can speak or cough, encourage him to cough to expel the obstruction. On the other hand, if he can't speak, cough, or breathe, respond at once. This person needs help to dislodge the obstruction.

1 Begin by asking the person, "Are you choking?" and then "Can I help?" If his airway is completely obstructed, he won't answer because airflow to his vocal cords will be blocked. But if he's making crowing sounds, his airway is only partially blocked. Encourage him to cough if he's indicated that you can help. Then, if the airway becomes completely blocked, proceed.

2 Tell the person that you'll try to dislodge the foreign body. Stand behind him, and put your arms around his waist. Make a fist with one hand. Place the top of your fist (thumb side) against the person's abdomen, slightly above the umbilicus and well below the breast bone (also called the xiphoid process). Now, grasp the bottom of your fist with your other hand.

3 Squeeze the person's abdomen 6 to 10 times with quick inward and upward thrusts. Each thrust should create an artificial cough with enough force to propel a foreign object from the person's airway.

When performing the thrusts, keep a firm grasp on the person. Also, be sure that you can provide support if he should lose consciousness and need to be lowered to the floor. Scan the floor for a clear, safe area where you can place the person, if necessary.

If the person loses consciousness, support him carefully. Gently lower him to the floor, using your leg as a sliding board. Remember to support his head and neck to prevent injury. Then take additional steps to clear his airway.

4 If the person is obese or pregnant, perform chest thrusts instead of abdominal thrusts. Place the top of your clenched fist (thumb side) against the middle of the person's breast bone. Put your other hand over the bottom of your clenched fist. Perform chest thrusts until the person expels the object or loses consciousness.

Performing CPR

An emergency procedure, cardiopulmonary resuscitation (CPR) seeks to restore and maintain the person's respiration and circulation after his heart stops beating and his breathing stops. It provides oxygen and blood flow to the heart, brain, and other vital organs until the person recovers or until advanced life support can begin.

Remember, the critical factor is time. If the person's heartbeat and respirations have been stopped for less than 4 minutes before intervention, he has a much better chance for complete recovery, provided CPR efforts succeed. If his circulation has been stopped for 4 to 6 minutes before intervention, he may suffer brain damage. If it has been stopped longer than 6 minutes, he'll almost certainly suffer brain damage.

When deciding whether to start CPR, follow this guideline: Give CPR if you have any doubt about how long the person has been without a pulse and respirations. Typically, you'll recognize a person in cardiopulmonary arrest by these signs: He is unconscious, appears ashen or gray, has no palpable carotid or femoral pulse, and has no breath sounds or air movement through the nose or mouth.

To follow the correct sequence for CPR, remember the

ABCs: open the *airway*, restore *breathing*, and restore *circulation*.

You can perform CPR quickly in almost any situation without assistance. You'll need a firm surface for the person to lie on so that you can deliver the most effective cardiac compressions.

1 Gently shake the person's shoulder and shout, "Are you OK?" in both ears, in case he has difficulty hearing. This simple action ensures that you don't start CPR on a conscious person.

Quickly scan the person for major injuries, particularly to the head or neck. Call for help and dial 911 for emergency assistance.

2 Position the person on his back on a hard, flat surface, such as the floor. If the person is in bed, use a board or put the bed's headboard under him. If you suspect a head or neck injury, move the person as little as possible to reduce the risk of paralysis. If you must move him, logroll him so that he lies flat (supine), supporting his head and neck to keep his backbone or spinal column from twisting.

Open the airway

3 To ensure an open airway, position yourself near the person's shoulders. (Unless you suspect a neck injury), place one hand on the person's forehead and the other hand on the bony portion of his chin near the jaw. Gently push his forehead back and pull upward on the chin, making sure the teeth are almost touching. This is called the head-tilt, chin-lift maneuver.

Pushing on the forehead and lifting the chin when you don't suspect a head or neck injury

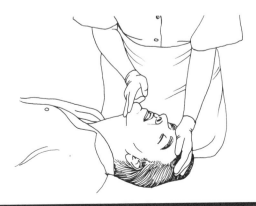

If you suspect a neck injury, open the airway using the jaw-thrust maneuver. Kneel behind the person's head. Rest your thumbs on his lower jaw near the corners of his mouth. Your thumbs should point toward the person's feet. Then place your fingertips around the lower jaw. With a steady, strong motion, lift the jaw upward and outward with your fingertips. This maneuver called the jaw-thrust maneuver, opens the airway without moving the neck.

Lifting the jaw upward and forward when you suspect a head or neck injury

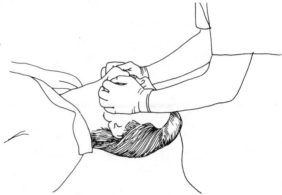

Restore breathing

4 Keep the person's airway open as you place your ear above his mouth and nose and look toward his feet.

Listen for the sound of moving air, and watch for chest movement. You may also feel air on your cheek. If you detect signs of breathing, keep the person's airway open and continue checking his breathing until help arrives.

Listening for air movement

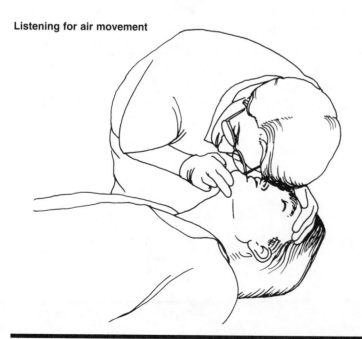

5 If breathing doesn't begin once the airway opens, start rescue breathing. Use the one-way valve mask, if available, placing the mask over the person's nose and mouth.

Using your hand that's closest to the person's chin,

maintain the chin-lift position to keep the airway open. Place the palm of your other hand on the person's forehead to stabilize the head. Use the index and middle fingers of this hand to seal the mask and hold it in position.

6 Without a mask, perform mouth-to-mouth rescue breathing. Once you've opened the person's airway, pinch his nostrils shut with the thumb and index finger of the hand you had on his forehead.

**Pinching the nostrils
shut**

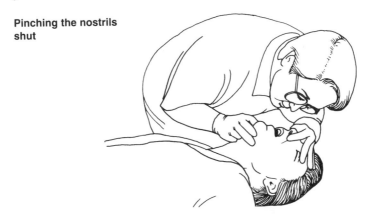

Take a deep breath, and cover the person's mouth with yours. Aim for a tight seal. Deliver two full ventilations (breaths), taking a deep breath after each to allow time for the person's chest to expand and relax and to prevent forcing air into the stomach. Each ventilation should last 1½ to 2 seconds. If this attempt fails, reposition the person's head and try again.

**Forcing air into the
person**

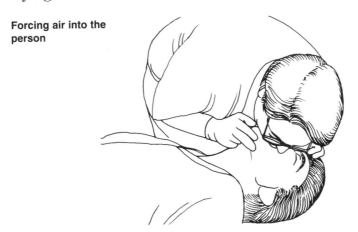

Restore circulation

7 Keep one hand on the person's forehead to keep the airway open. With your other hand, palpate the carotid artery closer to you by placing your index and middle fingers below the jaw and to the left or right of the Adam's apple. Press lightly on the artery for 10 seconds. If you detect a pulse, don't begin chest compressions. Instead, continue rescue breathing, giving 12 ventilations each minute (or 1 every 5 seconds). After every 12 ventilations, recheck the pulse.

Checking for a pulse

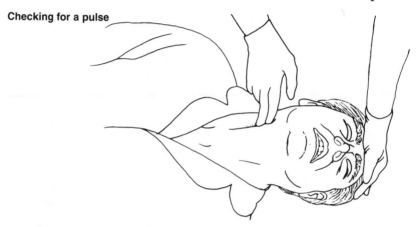

8 If you don't detect a pulse and help hasn't arrived yet, start chest compressions. Still kneeling, move to the person's side. Spread your knees apart for a wide base of support. Next, using the hand closer to the person's feet, locate the lower margin of his rib cage.

Locating the lower margin of the rib cage

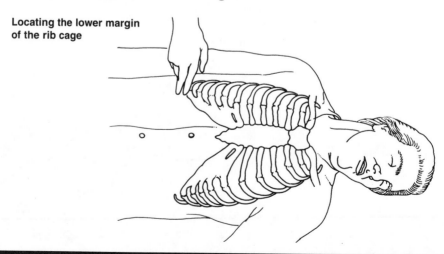

9 Move your fingertips along the margin to the notch where the ribs meet the breastbone (sternum). Place your middle finger on that notch (the xiphoid process) and your index finger next to it. Your index finger should be on the bottom of the person's sternum. Take care to find the correct hand position because improper placement can lead to complications.

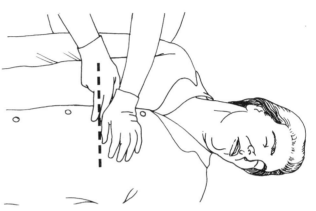

10 Put the heel of your other hand on the person's sternum, next to your index finger. The heel of your hand should align with the lower edge of the sternum, marked by the dotted line in the illustration.

11 Take your fingers off the notch, and place that hand directly on top of your other hand. Make sure the heel of your hand, not your fingers, rests on the person's chest.

**Positioning both
hands for chest
compression**

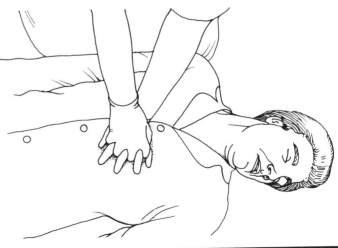

12 With your elbows locked, arms straight, and shoulders directly over your hands, you're positioned to start chest compressions. Using the weight of your upper body, compress the person's sternum 1½ to 2 inches (3.8 to 5 centimeters), delivering the pressure through the heels of your hands. Don't let your fingers rest on the person's chest.

After each compression, release the pressure and allow the chest to return to its normal position so that the heart can fill with blood. To prevent injuries, don't change your hand position during compressions.

Give 15 chest compressions at a rate that simulates 80 to 100 heartbeats per minute. Count "one and two and three and" up to 15, compressing on the number and releasing on the "and." After 15 compressions, move back up to the person's face and give two ventilations. Then, reposition your hands properly, and deliver 15 more compressions. Continue this pattern for four full cycles.

Compressing the chest

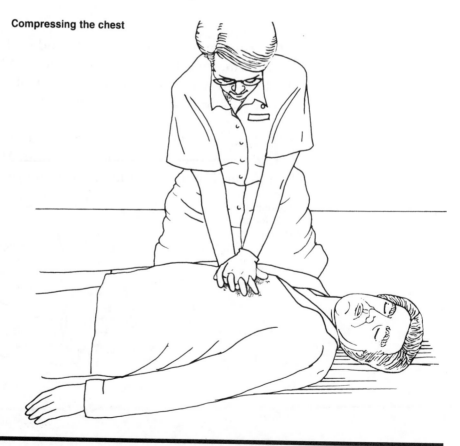

13 Check the carotid artery again for a pulse. If you still don't detect a pulse, give two quick breaths and continue CPR in cycles of 15 compressions and two ventilations. Perform CPR for 1 more minute, check for a pulse, and then call for help again.

Rechecking for a pulse

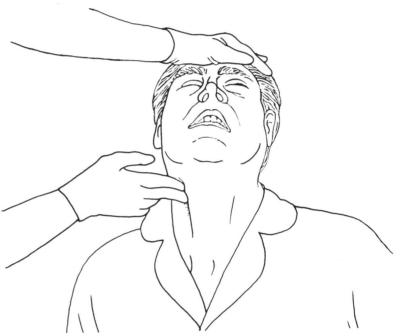

Without help, however, continue CPR. Check for breathing and a pulse. If you feel a pulse but no breath, give 12 ventilations per minute and monitor the pulse. Don't stop CPR until the person's breathing and pulse resume, someone takes over for you, or exhaustion halts your effort.

If you detect both a pulse and breathing, position the person on his side (turning his body as a unit) and monitor his condition.

Appendices and Index

Appendices

National Associations: A Resource Guide

AIDS Health Project
P.O. Box 0884
San Francisco, CA 94143-0884
(415) 476-6430

Allergy and Asthma Network
• Mothers of Asthmatics, Inc.
3554 Chain Bridge Road, Suite 200
Fairfax, VA 22030-2709
(703) 385-4403

Alzheimer's Association
919 North Michigan, 10th Floor
Chicago, IL 60611
(312) 335-8700

American Amputee Foundation
P.O. Box 250218, Hillcrest Station
Little Rock, AR 72225
(501) 666-2523

American Anorexia-Bulimia
Association
c/o Regents Hospital
425 East 61st Street, 6th Floor
New York, NY 10021
(212) 891-8686

American Association for Cancer
Education
P.O. Box 700
Birmingham, AL 35294
(205) 934-3054

American Association of Kidney
Patients
100 South Ashley Drive, Suite 280
Tampa, FL 33602
(800) 749-2257

American Association on Mental
Retardation
444 North Capitol Street, NW,
Suite 846
Washington, DC 20001
(202) 387-1968

American Association for
Respiratory Care
11030 Ables Lane
Dallas, TX 75229-4593
(214) 243-2272

American Cancer Society (ACS)
1599 Clifton Road
Atlanta, GA 30331
(800) ACS-2345; (404) 320-3333

American Chronic Pain Association
P.O. Box 850
Rocklin, CA 95677
(916) 632-0922

American College of Rheumatology
60 Executive Park South, Suite 150
Atlanta, GA 30329
(404) 633-3777

American Council of the Blind
1155 15th Street, NW, Suite 720
Washington, DC 20005
(202) 467-5081

American Deafness and Rehabilitation Association
P.O. Box 251554
Little Rock, AR 72225
(501) 868-8850

American Diabetes Association, National Center
1660 Duke Street
Alexandria, VA 22314
(800) 232-3472

American Foundation for the Blind
15 West 16th Street
New York, NY 10011
(212) 620-2000

American Foundation for the Prevention of Venereal Disease
(sexually transmitted diseases)
799 Broadway, Suite 638
New York, NY 10003
(212) 759-2069

American Foundation for Urologic Disease, Inc.
300 West Pratt Street, Suite 401
Baltimore, MD 21201-2463
(410) 727-2908; (410) 528-0550 (fax)

American Heart Association
7272 Greenville Avenue
Dallas, TX 75231
(214) 373-6300

American Kidney Fund
6110 Executive Blvd., Suite 1010
Rockville, MD 20852
(800) 638-8299

American Liver Foundation
1425 Pompton Avenue
Cedar Grove, NJ 07009
(201) 256-2550

American Lung Association
1740 Broadway
New York, NY 10019
(212) 315-8700

American Lupus Society
3914 Del Amo Blvd., Suite 922
Torrance, CA 90503
(310) 542-8891

American Paralysis Association
(spinal cord injury)
500 Morris Avenue
Springfield, NJ 07081
(201) 379-2690

American Parkinson Disease Association
60 Bay Street, Suite 401
Staten Island, NY 10301
(800) 223-2732

American Physical Therapy Association
1111 North Fairfax Street
Alexandria, VA 22314
(703) 684-2782

American Psychiatric Association
1400 K Street, NW
Washington, DC 20005-2492
(202) 682-6000

American Social Health Association
(sexually transmitted diseases)
P.O. Box 13827
Research Triangle Park, NC 27709
(919) 361-8400

American Society of Cataract and Refractive Surgery
4000 Legato Road, Suite 850
Fairfax, VA 22033
(703) 591-2220

American Urological Association, Allied
11512 Allecingie Parkway
Richmond, VA 23235
(804) 379-1306

Amyotrophic Lateral Sclerosis Association
21021 Ventura Blvd., Suite 321
Woodland Hills, CA 91364-2206
(818) 340-7500

Aplastic Anemia Foundation of America
P.O. Box 22689
Baltimore, MD 21203
(410) 955-2803

Arthritis Foundation
1314 Spring Street, NW
Atlanta, GA 30309
(404) 872-7100

Asthma and Allergy Foundation of America
1125 15th Street, NW, Suite 502
Washington, DC 20005
(202) 466-7643

Cancer Care
1180 Avenue of the Americas
New York, NY 10036
(212) 221-3300

Cancer Information Service
Building 31, Room 10A-07
9000 Rockville Pike
Bethesda, MD 20892
(301) 496-8664

Canine Companions for Independence
P.O. Box 446
Santa Rosa, CA 95402-0446
(707) 528-0830

Centers for Disease Control and Prevention (CDC) National AIDS Clearinghouse
P.O. Box 6003
Rockville, MD 20849-6003
(800) 458-5231; (301) 217-0023;
(301) 738-6616 (fax)

Center for Family Support
(mentally disabled)
386 Park Avenue South, Suite 1201
New York, NY 10016
(212) 889-5464

Centers for Disease Control and Prevention (CDC)
1600 Clifton Road, NE
Atlanta, GA 30333
(404) 639-3311

Chemotherapy Foundation
183 Madison Avenue, Room 403
New York, NY 10016
(212) 213-9292

Children's Blood Foundation (CBF)
333 East 38th Street, Suite 830
New York, NY 10016
(212) 297-4336

Citizens for Public Action on Blood Pressure and Cholesterol
7200 Wisconsin Avenue, Suite 10002
Bethesda, MD 20814
(301) 907-7790

Crohn's Disease and Colitis Foundation of America, Inc.
386 Park Avenue South
New York, NY 10016
(212) 685-3440

Cystic Fibrosis Foundation
6931 Arlington Road
Bethesda, MD 20814
(800) FIGHT CF; (301) 951-4422

Digestive Disease National Coalition
711 Second Street, NE, Suite 200
Washington, DC 20002
(202) 544-7497

Epilepsy Foundation of America
4351 Garden City Drive
Landover, MD 20785
(301) 459-3700

Health Education Resource Organization (HERO)
101 West Reed Street, Suite 825
Baltimore, MD 21201
(410) 685-1180

Help for Incontinent People
P.O. Box 544
Union, SC 29379
(803) 579-7900

High Blood Pressure Information Center
National Institutes of Health
4733 Bethesda Avenue
Bethesda, MD 20814
(301) 952-3260

Huntington's Disease Society of America
140 West 22nd Street, 6th Floor
New York, NY 10011-2420
(212) 242-1968

International Association for the Study of Pain
909 NE 43rd Street, Suite 306
Seattle, WA 98105-6020
(206) 547-6409

International Association of Laryngectomees
1599 Clifton Road, NE
Atlanta, GA 30029-4251
(404) 329-7651

Juvenile Diabetes Foundation International
432 Park Avenue South
New York, NY 10016-8013
(800) 533-2873

Leukemia Society of America
600 Third Avenue, 4th Floor
New York, NY 10016
(212) 573-8484

Look Good, Feel Better (LGFB)
(Cosmetic, Toiletry, and Fragrance Association Foundation)
1101 17th Street, NW, Suite 300
Washington, DC 20036
(202) 331-1770

Lupus Foundation of America
Four Research Place, Suite 180
Rockville, MD 20850-3226
(301) 670-9292

Make-A-Wish Foundation of America
100 West Claringdon Avenue
Suite 2200
Phoenix, AZ 85013
(602) 279-9474

Make Today Count
101½ South Union Street
Alexandria, VA 22314-3323
(703) 548-9674

March of Dimes Birth Defects Foundation
1275 Mamaroneck Avenue
White Plains, NY 10605
(914) 428-7100

Medic Alert Foundation International
P.O. Box 1009
Turlock, CA 95381-1009
(209) 668-3333

Muscular Dystrophy Association
330 East Sunrise Drive
Tucson, AZ 85718
(602) 529-2000

National Association of the Deaf
814 Thayer Avenue
Silver Spring, MD 20910
(301) 587-1788

National Association on Drug Abuse Problems
355 Lexington Avenue, 2nd Floor
New York, NY 10017-6683
(212) 986-1170

National Association of Home Care
519 C Street, NE
Washington, DC 20002
(202) 547-7424

National Association of People with AIDS (NAPWA)
1413 K Street, NW
Washington, DC 20005
(202) 898-0414

National Association for Sickle Cell Disease
3345 Wilshire Blvd., Suite 1106
Los Angeles, CA 90010-1880
(213) 736-5455

National Black Leadership Initiative on Cancer (NBLIC)
c/o Frank E. Jordan
NBLIC Program Director
Cancer Control Science Program
Bethesda, MD 20892
(301) 496-8680; (301) 496-8675 (fax)

National Chronic Pain Outreach Association (NCPOA)
7979 Old Georgetown Road,
Suite 100
Bethesda, MD 20814-2429
(301) 652-4948

National Coalition of Hispanic Health & Human Services
1501 16th Street, NW
Washington, DC 20036
(202) 387-5000

National Committee on the Treatment of Intractable Pain
c/o Wayne Coy, Jr.
Cohn and Marks
1333 New Hampshire Avenue, NW
Washington, DC 20036
(202) 452-4836

National Council on the Aging
409 Third Street, SW, #200
Washington, DC 20024
(202) 479-6665

National Digestive Diseases Information Clearinghouse
P.O. Box NDDIC
9000 Rockville Pike
Bethesda, MD 20892
(301) 468-6344

National Down's Syndrome Congress
1605 Chantilly Drive, Suite 250
Atlanta, GA 30324
(404) 633-1555

National Easter Seal Society
230 West Monroe Street, Suite 1800
Chicago, IL 60606
(312) 726-6200

National Head Injury Foundation
1776 Massachusetts Avenue, NW,
Suite 100
Washington, DC 20036
(202) 296-6443

National Heart, Lung, and Blood Institute (NHLBI) Information Center
P.O. Box 30105
Bethesda, MD 20824-0105
(301) 251-1222

National Hemophilia Foundation (NHF)
110 Green Street, Suite 303
New York, NY 10012
(212) 219-8180

National Hospice Organization
1901 North Moore Street, Suite 901
Arlington, VA 22209
(703) 243-5900

National Hypertension Association, Inc.
324 East 30th Street
New York, NY 10016
(212) 889-3557

National Institute of Allergy and Infectious Diseases
9000 Rockville Pike Building 31, Room 7A-50
Bethesda, MD 20892
(301) 496-5717

National Institute of Diabetes, Digestive, and Kidney Disorders
9000 Rockville Pike, Building 31, Room 9A-04
Bethesda, MD 20892
(301) 496-3583

National Institute of Neurological Disorders and Stroke
9000 Rockville Pike
Building 31, Room 8A-06
Bethesda, MD 20892
(301) 496-5751

National Jewish Center for Immunology and Respiratory Medicine
1400 Jackson Street
Denver, CO 80206
(303) 388-4461

National Kidney Foundation
30 East 33rd Street, Suite 1100
New York, NY 10016
(212) 889-2210

National Kidney and Urologic Diseases Information Clearinghouse
Three Information Way
Bethesda, MD 20892-3580
(301) 654-4415

National Leukemia Association
585 Stewart Avenue, Suite 536
Garden City, NY 11530
(516) 222-1944

National Lymphedema Network (NLN)
2211 Post Street, Suite 404
San Francisco, CA 94115
(800) 541-3259; (415) 921-4284 (fax)

National Marrow Donor Program
3433 Broadway, NE, Suite 400
Minneapolis, MN 55413
(612) 627-5800

National Mental Health Association
1021 Prince Street
Alexandria, VA 22314-2971
(703) 684-7722

National Multiple Sclerosis Society
733 Third Avenue
New York, NY 10017
(212) 986-3240

National Osteoporosis Foundation
1150 17th Street, NW, Suite 500
Washington, DC 20036
(202) 223-2226

National Parkinson Foundation
1501 NW Ninth Avenue
Miami, FL 33136
(800) 327-4545; (800) 433-7022
(Florida residents)

National Stroke Association
8480 East Orchard Road, Suite 1000
Englewood, CO 80111-5015
(303) 762-9922

Nutrition Education Association
P.O. Box 20301
3647 Glen Haven
Houston, TX 77225
(713) 665-2946

Occupational Safety and Health Administration (OSHA)
U.S. Department of Labor
200 Constitution Avenue, NW
Washington, DC 20210
(202) 219-8148

Oley Foundation
214 Hun Memorial, A23
Albany Medical Center
Albany, NY 12208
(800) 776-OLEY; (518) 262-5079

Parents Anonymous
(child abuse)
520 South Lafayette Park Place,
Suite 316
Los Angeles, CA 90057
(213) 388-6685

Parents Helping Parents, Family Resource Center
535 Race Street, Suite 140
San Jose, CA 95126
(408) 288-5010

Parkinson Support Groups of America
(neurologic disorders)
11376 Cherry Hill Road, #204
Beltsville, MD 20705
(301) 937-1545

Pediatric AIDS Foundation
1311 Colorado Avenue
Santa Monica, CA 90404
(310) 395-9051

Phoenix Society for Burn Survivors (PSBS)
11 Rust Hill Road
Levittown, PA 19056
(215) 946-BURN

Planned Parenthood Federation of America
810 Seventh Avenue
New York, NY 10019
(212) 541-7800

Prevent Blindness, America
500 East Remington Road
Schaumburg, IL 60173
(800) 331-2020

San Francisco AIDS Foundation
P.O. Box 426182
San Francisco, CA 94142-6182
(415) 864-5855

SIDS (Sudden Infant Death Syndrome) Alliance
10500 Little Patuxent Pkwy.
Suite 420
Columbia, MD 21044-3505
(410) 964-8000

Simon Foundation for Continence
P.O. Box 835
Wilmette, IL 60091
(708) 864-3913

Skin Cancer Foundation
245 Fifth Avenue, Suite 2402
New York, NY 10016
(212) 725-5176

Substance Abuse and Mental Health Services Administration (SAMHSA)
5600 Fishers Lane
Parklawn Building, Room 12-105
Rockville, MD 20857
(301) 443-4795

Thyroid Foundation of America
Ruth Sleeper Hall, Room 350
40 Parkman Street
Boston, MA 02114-1202
(617) 726-8500

United Cerebral Palsy Association
1522 K Street, NW, Suite 1112
Washington, DC 20005
(202) 842-1266

United Ostomy Association
36 Executive Park, Suite 120
Irvine, CA 92714
(714) 660-8624

United Parkinson Foundation
833 West Washington Blvd.
Chicago, IL 60607
(312) 733-1893

US TOO Prostate Cancer Survivor Support Group
US TOO International, Inc.
One Heritage Plaza Building
7501 Lemont Road
Woodridge, IL 60517
(800) 82-USTOO; (800) 828-7866

Women's Cancer Network
2413 West River Road
Grand island, NY 14072

Y-ME National Organization for Breast Cancer Information and Support
18220 Harwood Avenue
Homewood, IL 60430
(800) 221-2141 (patient hot line, 9 a.m. to 5 p.m. central time, week-days); (708) 799-8338; (708) 799-8228 (patient 24-hour hot line); (708) 799-5937 (fax)

Table of equivalents

Metric System equivalents

Weight (dry)

0.6 g = 600 mg

o.3 g = 300 mg

0.1 g = 100 mg

0.06 g = 60 mg

0.03 g = 30 mg

0.015 g = 15 mg

.001 g = 1 mg

1 milligram (mg) = 1,000 micrograms (mcg)

1,000 milligrams = 1 gram (g or gm)

1,000 grams = 1 kilogram (kg)

Volume (liquid)

1 liter (l or L) = 1,000 milliliters (ml)*

1 milliliter = 1,000 microliters (µl)

Conversions

1 oz = 30 g

1 pound (lb) = 453.6 g

2.2 lb = 1 kg

Liquid and dry measure equivalents

1 teaspoon = 4 or 5 ml

30 ml = 1 ounce (oz)

3 teaspoons (tsp) = 1 tablespoon (T or Tbs)

2 tablespoons = 1 ounce = 30 grams

4 tablespoons = ½ cup

1 cup = 240 ml

2 cups = 1 pint = 16 ounces

16 ounces = ½ quart = 459 grams = 473 ml

473 ml = ½ liter

4 cups = 2 pints = 32 ounces

32 ounces = 1 quart = 946 ml

946 ml = 1 liter

4 quarts = 3¾ liters = 1 gallon

8 quarts = 7¼ kilograms = 1 peck

4 pecks = 1 bushel

*1 ml = 1 cubic centimeter (cc); however, ml is the preferred term.

Index

A

Abdominal binder, how to apply, 241-242
Abdominal breathing, 349-350
Abdominal pain as danger sign, 58
Activities
  organizing, 11
  strenuous, scheduling, 10
Activity level, observing changes in, 45
Acupuncture as pain-control technique, 94
Aerobic exercises, 354
Aerochamber system, how to use, 361-362
Aerosol equipment
  cleaning parts of, 358
  maintaining, 358-359
  troubleshooting problems with, 359
Aerosol treatment, how to perform, 359
Affection, direct expression of, 6, 8
AIDS, caring for person with, 487-481
Airflow through lungs, exercises for improving, 351-354
Airway, obstructed, clearing, 503-504
Alzheimer's disease, caring for person with, 472-476
Anaphylaxis kit, how to use, 500-503
Appetite
  loss of, as danger sign, 45
  stimulating, 131-132
Arteriovenous fistula site, caring for, 425-426
Artificial nose, 342
Assistance, arranging for, 11-12

B

Back massage, how to give, 83-84. *See also* Massage techniques.
Backrest, 106-107
  how to make, 106-107
Back-strengthening exercises, 275-280
Backward-sitting transfer to wheelchair, 295-296
Bandages
  reasons for using, 236
  types of, 236
Bathroom, safety precautions in, 23
Bed bath, how to give, 62-64
Bed board, 100-101
Bed cradle, 103-105
  how to make, 104-105
  types of, 104
Bedding, 111-112
Bed-making techniques, 109-111
  for occupied bed, 112-115
  for unoccupied bed, 115

Bedpan, how to use, for person confined to bed, 36-37
Bedroom, safety precautions in, 22-23
Bedside drainage bag, attaching, 411-412
Bedside table, 108
Bed tray, 108
Biofeedback as pain-control technique, 93-94
Bladder habits, changes in, 44
  as danger sign, 59-60
Bladder incontinence, 200
Bladder infection, preventing, 413-414
Bladder retraining, 202-203
Blood glucose levels, testing, 466-468
Blood in the stool as danger sign, 59
Blood pressure, 33-35
  taking another person's, 34-35
  taking your own, 34
  using digital monitor to measure, 34
Bone healing
  average time for, 394t
  stages of, 392-393
Bowel habits, noting changes in, 44
Bowel incontinence, 201-202
Bowel retraining, 209-210
Bowel stimulation, how to perform, 210-211
Breathing, observing, 44. *See also* Respirations.
Breathing difficulty as danger sign, 55
Breathing exercises, 351
Breathing relaxation exercises as pain-control technique, 90-91
Brushing and combing hair, 69-70
Buccal medications, how to give, 143, 144

C

Calcium-rich diet, 126-127
Calories, addition of, to diet, 122-123, 124-125t
Cane
  carrying objects when using, 257
  climbing stairs with, 255-256
  getting into and out of chair with, 257
  how to choose, 251
  types of, 252
  walking with, 253-254
Capsules
  storing, 141-142
  swallowing, 141
  types of, 140
Caregiver, home care and, 2-20
Caregiver burnout, avoiding, 12-15

Caregiver goals, setting, 10
Cast
  caring for, 394-397
  reasons for applying, 392
  removal of, 403
Casted arm or leg,
  exercises for, 400-402
  troubleshooting problems with, 397-400
Central venous catheter, caring for, 186-188
Chemotherapy, controlling side effects of, 481-485
Chest mobility exercises, 353-354
Chest pain as danger sign, 56
Chest physiotherapy, 354-356
  when to perform, 355
Chewing problems, feeding person with, 136-137
Cold therapy as pain-control technique, 93
Colostomy
  how to irrigate, 444-447
  living with, 448-451
  troubleshooting tips for, 448
Comfort
  household changes required for, 22-24
  importance of, 79
Concussion, caring for person after, 476-478
Condition of person, finding out about, 3
Condom catheter, how to use, 206-208
Confusion as danger sign, 53
Constipation as danger sign, 59
Continuous positive airway pressure
  mechanics of, 365
  setting up machine for, 365
  troubleshooting equipment problems with, 366
Cooking, nutrient preservation and, 121-122
Coughing
  as part of chest physiotherapy, 356. *See also* Chest physiotherapy.
  benefits of, 315, 316
CPR, how to perform, 504-511
Cream, how to apply, 145
Crutches
  carrying objects when using, 257
  climbing stairs with, 248
  getting back on feet after fall with, 250-251
  getting into and out of chair with, 249-250
  how to choose, 244-245
  walking with, 246-248

t refers to a table

t refers to a table

t refers to a table

t refers to a table